Practical Management of Urinary Stone

Anthony C.F. Ng • Michael Y.C. Wong
Shuji Isotani
Editors

Practical Management of Urinary Stone

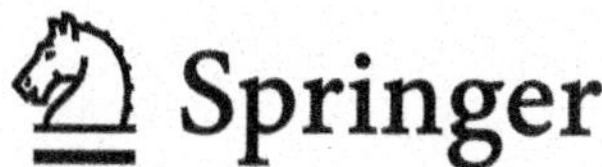

Editors
Anthony C.F. Ng
Department of Surgery
Chinese University of Hong Kong
Hong Kong
Hong Kong

Michael Y.C. Wong
International Urology, Fertility and
Gynecology Centre
Mount Elizabeth Hospital
Singapore
Singapore

Shuji Isotani
Department of Urology
Juntendo University
Tokyo
Japan

ISBN 978-981-16-4195-4 ISBN 978-981-16-4193-0 (eBook)
https://doi.org/10.1007/978-981-16-4193-0

This Springer imprint is published by the registered company Springer Nature Singapore Pte Ltd.
The registered company address is: 152 Beach Road, #21-01/04 Gateway East, Singapore 189721, Singapore

Foreword

Urolithiasis is a very common clinical problem which uses a lot of medical and society resources since ancient times. The lifetime prevalence of urinary tract stone is estimated to be around 10%. It means 1 out of 10 population needs medical care for urinary tract stone sooner or later. Furthermore, the incidence of stone disease is rising gradually attributed to changing climate and lifestyle modification. The management of urinary stone is becoming more important clinically. It is my honor to be invited to share my opinions in the preface for the book entitled *Practical Management of Urinary Tract Stone*. The authors are internationally renowned urologists, Professor Anthony C.F. Ng, Michael Y.C. Wong, and Shuji Isotani; all have abundant experience and knowledge on urolithiasis. They invited many outstanding scholars in Asia to publish this book. This is a comprehensive book covering many important topics from "basic principle and management of urinary calculi, instruments for endourological treatment of urinary calculi, and ureteroscopy to percutaneous nephrolithotomy and other approaches. It also addresses many novel surgical techniques such as intrarenal flexible ureteroscopy with laser or non-laser intrarenal lithotripsy, mini-PCNL, supine PCNL, tubeless percutaneous nephrolithotomy, and endoscopic combined intrarenal surgery. This is a practical tool and handy book, which is very useful for urologists in their daily practice such as how to treat urinary stones in patients with challenging intrarenal anatomy, patients with special medical condition, patients with special anatomy, etc. As the Secretary General of Urological Association of Asia whose main purpose is to elevate the horizon of urologists in this region through education, I truly believe you will benefit a lot after reading this book, especially for urologists who are practicing urinary stone management in Asia.

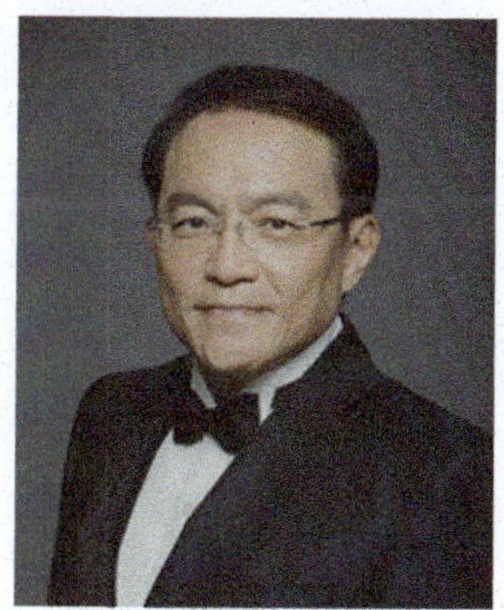

Allen W. Chiu, MD, PhD
Secretary General, Urological Association of Asia
Taipei, Taiwan

National Yang-Ming University, Mackay Medical University
Taipei, Taiwan

Preface

Urinary calculi is an ancient disease and has affected millions of patients in the world. Although bladder stone was the predominant stone described in history, the improvement in medical technology and healthcare system has changed the scene. Currently, renal and ureteric stones are the most common urinary stones occurring in the modern world, with an incidence of up to 10% in their lifetime. The prevalence of urinary stone varies in regions, and people in the so-called stone belt regions are at highest risk of stone formation. This may be related to the climate and lifestyle in these regions. In Asia, the stone belt has covered various countries, including Southern China, India, Japan, and Korea. Not surprisingly, patients with urinary stones are one of the main workloads for Asian urologists. Meanwhile, this also helps to nourish the experience in managing urinary stones in the region.

With the aim of training young urologists for increasing demand from our Asian patients, a group of Asian urologists have formed the Asian Urological Surgery Training and Education Group (AUSTEG) in 2015. The mission of the group is to advance the standard of urological surgery in Asia and develop next-generation leaders in Asia. AUSTEG has a unique focus on training of operation skills, through didactic lectures, experience sharing, case discussion, and hands-on workshops. This was particularly important for the training of stone management, as stone cases vary from one another, with different stone size, location, composition, and management further complicated by diverse patients' anatomical and medical factors. Moreover, the rapid development in technologies related to endoscopy, lithotripsy, and other accessories has also changed the landscape of stone management in recent years. Therefore, there is a continuous gap in the demand for stone treatment training and the availability of workshops that we could provide in the past few years. As a result, we have gathered a team of experienced "stone surgeons" in Asia to prepare this book *Practical Management of Urinary Stone*. We aimed to provide not only the most up-to-date knowledge in the field but also experience sharing on practical tips in different procedures. Moreover, we also provide advice on the management of challenging stone conditions, such as stones in various anatomical anomalies and patients with complicated medical conditions. In line with our group's mission, we want to make the content as practical as possible to meet the needs of our young surgeons.

The planning of the book was made before the COVID-19 pandemic, which has changed the mode of training completely in the past one year.

While face-to-face experience sharing and hands-on workshop might not be feasible at this moment, we hope our book could help to bridge this knowledge gap and help the continuous development of stone management in Asia and the world.

Hong Kong, Hong Kong — Anthony C.F. Ng
Singapore, Singapore — Michael Y.C. Wong
Tokyo, Japan — Shuji Isotani

Contents

Part I

Basic Principle and Management of Urinary Calculi

1 Symptoms, Signs and Basic Investigations for Urinary Calculi

Nitesh Ranasinha and Srinath Chandrasekera

1.1 Introduction

'Listen to your patient, (s)he is telling you the diagnosis'—Sir William Osler, 1849–1919.

A thorough clinical history is fundamental to patient assessment in any clinical context. A diagnosis of urinary stone may be suspected based on the clinical history and physical exam findings, strengthened by laboratory results, and ultimately confirmed with imaging studies. However, a thorough clinical history informs not merely diagnosis but can also suggest underlying aetiology, appropriate management strategies and risk of recurrence, in patients with urinary stone disease.

This chapter offers the basic principles of a focused history and physical examination and an overview of biochemical investigations to aid the practical management of urinary stone.

1.2 History

1.2.1 Demographics

The lifetime prevalence of urinary stone formation is estimated to be around 10% [1], with the probability of having a stone affected by a number of factors:

Gender. Urinary stone typically affects adult men more commonly than adult women, with a male-to-female ratio between 2:1 and 3:1 [2]. However, there is now evidence that this difference in incidence between men and women is narrowing [3].

Race. In US men, the highest prevalence of urinary stone is found in white men, followed by Hispanic, Asian and black men [2]. Among US women, the prevalence is highest among white women but lowest among Asian women [4].

Age. Historically, urinary stone occurrence was relatively uncommon before age 20 years, but the incidence of stones in children and adolescents is rising [5]. In adults, stone incidence peaks in the fourth to sixth decades of life [6]. When children present with stones, they fall into the 'high-risk' category and should be investigated extensively for an underlying cause.

Geographic location. Urinary stone has a higher prevalence in hot, arid or dry climates, such as mountains, desert or tropical areas. Worldwide regions of high stone prevalence include the United States, British Isles and Scandinavian and Mediterranean countries. The Afro-Asian stone belt, encompassing North Africa, the Middle East and South and East Asia, has a particularly high prevalence of urinary stone, estimated at 4–20% [7]. Indeed, these areas offer rich historical evidence of early medi-

N. Ranasinha
Medical Sciences Division, University of Oxford, Oxford, United Kingdom

S. Chandrasekera (✉)
Faculty of Medical Sciences, University of Sri Jayewardenepura, Nugegoda, Sri Lanka

A. C.F. Ng et al. (eds.), *Practical Management of Urinary Stone*,
https://doi.org/10.1007/978-981-16-4193-0_1

cal literature on urinary stone; a study of ancient Egyptian mummies shows evidence of urethral catheterisation for bladder stones, while Mesopotamian and ancient North Indian stone tablets detail how pulverised ostrich egg shell, with a high content of calcium carbonate, was ingested to bind lithogenic substances [1].

1.2.2 Presenting Complaint

The clinical presentation of urinary stones depends largely on the site of stone location/ impaction, infection status and specific patient-related factors, such as renal functional status of the contralateral kidney.

Classically, obstructed ureteric stones cause a ureteric colic: severe, acute flank pain that may radiate to the ipsilateral groin, commonly associated with nausea and vomiting. Frequently, this is accompanied by haematuria [8]. The triad of acute loin to groin pain, nausea and vomiting and haematuria are typical of a ureteric colic. Obstruction of the collecting system leads to an increase in intraluminal pressure, stretching nerve endings to cause the sensation of a ureteric colic. Pain from urinary calculi can also be attributed to local inflammatory mediators, oedema and hyperperistalsis. As stones pass and get lodged in the distal ureter or intramural tunnel, this can lead to bladder mucosal irritation manifested as urinary frequency or urgency. Ipsilateral testicular and groin pain may occur in men with obstructive stones where the stone is impacted in the lower ureter or classically in the vesico-ureteric junction. Fever, accompanied by urinary obstruction, indicates an obstructed infected kidney, which requires urgent resuscitation and decompression. Furthermore, recurrent upper urinary tract infections may indicate struvite stones [9]. However, in the absence of obstruction, calculi may frequently be asymptomatic. Such stones may grow to large size resulting in chronic obstruction and subsequent impairment of renal function.

It is important to exclude a broad range of differential diagnoses for ureteric colic. Other causes of abdominal pain, such as biliary and intestinal colic, have different characteristics (Fig. 1.1), though these differences are clearer in theory than in practice. In contrast to patients presenting with ureteric colic who find constant movement mitigates discomfort, peritonitic patients typically lie motionless, as movement exacerbates peritonism. Gynaecological causes, especially ectopic pregnancy and twisted ovarian cysts, should always be excluded in female patients presenting with flank or lower abdominal pain.

As a general rule, pregnancy and associated complications should be foremost in the differential diagnosis of females of the childbearing age presenting with abdominal pain. Occasionally, severe strangury, the painful desire to pass urine when stones are impacted at the vesico-ureteric junction, can be misinterpreted as acute urinary retention. Radiating loin to groin pain may also result from radiculopathy and, on occasions, neu-

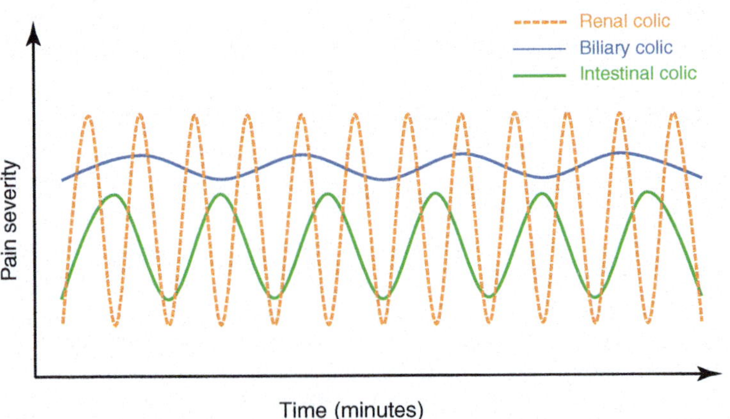

Fig. 1.1 Characteristic profiles of abdominal colics

ritis due to varicella zoster, manifesting with a typical rash along the dermatome several days after the onset of pain. Dissecting aortic aneurysm is another rare but important cause of radiating left-sided loin to grain pain, presenting sometimes even with haematuria.

In patients with a single kidney, the complete obstruction to the only functioning kidney will present as anuria and acute kidney injury. Larger ureteric stones may pass through the ureter and impact at the bladder neck causing acute urinary retention. This is a frequent cause of acute urinary retention in young males in the tropics [10].

Stones in the bladder typically present with filling-type lower urinary tract symptoms (LUTSs), supra-pubic pain and haematuria. Very rarely, long-standing, untreated urinary stones may result in malignant transformation of the urothelium, resulting in squamous carcinoma of the bladder or kidney [11].

1.2.3 Past History

1.2.3.1 Urological

Previous episodes. Details of any previous episodes of ureteric colic or stone disease are important to ascertain as this increases the likelihood of reaching a urinary stone diagnosis and suggests the patient's risk of recurrence. More than 50% of patients with urinary stones will have another episode within 10 years [12]. Visual features of previously sieved stones can provide useful clues to stone composition. Patients may recall, for example, whether a previously passed stone was dark brown (suggestive of calcium oxalate), bright yellow (suggestive of uric acid) or white (suggestive of struvite or calcium phosphate) [13].

Solitary or transplanted kidney. This is important as the single kidney by itself increases the risk of stone formation; prevention of stone recurrence is of more importance in protecting such a 'precious' kidney. Significantly, transplanted kidneys are surgically denervated, and ureteric obstruction therefore will not cause pain. Instead, the clinical manifestations would be due to other factors such as obstruction (anuria/AKI) or sepsis.

Renal disease. Structural renal diseases, such as medullary sponge kidney [14], horseshoe kidney [15], polycystic kidney disease [16], pelvicoureteric junction obstruction and ureteric strictures, can result in urinary stasis and are associated with stone formation. Moreover, in all forms of chronic kidney disease, renal stones are an important preventable cause of 'acute-on-chronic' deterioration of renal function.

Urological surgery. History of urological surgeries, such as continent urinary diversion and ileal conduit formation, predispose to turbulent urinary flow, stasis and stone formation. Moreover, history of any abdominal surgery increases the risk of urological scarring, adhesions, strictures and diverticula, which may also predispose to urinary stasis and stone formation. The presence of foreign bodies from previous interventions, such as forgotten stents and inappropriately used non-absorbable sutures, predisposes to infection and the formation of struvite stones.

1.2.3.2 Medical

Hypercalcaemia. Hyperparathyroidism, sarcoidosis and increased levels of vitamin D [17] predispose to hypercalcaemia and to the formation of calcium stones [18]. The relationship of low vitamin D to stone risk is not well established.

Hyperuricosuria. Myeloproliferative disorders, tumour lysis syndrome and gout predispose to hyperuricosuria and uric acid stone formation [19].

Metabolic syndrome. Diabetes and obesity are also associated with urinary stone formation, with the magnitude of association higher in women than in men [20, 21]. Evidence linking obesity with low urine pH and hypercalciuria may account for an increased risk of uric acid and calcium oxalate stones in these patients [22].

Malabsorptive conditions. Gastrointestinal disease, such as inflammatory bowel disease [23], and surgery, such as jejuno-ileal bypass, intestinal resection and bariatric surgery [24], can impair gut absorption leading to biochemical abnormalities. For example, malabsorbed fat

Table 1.1 Pharmacological compounds associated with urinary stone formation

Active compounds crystalising in urine	Substances impairing urine composition
Allopurinol/oxypurinol	Acetazolamide
Amoxicillin/ampicillin	Allopurinol
Ceftriaxone	Aluminium magnesium hydroxide
Quinolones	Ascorbic acid
Ephedrine	Calcium
Indinavir	Furosemide
Magnesium trisilicate	Laxatives
Sulphonamides	Methoxyflurane
Triamterene	Vitamin D
Zonisamide	Topiramate

sequesters calcium in the gastrointestinal tract, generating excess free oxalate for absorption [24]. The ensuing hyperoxaluria predisposes to oxalate stone formation.

1.2.4 Drug History

Pharmacological treatments can induce stone formation. These drugs can be categorised into two groups: stones formed by crystalised drug compounds and stones formed due to unfavourable changes in urine composition under drug therapy [25] (Table 1.1).

Drug allergies are also important to note; particularly relevant in the context of suspected urinary stones are allergies to non-steroidal analgesics, anti-emetics and antibiotics, frequently employed in acute management.

1.2.5 Family History

A positive family history is associated with an increased risk of stone formation. Twin studies have estimated the heritability of stone formation as 56% [26]. Patients with a family history of urinary stones also have a higher incidence of multiple stones and early recurrence [27].

A number of inherited metabolic conditions, including cystinuria, primary hyperoxaluria, renal tubular acidosis type 1 and cystic fibrosis, can cause urinary stone formation [28, 29]. While rare, these conditions should be considered, particularly in children and adolescents where stone formation is less common. With early recognition, appropriate treatments can be instigated, and genetic risks to other family members can be evaluated.

1.2.6 Social/Dietary History

Assessment of diet can reveal several modifiable risk factors for urinary stone formation.

Dehydration. An inverse relationship between high fluid intake and stone formation has been clearly demonstrated [30, 31]. Dehydration reduces urinary volume, promoting urinary supersaturation and crystallisation, leading to stone formation. An accurate estimation of fluid intake is an important component of a urinary stone history. Several approaches, including hydration diaries and fluid questionnaires, can be utilised in clinics to improve the accuracy of fluid intake assessments. Circadian fluid intake of 2.5–3 L/day of pH neutral beverage and diuresis of 2–2.5 L/day are recommended. Occupational dehydration and heat exposure are risk factors for urinary stone formation, and as such manual workers in hot environments should be identified and counselled on the importance of hydration [32, 33].

Calcium. A demonstrable positive relationship between ingested calcium and hypercalciuria would suggest that a high calcium diet might promote stone formation [34]. Interestingly, the opposite effect is seen, with the risk of calcium oxalate stone formation reduced in men and women on a high calcium diet [21]. This phenomenon may relate to the timing of calcium intake since dietary calcium sources, such as dairy products, broccoli, cabbage and sardines, are typically ingested at mealtimes alongside other foods containing oxalate. This provides an opportunity for dietary calcium to bind oxalate in the gut, resulting in decreased oxalate absorption and urinary excretion. The resultant reduction in net calcium-oxalate urinary super-saturation (despite an increase in urinary calcium) may explain reduced calcium oxalate stone formation [34].

Oxalate. The relative contributions of dietary and endogenous oxalate to urinary oxalate remain controversial, with dietary oxalate estimated to account for 10–50% of urinary oxalate [35]. Oxalate-rich foods, including spinach, chocolate, beetroot and peanuts, contribute to a moderately increased risk of calcium oxalate stone formation, particularly in the older population [36]. However, malabsorptive conditions, like inflammatory bowel disease and intestinal surgery, are typically more significant causes of secondary hyperoxaluria than dietary factors alone.

Protein. Excessive consumption of animal protein has several biochemical effects that favour stone formation, including hypercalciuria, hypocitraturia, low urinary pH, hyperoxaluria and hyperuricosuria [37].

Salt. Excessive salt intake is associated with higher urinary sodium and calcium levels and decreased urinary citrate, promoting calcium crystallisation. Salt excess can also contribute to bone degradation, thereby worsening hypercalciuria [37].

Beverages. Carbonated drinks may increase the risk of stone formation [38]. Besides its dehydrating effect, alcohol is thought not to have an independent effect on the risk of urinary stone formation.

1.3 Physical Examination

Physical examination of patients with renal colic is non-specific and minimal despite severe pain. The presence of tenderness or other clinical signs may be due to further sequelae such as extravasation of urine (urinoma) following calyceal rupture. Importantly, alternate diagnoses must also be considered when a patient with a presumed ureteric colic has unusual physical signs. Systemic signs of sepsis, including fever, tachycardia and hypotension, may indicate an obstructing stone with infection, warranting urgent assessment and intervention.

1.4 Investigations

All first-time presentations and low-risk cases need a basic workup, which includes urine analysis and a renal profile. Retrieved stones must be sent for analysis using infra-red spectrometry. These measures constitute the 'basic assessment' required in all stone patients.

Recurrent stone formers and others with increased predisposition (high-risk categories) must have a 'comprehensive assessment'.

1.4.1 Basic Assessment

1.4.1.1 Urinalysis

A simple *urine dipstick* and *urine microscopy, culture and sensitivity* are helpful in confirming a diagnosis of urinary stone as microscopic haematuria is present in the majority of patients. However, the absence of haematuria does not exclude urinary stones. The presence of >5–10 WBCs per high-powered field or pyuria is not infrequent and may indicate the presence of urinary tract infection or be secondary to stone-related inflammation. The presence of nitrite raises the high possibility of concomitant infection or the primary diagnosis to be infective (pyelonephritis).

Urinary crystals of calcium oxalate, uric acid or cysteine may indicate stone composition; however, only cysteine and uric acid crystals are pathognomonic for the underlying stone type [39].

Urine pH influences the formation of various types of urinary stone. Alkaline pH favours crystallisation of struvite and phosphate stones, whereas acidic pH promotes calcium oxalate, uric acid and cysteine stones [40]. Consequently, acidification agents (e.g. L-methionine) and alkalinisation agents (e.g. sodium bicarbonate and alkaline citrates) can be used to manipulate urinary pH and reduce the risk of recurrence in patients with struvite or phosphate stones and calcium oxalate, uric acid or cysteine stones, respectively. A urine pH greater than 7 suggests the presence of urea-splitting organisms, such as *Proteus*, *Pseudomonas* and *Klebsiella* [41].

1.5 Biochemical Investigations

Prior to imaging, all urinary stone patients need a succinct biochemical workup of urine and blood.

1.5.1 Serum Analysis

Serum electrolytes, urea and creatinine are important in assessing renal function. Abnormalities in serum calcium, phosphate and uric acid can point towards different stone compositions. For example, hyperuricaemia may suggest gout as an underlying aetiology, while hypercalcaemia may suggest hyperparathyroidism (further investigated by serum parathyroid hormone levels). It is noteworthy that the majority of patients with uric acid stones have high urinary uric acid excretion (uricosuria) rather than elevated serum uric acid levels (hyperuricemia).

Standard surgical blood tests, including FBC and CRP, are routine parameters if intervention is planned, and a raised WBC count can indicate pyelonephritis or urinary tract infection secondary to an obstructed system. Frequently, serum creatinine level and leucocyte count are marginally elevated in the acute setting of ureteric colic and return to baseline within 24–48 h. It is speculated that the acute obstruction to one kidney transiently impairs GFR until the contralateral kidney compensates in response. The marginal rise in the leucocyte count may be due to the local acute inflammatory response.

In all women of childbearing age, a serum hCG test should be done for the dual purpose of excluding ectopic pregnancy as the cause of symptoms and prior to imaging with ionising radiation.

1.5.2 Stone Analysis

The most accurate method for determining stone composition is, unsurprisingly, analysis of the stone itself [42]. Stone analysis should be conducted in all first-time stone formers. Stones can be retrieved following surgical extraction or spontaneous expulsion. Patients should be instructed to filter their urine to retrieve concrement for analysis. Stone passage and restoration of renal function should be confirmed radiologically and biochemically, respectively, as the mere absence of pain is not a reliable indicator of stone passage. The preferred analytical procedures for retrieved stones are infrared spectroscopy or X-ray diffraction [43]. Equivalent results can be obtained by polarisation microscopy. Chemical analysis (wet chemistry) is increasingly deemed to be obsolete [44].

In clinical practice, repeat stone analysis is indicated in certain cases:

- Recurrence under pharmacological prevention
- Early recurrence after interventional therapy with complete stone clearance
- Late recurrence after a prolonged stone-free period

Further urinary or serum metabolic workup is not usually necessary for first-time stone formers with a low risk of recurrence.

1.5.3 Comprehensive Assessment

The European Association of Urology (EAU) guideline on urolithiasis has described categories of patients who are at higher risk of recurrence. These include children; recurrent stone formers; and those with bilateral or multiple stones, a history of bowel surgery or malabsorption, hyperparathyroidism, gout, renal tubular acidosis or nephron calcinosis and stones formed from cysteine, uric acid or calcium phosphate.

In such patients, a 24-h urine collection should be evaluated: volume, pH, creatinine, calcium, phosphate, sodium, oxalate, uric acid and citrate. The 24-h urine collection is best done at least 4–6 weeks after a stone episode and in the absence of infection. Also, medications prescribed to control the recurrence of stones should be withheld for 2 weeks prior to the study. Most importantly, patients must be counselled not to deviate from their normal dietary and social habits during this study as often, the tendency is for patients to 'behave better' during medical assess-

Table 1.2 Distinctive risk factors for urinary stone types

Stone type	Risk factors
Calcium stones	Hyperparathyroidism, granulomatous disease, family history of renal tubular acidosis
Uric acid stones	High purine diet, gout, myeloproliferative disorders, tumour lysis syndrome
Infection (struvite) stones	Neurogenic bladder, spinal cord injury, continent urinary diversion, ileal conduit, foreign body, indwelling urinary catheter, urethral stricture, benign prostatic hypertrophy, bladder diverticulum, cystocoele, calyceal diverticulum
Genetic stones	See Sect. 1.2.5
Drug stones	See Table 1.2

ments. Serum parathormone levels are recommended only if there is a clinical suspicion.

1.6 Conclusion

A comprehensive urinary stone history is a key step in a complete diagnosis. It can also yield clues as to the type of stone (Table 1.2), severity of the problem and underlying aetiologies. This, following a physical examination, guides informed biochemical and imaging investigations.

References

1. Shah J, Whitfield HN. Urolithiasis through the ages. BJU Int. 2002;89:801–10.
2. Soucie JM, Thun MJ, Coates RJ, McClellan W, Austin H. Demographic and geographic variability of kidney stones in the United States. Kidney Int. 1994;46:893–9.
3. Lieske JC, et al. Renal stone epidemiology in Rochester, Minnesota: an update. Kidney Int. 2006;69:760–4.
4. Sarmina I, Spirnak JP, Resnick MI. Urinary lithiasis in the black population: an epidemiological study and review of the literature. J Urol. 1987;138:14–7.
5. Tasian GE, et al. Annual incidence of nephrolithiasis among children and adults in South Carolina from 1997 to 2012. Clin J Am Soc Nephrol. 2016;11:488–96.
6. Marshall V, White RH, De Saintonge MC, Tresidder GC, Blandy JP. The natural history of renal and ureteric calculi. Br J Urol. 1975;47:117–24.
7. Robertson WG. Renal stones in the tropics. Semin Nephrol. 2003;23:77–87.
8. Yeoh M, Lai NK, Anderson D, Appadurai V. Macroscopic haematuria—a urological approach. Aust Fam Physician. 2013;42:123–6.
9. Gettman MT, Segura JW. Struvite stones: diagnosis and current treatment concepts. J Endourol. 1999;13:653–8.
10. Ahmed A, Saeed NM. Experience with the management of urethral stones presenting with urinary retention at Gusau. Niger J Clin Pract. 2008;11:309–11.
11. Yu Z, et al. The risk of bladder cancer in patients with urinary calculi: a meta-analysis. Urolithiasis. 2018;46:573–9.
12. Worcester EM, Coe FL. Clinical practice. Calcium kidney stones. N Engl J Med. 2010;363:954–63.
13. Khan SR, et al. Kidney stones. Nat Rev Dis Prim. 2016;2:16008.
14. Yagisawa T, Kobayashi C, Hayashi T, Yoshida A, Toma H. Contributory metabolic factors in the development of nephrolithiasis in patients with medullary sponge kidney. Am J Kidney Dis. 2001;37:1140–3.
15. Pawar AS, et al. Incidence and characteristics of kidney stones in patients with horseshoe kidney: a systematic review and meta-analysis. Urol Ann. 2018;10:87–93.
16. Mufti UB, Nalagatla SK. Nephrolithiasis in autosomal dominant polycystic kidney disease. J Endourol. 2010;24:1557–61.
17. Hu H, et al. Association between circulating vitamin D level and urolithiasis: a systematic review and meta-analysis. Nutrients. 2017;9:301.
18. Rodman JS, Mahler RJ. Kidney stones as a manifestation of hypercalcemic disorders. Hyperparathyroidism and sarcoidosis. Urol Clin North Am. 2000;27:275–85. viii.
19. Cameron MA, Sakhaee K. Uric acid nephrolithiasis. Urol Clin North Am. 2007;34:335–46.
20. Curhan GC, Willett WC, Rimm EB, Stampfer MJ. A prospective study of dietary calcium and other nutrients and the risk of symptomatic kidney stones. N Engl J Med. 1993;328:833–8.
21. Curhan GC, Willett WC, Speizer FE, Spiegelman D, Stampfer MJ. Comparison of dietary calcium with supplemental calcium and other nutrients as factors affecting the risk for kidney stones in women. Ann Intern Med. 1997;126:497–504.
22. Rendina D, De Filippo G, D'Elia L, Strazzullo P. Metabolic syndrome and nephrolithiasis: a systematic review and meta-analysis of the scientific evidence. J Nephrol. 2014;27:371–6.
23. Gaspar SR, Mendonça T, Oliveira P, Oliveira T, Dias J, Lopes T. Urolithiasis and crohn's disease. Urol Ann. 2016;8(3):297–304.
24. Gonzalez RD, Canales BK. Kidney stone risk following modern bariatric surgery. Curr Urol Rep. 2014;15:401.
25. Matlaga BR, Shah OD, Assimos DG. Drug-induced urinary calculi. Rev Urol. 2003;5:227–31.

26. Goldfarb DS, Fischer ME, Keich Y, Goldberg J. A twin study of genetic and dietary influences on nephrolithiasis: a report from the Vietnam Era Twin (VET) Registry. Kidney Int. 2005;67:1053–61.
27. Basiri A, et al. Familial relations and recurrence pattern in nephrolithiasis: new words about old subjects. Urol J. 2010;7:81–6.
28. Rumsby G. Genetic defects underlying renal stone disease. Int J Surg. 2016;36:590–5.
29. Gibney EM, Goldfarb DS. The association of nephrolithiasis with cystic fibrosis. Am J Kidney Dis. 2003;42:1–11.
30. Borghi L, et al. Urinary volume, water and recurrences in idiopathic calcium nephrolithiasis: a 5-year randomized prospective study. J Urol. 1996;155:839–43.
31. Bao Y, Wei Q. Water for preventing urinary stones. Cochrane Database Syst Rev. 2012:CD004292. https://doi.org/10.1002/14651858.CD004292.pub3.
32. Borghi L, et al. Hot occupation and nephrolithiasis. J Urol. 1993;150:1757–60.
33. Atan L, et al. High kidney stone risk in men working in steel industry at hot temperatures. Urology. 2005;65:858–61.
34. Lemann JJ. Composition of the diet and calcium kidney stones. N Engl J Med. 1993;328:880–2.
35. Holmes RP, Goodman HO, Assimos DG. Contribution of dietary oxalate to urinary oxalate excretion. Kidney Int. 2001;59:270–6.
36. Taylor EN, Curhan GC. Oxalate intake and the risk for nephrolithiasis. J Am Soc Nephrol. 2007;18:2198–204.
37. Borghi L, et al. Comparison of two diets for the prevention of recurrent stones in idiopathic hypercalciuria. N Engl J Med. 2002;346:77–84.
38. Shuster J, et al. Soft drink consumption and urinary stone recurrence: a randomized prevention trial. J Clin Epidemiol. 1992;45:911–6.
39. Daudon M, Frochot V. Crystalluria. Clin Chem Lab Med. 2015;53(Suppl 2):s1479–87.
40. Wagner CA, Mohebbi N. Urinary pH and stone formation. J Nephrol. 2010;23(Suppl 16):S165–9.
41. Bichler K-H, et al. Urinary infection stones. Int J Antimicrob Agents. 2002;19:488–98.
42. Kourambas J, Aslan P, Teh CL, Mathias BJ, Preminger GM. Role of stone analysis in metabolic evaluation and medical treatment of nephrolithiasis. J Endourol. 2001;15:181–6.
43. Abdel-Halim RE, Abdel-Halim MR. A review of urinary stone analysis techniques. Saudi Med J. 2006;27:1462–7.
44. Gilad R, et al. Interpreting the results of chemical stone analysis in the era of modern stone analysis techniques. J Nephrol. 2017;30:135–40.

Imaging for Urinary Calculi

2

Kay-Seong Ngoo and Selvalingam Sothilingam

Abstract

The accurate diagnosis of urinary calculi is essential for treatment planning. Non-contrast-enhanced computed tomography (NCCT) is considered the gold standard for adults to diagnose urolithiasis in acute flank pain. Generally, CT has also overtaken the role of intravenous urography in stone diagnosis and treatment planning. Lower dose CT seems to be as accurate as NCCT for the same purpose. Ultrasonography (US) is considered first-line imaging for urolithiasis in paediatric and pregnancy groups of patients. Various iterations of US, especially with the Doppler setting, can improve diagnostic accuracy, whereas magnetic resonance imaging may be an alternative investigation tool for pregnant women. Plain radiographs and US scans can be combined for stone surveillance purposes. The study of stone composition can be inferred from double-energy CT scans. Differential kidney function is conventionally derived from nuclear renogram, but recently, CT-derived parameters have been shown to be a promising alternative.

Keywords

Computed tomography · Imaging
Urolithiasis · Ultrasonography

2.1 Introduction

The prevalence of urolithiasis is increasing worldwide, and in Asia, it is estimated to be around 1–5% [1]. The rising incidence of stone disease is largely attributable to changing climate and lifestyle modification. Consequently, there has been a rise in emergency department visits due to acute urolithiasis complications, while stone recurrence is also not uncommonly encountered [2].

Therefore, it is imperative that appropriate imaging is selected to accurately diagnose urinary calculi as it not only helps with treatment planning but also reduces the harm of ionising radiation to the patient. Imaging modalities are also used to help follow-up patients after conservative measures or definitive treatment. Finally, the output from imaging techniques can be used as a surrogate for renal function.

2.2 Utility of Imaging

The radiological diagnosis of urolithiasis in an emergency setting helps to confirm the presence of stones in acute abdomen presentations.

K.-S. Ngoo
Department of Surgery, Hospital Angkatan Tentera Tuanku Mizan, Kuala Lumpur, Malaysia

S. Sothilingam (✉)
Pusat Perubatan Sunway Velocity, Kuala Lumpur, Malaysia

A. C.F. Ng et al. (eds.), *Practical Management of Urinary Stone*,
https://doi.org/10.1007/978-981-16-4193-0_2

Non-contrast-enhanced computed tomography (NCCT) is now considered the gold standard in the diagnosis of urolithiasis in adults with acute renal colic. Ultrasonography (US) is preferred for the paediatric and pregnant groups of patients. In the elective setting, treatment planning for stones utilises various imaging modalities for stone localisation, assessment of stone fragility and estimating differential renal function. Plain radiographs, along with intravenous urography (IVU), still play a role in identifying stones and outlining the upper urinary tract. Magnetic resonance imaging (MRI) is usually reserved for situations where ionising radiation and intravenous contrast studies are contraindicated. Radio-isotope scans provide information about the relative renal function, which can aid in decision-making for urolithiasis intervention. Lately, many new iterations from plain radiograph, CT and US scans have been developed to increase the accuracy of stone detection whilst reducing exposure to ionising radiation.

2.3 Hazards of Imaging

There are risks associated with the use of imaging modalities, particularly those emitting ionising radiation. Risks can be divided into deterministic or stochastic effects. Deterministic effects of ionising radiation occur at a given threshold, and the effect is therefore proportional to the dose. Examples include skin erythema and cataract generation [3]. Stochastic effects relate to the induction of secondary cancers or hereditary effects. This can occur at any dose of radiation. Thus, the probability for the stochastic effect to occur increases with the dose. The severity, however, is dose-independent. In general, deterministic effects are rarely encountered in diagnostic imaging radiation doses [3].

The effective dose (measured in milli-Sievert, mSv) is a way of quantifying the risk of radiation exposure to human beings. It estimates the potential adverse biologic effect of the sum of equivalent doses of radiation to the exposed organs [3, 4].

Imaging modalities that utilise intravenous contrast (iodine or gadolinium) also have associated risks such as allergic reactions, impaired renal function, nephrogenic systemic fibrosis and death. It is therefore prudent that imaging studies are selected based on the As Low As Reasonably Achievable (ALARA) principle, i.e. using the lowest ionising radiation modality to answer a clinical question [3].

2.4 What Do the Guidelines Say?

Guidelines from the American College of Radiology (ACR) [4], American Urological Association (AUA) [3, 5], European Association of Urology (EAU) [6] and *Societe Internationale d'Urologie*–International Consultation of Urological Disease (SIU-ICUD) [7] provide recommendations on the utility of imaging in urolithiasis. For children, additional recommendations are available from the European Society for Paediatric Urology (ESPR) [8].

2.4.1 Adults

- For acute flank pain suspicious of urolithiasis, all guidelines recommend performing an NCCT [Level A]. The EAU guidelines advocate NCCT after the initial US assessment.
- Low-dose NCCT should be performed when evaluating for ureteral and renal stones [ACR], especially in patients with BMI <30 [SIU-ICUD: Level A].
- For a young patient and known stone former with previous radio-opaque stones, the AUA and ACR recommend US combined with kidney–ureter–bladder radiography (KUBXR) [Level C].
- In complex stones or anatomy, additional contrast imaging can be obtained if the further definition of the collecting system and ureteral anatomy is needed [AUA: Grade C].
- A focused area re-imaging can be performed prior to surgery if the passage of stone is suspected or stone movement will change management [AUA: Principle].

2.4.2 Pregnancy

- US is the preferred method for imaging a pregnant woman with suspected urolithiasis.
- The second-line option would be magnetic resonance imaging [AUA/EAU: Level 3].
- Low-dose NCCT should be used as the last option in pregnant women [AUA/EAU].

2.4.3 Paediatrics

- US is the first-line imaging modality for children with suspected urolithiasis, but it should include kidneys, fluid-filled bladder and ureter [EAU/AUA/ACR/ESPR: Level 2b].
- KUBXR or low-dose NCCT is an option if US does not provide the relevant information [EAU/AUA Level 2b].
- For non-obstructing renal stones, active surveillance can be pursued using periodic ultrasonography [AUA: Expert Opinion].
- Prior to performing PCNL, a low-dose NCCT should be obtained [AUA: Grade C].
- However, ESPR is unable to recommend the general use of low-dose NCCT in paediatric patients.

2.4.4 Surgical Planning

- A functional imaging study (DTPA or MAG-3) may be obtained if clinically significant loss of renal function in the involved kidney or kidneys is suspected [AUA: Level C].
- In planning for stone surgery, a contrast study can be performed to evaluate the anatomy of the renal collecting system [EAU].
- For shockwave lithotripsy (SWL), careful fluoroscopic and/or ultrasonographic monitoring during SWL facilitates good outcomes [EAU: Level 2a].
- In planning for endourological procedures, pre-procedural imaging of the kidney with US or CT scan, including contrast medium where possible or retrograde pyelographic study when starting a procedure, can be performed to assess stone comprehensiveness and anatomy of collecting system [EAU: Level 1a].
- A low-dose NCCT may be obtained prior to performing percutaneous nephrolithotomy on paediatric patients [AUA: Level C].
- Deferred imaging is performed after SWL, ureteroscopy or percutaneous antegrade lithotripsy to determine the presence of residual fragments [EAU: Level 3].
- Paediatric patients with asymptomatic or non-obstructing renal stones may be actively surveyed with periodic US [AUA: Expert Opinion].

2.4.5 Stone Workup

- In patients with unknown stone composition, US is performed in the case of suspected urolithiasis, which is then followed by NCCT with determination of Hounsfield units to provide information about stone composition [EAU].

2.5 Imaging Modalities

2.5.1 Plain Radiograph/X-Rays

Plain X-ray involves the use of a single energy source to produce photons. These pass through tissues, which then encounter a contralateral receiver. Historically, kidney–ureter–bladder radiograph (KUBXR) was used to complement intravenous urography studies [9].

A plain KUBXR is commonly used in patients with renal colic, as most stones contain calcium salts and hence are radio-opaque. It can reveal the cause of renal colic if radiopacity is detected at the expected location of the kidney or ureter based on the patient's symptoms. Nevertheless, not all stones are radio-opaque and not all calcifications are phleboliths. The sensitivity and specificity of KUBXR have been reported to be 57% and 76%, respectively [9]. When assessing for new stones, the effective radiation dose per KUBXR study ranges between 0.7 and 1.5 mSv [10].

The advantages of KUBXR include (a) low ionising radiation exposure, (b) widespread availability, (c) not dependent on the expertise and (d) low cost (it is about 10% of the cost of an ultrasound study) [9].

In addition to its relatively low accuracy in diagnosing urinary calculi, KUBXR also does not detect all stones (radiolucent) such as uric acid, xanthine and drug stones [6].

Nevertheless, KUBXR remains useful in (a) the treatment planning for radiopaque stones in extra-corporeal shockwave lithotripsy (ESWL), (b) the evaluation of ureteral stent placement and (c) the follow-up of residual stone burden after treatment [11].

To improve its accuracy, when combined with abdominal US for initial evaluation of acute colic, the sensitivity and specificity for the diagnosis of ureteral stones are 96% and 91%, respectively [12]. One study on 66 patients comparing US–KUBXR with NCCT found that the combination affords a sensitivity of 79% versus 93% of NCCT in detecting stone. All the missed cases had reported spontaneous stone passage. Therefore, it was suggested that after a negative combined US–KUBXR evaluation, NCCT would not add further information [13]. Lipkin and Ackerman suggested that KUBXR should be done before the US as the former can detect calcifications, direct the US examination and confirm the diagnosis [14]. The American College of Radiology proposed that this combined imaging modality may be able to detect all clinically significant stones and hence should be considered in young patients and those with known stone diseases [4].

Scout films on CT are performed at a lower mA than a standard KUBXR. However, NCCT scout image is not equivalent to a KUBXR [3]. The former can miss up to 25–51% of stones detected on KUBXR [10]. When a ureteral stone is detected on NCCT, the stone is only visualised on CT scout images about half the time. Thus, KUBXR should still be used if the stone is not seen on CT scout, as the stone will be detected in 10% of these patients [3]. For ureteral stone, the AUA recommends that KUBXR has a role for follow-up, for stones seen on CT scout image or initial KUBXR, in those patients undergoing medical expulsion therapy [11]. Surveillance oblique KUBXR films may be considered in stones located in the sacro-iliac area, which was not visible on CT scout or initial KUBXR [3].

KUBXR findings were also found to be able to significantly change the surgical management in 17% of renal stones initially detected on NCCT [15].

When assessing for new stones, KUBXR was found to have a sensitivity of 37.0% for stones <5 mm, and this increased to 87.5% for larger stones. Therefore, in the follow-up of stone formers, this may be a cost-effective modality for monitoring stone size [9].

Overall, although KUBXR may confer a lower ionising radiation dose, multiple radiographs performed over time, especially for young stone formers, may expose a patient to an effective dose similar to a low-dose CT scan [4].

2.5.2 Digital Tomosynthesis

This modality of imaging integrates KUB radiograph scout films taken via a 60-degree arc around the patient, with a digital detector and special computational software system for integration of imaged data on the opposing end detector [9, 14, 16]. Coronal section images are taken whilst overlying structures are subtracted to produce an image for the area of interest [9, 14]. The enhanced visualisation of digital tomosynthesis (DT) in the antero-posterior axis is of advantage over conventional KUBXR [16]. DT has a lower resolution than a CT but at a reduced dose of radiation compared with standard or low-dose CT. It outperforms KUBXR or intravenous urography in diagnostic accuracy whilst preserving image quality regardless of the patient's BMI [16]. DT is also less costly compared to conventional CT [14].

There is emerging evidence that DT is more sensitive in detecting renal rather than ureteral stones in ex vivo studies [16]. In an in vivo study, DT was found to be significantly more sensitive than digital radiography for detecting kidney stones but not ureteral stones. The sensitivity of detection for stone sizes between 2 and 5 mm was reported as 64% and for larger stones, 76%. Radiation dose was only slightly increased when compared to digital radiography but substantially lower than standard and low-dose CT [14].

2.5.3 Intravenous/Intraluminal Urography and Pyelography

Before the widespread availability of CT scans, intravenous urography (IVU) was the standard imaging technique for diagnosing and planning stone surgery. It provides information on renal function, anatomy of the collecting system and the level of obstruction [6]. Each examination confers an effective radiation dose between 1.5 and 3.5 mSv [10].

In acute flank pain assessment, IVU has a sensitivity of 85.2% and specificity of 90.4% in detecting stone [14]. The advantages of IVU are its ability (a) to delineate challenging renal anatomy, particularly before percutaneous nephrolithotomy (PCNL), and (b) to provide relative renal function information, in addition to evaluating for obstruction. All these pieces of information are useful for surgical planning [10].

However, IVU has the disadvantages of (a) higher effective radiation dose compared to standard radiograph, (b) longer acquisition time than CT, especially in the evaluation of obstruction, (c) inability to identify alternative diagnoses compared to CT scan, (d) higher cost and (e) higher risk due to contrast use [4].

IVU is also useful in equivocal situations of calcific density, which may represent a phlebolith or ureteral stone [4]. It has been shown that when IVU is added to DT, the diagnostic quality of standard IVU for urolithiasis rises from 46.5% to 95.5%, with a mean radiation dose reduction of 56% [17]. IVU along with an excretory CT scan can help to characterise the lower pole anatomy in urolithiasis to prognosticate the success of ESWL [10].

IVU is contraindicated in renal insufficiency, dehydration, pregnancy and in patients with past reactions to iodinated contrast agents. Currently, the availability of non-iodinated contrast material has reduced the risk of contrast allergies [4].

Retrograde pyelography performed prior to percutaneous nephrolithotomy (PCNL) or flexible ureteroscopy procedures in an anaesthetised patient helps to provide an on-table assessment of the upper urinary tract collecting system. This review may lead to a change in operative strategy [5, 10]. In addition, the placement of the nephrostomy tube after PCNL can be facilitated by antegrade pyelography.

In general, NCCT and contrast-enhanced CT have supplanted the use of IVU in the management of nephrolithiasis.

2.5.4 Ultrasonography

Ultrasonography (US) is commonly used as first-line imaging for suspected urolithiasis. Generally, it visualises the renal parenchyma, renal collecting systems and the bladder well but is poor in delineating the ureter due to overlying bowel gas or thick adipose tissue [11]. Apart from kidney and bladder stones, US is also able to detect calculi at pyelo-ureteral and vesico-ureteral junctions, as well as to detect upper urinary tract dilatation [6]. The sensitivity and specificity for the detection of ureteral stone are 45% and 94%, respectively. For renal stones, the accuracy is 45% and 88%, respectively [9, 16]. However, sensitivity can be reduced if the stone size is <3 mm, as it may not produce a shadow or miss out due to a decompressed urinary system [9]. In addition, US is useful in picking up secondary signs of urinary obstruction (i.e. hydronephrosis, hydroureter and perinephric fluid) and identifying other sources of flank or abdominal pain [3, 4].

The advantages of US include (a) its portability, (b) its ubiquitousness, (c) no radiation exposure (hence it is suitable for subsets of patients, i.e. pregnant women and paediatric patients) and (d) its reproducibility [6, 14].

However, US is disadvantageous because of (a) reduced sensitivity and specificity compared to CT scan, (b) inaccuracy in stone size determination, (c) reduced accuracy in stone detection for obese patients [14], (d) the need for skilled/medical personnel to perform, (e) significantly more time-consuming and (f) its variable findings as it is operator-dependent [10].

In obese patients, US can overestimate stone sizes compared to NCCT, up to 1 mm in stones smaller than 5 mm [10, 16]. Furthermore, US cannot differentiate dilatation without obstruction from true obstruction [4].

In a randomised controlled study comparing the role of US and CT in the assessment of suspected obstructive urolithiasis, no differences were reported in the sensitivity (~85%) and specificity (~50%), or complication rates, between the two intervention arms, at the time of discharge from the emergency department. However, a follow-up CT scan was performed for 40.7% of patients who had initial point-of-care US scan and in 27% of those who had radiology departmental US. Overall healthcare costs were also not significantly different between the groups [18]. Therefore, it has been proposed that US can be safely used as first-line imaging in emergency settings for patients with symptoms of urolithiasis [19].

Furthermore, for patients presenting to the emergency department, especially with solitary kidney, fever or doubt regarding the diagnosis of renal colic, the EAU recommends US as the initial evaluation [6].

There are many iterations to an US study that can potentially improve its accuracy in detecting stone and obstruction. Colour Doppler US adds value to grey-scale US alone in the evaluation of urolithiasis [11, 16].

When the urinary bladder is visualised in the transverse view using colour Doppler, *ureteral jets* appear as intermittent bursts of fluid on each side of the bladder. The unilateral absence or reduced jet flow rate with continuous jet flow pattern due to decreased peristalsis is specific for the presence of an obstructing ureteral stone [9, 14, 20].

The sonographic *twinkling artefact* is characterised by the appearance of alternating colours located deep to the stone on colour Doppler (typically seen as shadows on grey-scale US). Imaging with high pulse repetition frequency has been shown to increase the sensitivity of urolithiasis diagnosis from 66% on grey-scale to 97% as compared to NCCT [10]. Nevertheless, there is a high false-positive rate of about 50% [10, 11], which, in the acute setting, may have implications for confirmatory NCCT scan [16]. Therefore, the artefact should be evaluated with other parameters.

Doppler US can also be used to calculate the *resistive index* (RI) of the renal artery in a kidney with hydronephrosis. This measurement has been proposed as an indicator of ureteral obstruction when elevated unilaterally in a hydronephrotic kidney. Typically an RI value of 0.70 or a RI difference of ≥10% between the two kidneys indicates obstruction [10, 11]. However, the estimated RI has not been widely accepted due to conflicting results [11].

In patients presenting with acute flank pain, US has been found to be up to 100% sensitive and 90% specific for the diagnosis of ureteral obstruction. However, it is worth noting that about 11–15% of patients with urolithiasis may not show hydronephrosis on US [20]. This may be due to dehydration or that the hydronephrosis has not developed, typically only visible within 2 h of clinical presentation [4].

Another role of US is providing sonographic guidance for percutaneous access for nephrolithotomy procedures. In experienced hands, the success rate of access is as high as 88–99% with US guidance. For obese patients who require higher effective radiation dose under fluoroscopic guidance for comparable image quality, US is more advantageous [16].

Given its performance in detecting renal stones, US can be used as an alternative to CT as a follow-up imaging for patients with distal ureteric stones or renal stones undergoing conservative management [6, 7, 10].

2.5.5 Multidetector Computed Tomography

Helical/spiral non-contrast-enhanced CT (NCCT) was initially studied for flank pain by Smith et al. in the early 1990s [21]. This imaging technique relies on the relative absorption of radiation by body tissues and stones, where the

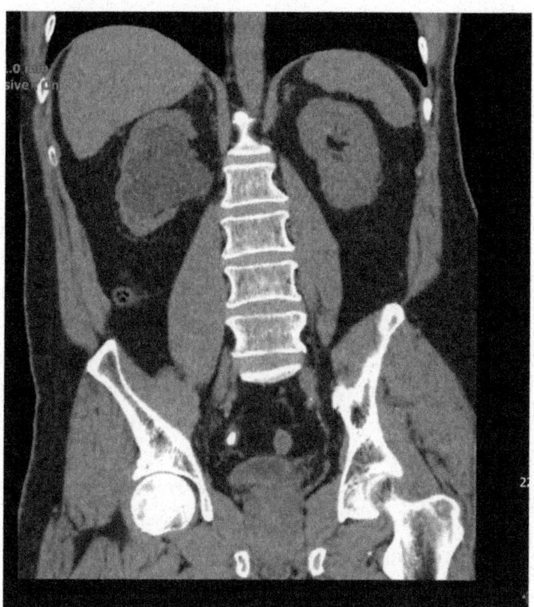

Fig. 2.1 NCCT demonstrating right gross hydronephrosis with a distal ureteric stone

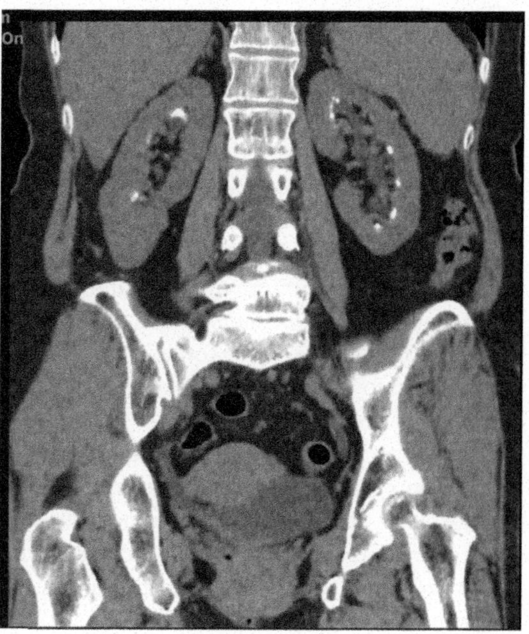

Fig. 2.2 NCCT demonstrating bilateral medullary nephrocalcinosis in a patient presenting with flank pain

3-D image of stone and the surrounding anatomy are then reconstructed into multi-planar views [9]. Thinner transverse slices (1–3 mm) are usually preferred with improved sensitivity in stone detection. However, 5 mm axial slices with 3 mm coronal and sagittal re-formatted images also provide adequate stone detection with a lower radiation dose [11].

The most commonly applied iteration of CT scan for urolithiasis is NCCT or CT-KUB. It is now regarded as the first-line imaging for acute flank pain suspicious of urolithiasis in the emergency department. NCCT confers high sensitivity (95–100%) and specificity (96–98%) in detecting stones [5, 6, 10]. Furthermore, it is useful in detecting secondary signs of obstruction due to ureteral stones such as hydronephrosis, hydroureter, periureteral oedema and renal enlargement (Fig. 2.1) [4]. It can also demonstrate other organic causes of flank pain in 9–15% of scans (Fig. 2.2). NCCT is also considered the gold standard for detecting residual stone fragments post-therapy [11].

Apart from stone diagnosis, NCCT provides other qualitative measurements such as stone size and location, as well as inference on stone composition and density, expressed in Hounsfield units (see later) [4–6]. Coronal views of CT accurately provide maximal stone size estimation, which may be a factor in treatment decision and predicting stone passage [4, 22].

NCCT also conveys skin-to-stone distance (SSD) measurement, which is useful in treatment planning using extra-corporeal shockwave lithotripsy (ESWL). SSD greater than 9–11 cm has been associated with lower stone-free rates [10]. This parameter is derived from the mean of three measurements (lateral skin-to-stone, posterior skin-to-stone and 45 degrees between the initial two measurements) [11]. Other anatomical parameters derived from NCCT, which are predictive of successful ESWL stone treatment, include unfavourable factors such as narrow infundibulo-pelvic angle (<70°), long infundibular length (>3 cm) and narrow infundibular width (<5 mm) [10].

Differentiating stones that are intramural or have already passed into the bladder in supine NCCT during acute renal colic can be challenging [22]. In symptomatic patients who are suspicious of having distal ureteral stones, a prone NCCT can be very helpful [10]. Furthermore, prone positioning allows for anatomic determination of kidneys with surrounding organs and pleura in planning for PCNL [14].

NCCT can also be used to estimate stone volume in relation to the pelvicalyceal system and surrounding organs. This can be calculated from the water displacement method, which is comparable to volumetric stone measurement using software [22]. Such information is vital for pre-operative evaluation of the site and direction of percutaneous renal access, for example. It can also be used to predict the success of ESWL and flexible ureteroscopy [10].

The advantages of NCCT include (a) the ease of performing in the emergency department with faster image acquisition by non-medical staff [10], (b) no requirement for IV contrast, (c) ability to assess other abdomino-pelvic viscera and pathologies [14] and (d) ability to identify radiolucent stone [16]. Interestingly, about one-third of NCCT scans for urolithiasis resulted in observations for other findings, while up to 70% of acute flank pain requiring NCCT resulted in non-urolithiasis aetiologies [14].

The disadvantages include (a) the use of ionising radiation, which is of concern in those at risk of stone recurrence, thus requiring multiple lifetime imaging, and (b) the inability to image protease-inhibitor-related stones such as indinavir.

At times, delineation of the collection system using contrast-enhanced CT with excretory phase is useful when stone removal is planned [5, 6, 11]. This is recommended for complex renal or ureteral anatomy (e.g. horseshoe kidney, cross-fused ectopia) and unusual patient body habitus (refer to Chap. 25) [5]. Although IVU can provide this information, a randomised clinical trial found that, for supine PCNL planning, CT scan resulted in easier access into the pelvicalyceal system and reduced operating time [23].

There are valid concerns regarding cumulative exposure to radiation, especially in young patients with urolithiasis who may undergo repeat scans over the years, as well as obese patients who may require three times the effective radiation dose compared with non-obese patients [16]. Another relevant concern is the induction of secondary cancer, with one case in every 660 patients having received a single CT of the abdomen [22].

2.5.6 Measures That Are Taken to Lower the Emission of Ionising Radiation During CT

Several advancements have been made in CT technology to address the radiation dose concern. This includes modification of scan parameters, modulation of scan parameters according to the patient's characteristics and the use of automatic dose-modulation software or X-ray filters, which adjust the radiation based on the scout images and according to the thickness and density of various anatomic regions [10, 16]. Limiting the range of view to the kidney, ureter and bladder also reduces radiation dose [4].

Standard CT evaluation involves radiation dose of up to 9.6 mSv for men and 12.6 mSv for women, per examination. Recent advancements in CT technology allow for low-dose CT (LDCT) to be performed (with effective radiation doses of 0.7–2.3 mSv) per examination. Even low-density stones such as uric acid stone are well detected by LDCT [14]. Similar sensitivities and specificities have been reported between standard- and low-dose CT regimens for the diagnosis of urolithiasis [10]. A meta-analysis of prospective studies found a pooled sensitivity of 93.1% and pooled specificity of 96.6% for LDCT detection of urolithiasis [24]. LDCT has been shown to produce equivalent stone measurements as compared to standard-dose CT [4]. However, LDCT performs poorly for obese patients (BMI > 30 kg/m^2) and smaller stones (<3 mm) [14]. Thus, LDCT is preferred for BMI $\leq$ 30, while reducing ionising radiation dose and maintaining both sensitivity and specificity at 90% and higher [3, 6].

Advances in ultra-LDCT (i.e. effective radiation dose ~1 mSv) showed that combined with model-based iterative reconstruction, stones of 3 mm or larger can be detected [14, 22]. The sensitivity and specificity of this modality are 74% and 77% for stone size <3 mm and 92% and 82%

for stones ≥3 mm, respectively. Ultra-LD CT was also inferior to LDCT in detecting secondary signs [14].

Limitations of ultra-LDCT are the detection of stones less than 3 mm and patients with BMI > 30 [22]. An in vivo study by Rob et al. compared ultra-LDCT (effective dose ≤1.9 mSv) or LDCT (<3.5 mSv) versus standard-dose CT (4.5–5 mSv). They reported sensitivity of 90–100% and specificity of 86–100% for ultra-LDCT and LDCT, respectively [25].

Despite the benefits of low-dose CT, the uptake of LD protocol has been less than 10% based on cross-sectional studies performed in the United States [22].

2.5.7 Magnetic Resonance Imaging

This imaging modality provides a comprehensive review of soft tissues in the abdomino-pelvic region. However, magnetic resonance urography (MRU) cannot be used to directly detect urolithiasis [6, 10]. Using standard magnetic resonance imaging (MRI) sequences, stones will appear as non-specific signal void [9].

MRI is able to detect secondary effects of obstruction due to urolithiasis, but this could be non-specific, as filling defects in the ureter could be due to a blood clot or tumour [10]. The T2-weighted sequences are able to reveal signs of obstruction such as hydronephrosis and perinephric oedema [4, 10]. Compared to CT scan, MRI performed in acute ureteral obstruction has a greater sensitivity (77%) in detecting perinephric fluid compared to perinephric stranding on CT scan (45%) [14]. Diffusion-weighted sequence allows for the detection of pathophysiological changes to renal perfusion and diffusion in patients with unilateral ureteral obstruction and for monitoring treatment progress [10]. Nevertheless, MRI does not provide quantitative information on the renal function that could assist management in the setting of obstructive uropathy [14].

The sensitivity of MRI for urolithiasis detection is variable. It has a reported median sensitivity of 82%, which is higher than that of US and KUBXR but lower than CT scan [3]. In diuretic-enhanced excretory MRU in patients with obstructive uropathy, MRI accuracy was reported as 93% [20].

One utility of MRI is the detection of protease-inhibitor (Indinavir) stones in HIV patients, which is radiolucent and not visible on CT or KUBXR [14].

The advantages of MRI include (a) no ionising radiation, thus making it desirable for paediatric patients, pregnant women and nephropathy patients who must avoid contrast [14]; and (b) its ability to provide 3-D images without radiation [9].

The disadvantages of MRI are (a) restricted access, (b) higher cost (i.e. three times more than a CT scan), (c) lower accuracy and (d) longer image acquisition time [9]. In addition, the use of high-dose paramagnetic contrast may be teratogenic, as shown in animal studies [10].

2.6 Imaging in Special Groups

2.6.1 Pregnancy

The risk of ionising radiation for investigative procedures during pregnancy is dependent on the gestational age of the foetus (the lowest risk is before 8th and after 23rd week) and radiation dose (<50 mGy is considered safe) [6]. Radiological exposure carries a risk of <1 in 5000 (1 in 33,000 per mGy) for fatal childhood cancers and <1 in 10,000 (1 in 40,000 mGy) for induced heritable diseases. Hence, stochastic effects of ionising radiation on the foetus are of particular concern. In pregnancy, radiation harm can be reduced further by (a) imaging only the affected side, (b) shielding the maternal pelvis and (c) keeping the exposure time or number of radiographs to a minimum [26].

In pregnant women with flank pain suspicious of urolithiasis, transabdominal or transvaginal US is regarded the best initial study [4–7]. To increase the accuracy in US detection, Doppler US measurement of the resistive index (RI), using a cut-off of 0.70 or a change in RI of 0.06, is useful in the diagnosis of acute unilateral ureteric obstruction if the scan is performed within

6–48 h of presentation [26]. However, detection rates can be compromised if done outside this time window in patients with renal disease and with non-steroidal anti-inflammatory drugs on board [26].

The twinkling artefact of US, using B-mode and Doppler, can improve the sensitivity of stone detection by differentiating stones from other echogenic structures [9]. Colour Doppler can be utilised to detect ureteral jets, or the passage of urine, at the uretero-pelvic junction where an absence of jets represents complete ureteral obstruction. However, false positives can occur due to the ureteral compression by a gravid ureter. Hence, this study should be confirmed in contralateral decubitus patient position [26].

If US is equivocal in detecting stones, MRI is proposed as the second-line imaging modality. This investigation defines the level of obstruction, and in some situations, it provides an estimate of stone size [6]. Although it has no harmful ionising radiation to the foetus, MRI should be avoided in the first trimester of pregnancy due to limited data on safety during foetal organogenesis [26]. Nevertheless, there is inadequate data to prove the deleterious effects of MR exposure to a developing foetus. Non-contrast MRI at 1.5 T should be used on the basis that medical benefits outweigh any unknown potential risks [27]. Furthermore, there is widespread consensus that gadolinium-based contrast agents should be avoided during pregnancy [27].

The MRI also serves as a useful adjunct for US in pregnant women. Kidneys do undergo physiological dilatation 90% of the time, especially on the right side, usually seen as early as 6 weeks gestation and resolves by 6 weeks postpartum [9]. Hydronephrosis can be attributable to a compressed ureter between the gravid uterus and the linea terminalis [4]. Hence, MRI is useful if stones cannot be visualised on US, but clinical suspicion of obstructing urolithiasis persists [9].

In the second and third trimesters of pregnancy, low-dose CT (LDCT) scan can be considered the last option for stone detection if US and MRI cannot achieve a diagnosis [4–6]. LDCT has a higher positive predictive value (95.8%) than MRI (80%) and US (77%); thus this can potentially avoid unnecessary negative interventions such as ureteroscopy [6]. The American College of Obstetrics and Gynaecology stated that radiation exposure of less than 50 mGy, which is well below the average for low-dose CT, is not associated with the development of foetal anomalies or foetal loss [3, 5].

2.6.2 Paediatrics

Children with urolithiasis represent a group with a higher risk of stone recurrence. Hence, with the prospect of repeated imaging throughout their lifetime, the ALARA principle should be adhered to [6, 9]. Furthermore, imaging procedures may require their co-operation, anaesthesia and exposure to ionising radiation. Adult protocols cannot be applied to children because (a) their stones are small and poorly calcified, (b) they have smaller ureters surrounded by fat, which can reduce the diagnostic accuracy of CT scan [6, 8], and (c) they have 10 times higher sensitivity to radiation than adults, thus higher chance of developing malignancies later in life [10].

US scan should be the first choice in investigating urolithiasis in children. This modality can visualise the kidney and the rest of the urinary tract rather well, with adequate hydration and good bladder volume. Most of the stones in children are located in the pelvicalyceal junction or in the proximal and/or distal ureter. Sometimes, small concretions are detected by US, which may be missed by IVU or low-dose CT [8]. US also has a higher accuracy in stone detection in children due to small body size and shorter stone to probe distance [8].

The US features for stones in children include echogenic foci with posterior shadowing, ureteral and pelvicalyceal system dilatations, and increased renal echogenicity and size, which are more conspicuous than in adults [8]. Nevertheless, small stones and modern US machines with harmonic and spatial compounding imaging features may fail to cast an acoustic shadow [28]. Although less sensitive (70%) than CT, it is an adequate screening tool to diagnose most clinically significant stones [28]. In addition, US can be used for surveillance for asymptomatic and non-obstructive renal stones in children [5]. US detection of stones during acute obstruction can be enhanced by the twinkling artefact and measurement of the resistive index using colour Doppler, such as in pregnant women [8]. However, US fails to detect >40% of stones in children, and it provides limited information regarding renal function [6]. US is advantageous as it does not require anaesthesia and no radiation is involved.

The use of plain X-ray can assist in localising stone before lithotripsy procedures, and it is useful for follow-up, too [6, 8]. IVU should be used judiciously for specific indications, and usually it supplements US findings. The IVU should be limited to three or four views, including KUBXR, and with adequate coning, this should be adequate for diagnosis with a lowered radiation dose [8].

There is now widespread use of CT as a first-line study given its wide availability in the United States. Between 2003 and 2011, about 63% of children underwent CT scans compared to US (24%) as first-line imaging in the United States. NCCT confers near 100% sensitivity and specificity for urolithiasis. Low-dose CT (radiation dose <3 mSv) using stone protocol has been introduced, and this achieved a diagnostic sensitivity of 96.6% for nephrolithiasis. Nevertheless, the accuracy of low-dose CT for paediatric nephrolithiasis has not been confirmed [28]. Thus, low-dose CT can be considered an alternative if US cannot provide information on urolithiasis [6].

2.7 Stone Composition and Fragility

Pre-procedural determination of stone composition can assist in optimal stone management. Traditionally, the stone composition is deduced from chemical analysis utilising sophisticated spectrometry, which can be costly and is not widely available. No other chemical analysis can determine in vivo stone composition. Stone fragility can be assessed to predict the likelihood of fragmentation.

Historically, stone density has been regarded as a surrogate of its composition. This is measured using NCCT and expressed in Hounsfield units (HU). In addition, HU can be used to predict success rates for stone treatment [16]. For ESWL treatment, stones with HU of between 900 and 1200 were found to be independent factors for treatment failure. In practice, the association between ESWL failure rate and HU values is not linear. Furthermore, most stones have mixed composition, resulting in overlap in their attenuation values, thus making the response to ESWL less predictable [16]. Other limitations of HU values include variability between CT scanner models and the high radiation dose involved in deriving its value [29].

A Turkish study on 115 patients with renal stones who had HU measurements and subsequent stone analyses found that HU_{diff} (the difference between maximal and minimal HU for a particular stone) and the mean HU value (HU_{ave}) can reliably predict stone mineral complexity. $HU_{diff} < 341.5$ showed 81.8% sensitivity and 67.2% specificity for identifying mono-mineral stones [30]. Other studies identified that $HU_{ave} < 900$ predicts uric acid stone, $HU_{ave} > 1000$ favours a calcium-based stone, whilst HU of 900–1000 is associated with other stones (cystine, struvite and calcium oxalate monohydrate–uric acid) [30].

Double-energy CT (DECT), which is performed by scanning an object with two scanners at two different energies (80 and 140 kV), thus producing two sets of data, which are then merged into a CT image, is an alternative method to predict in vivo stone composition [16]. The different X-ray attenuation obtained from the two scanners for various stone elements with different atomic numbers can be used to infer stone composition by measuring their differences [11, 16].

In vivo characterisation of urinary stones and sub-characterisation of calcium stones are now possible with DECT. It has been shown that DECT is better than conventional CT in differentiating uric acid from non-uric acid stones [11]. Lately, the distinction between struvite and cysteine stone has also been made by DECT. This will facilitate the selection of struvite stone patients for ESWL who are more likely to achieve treatment success [11]. DECT can also generate a low-to-high energy ratio. Differences in the ratios of different stone types can be used to predict its composition. For example, a ratio of 1.13 to 1.24 predicts cysteine stone, whereas a ratio more than 1.24 is likely to be a calcium salt [16].

Initially, DECT required a higher effective radiation dose. Thus, Nestler et al. proposed stratifying patients with uric acid stone in which patients with urine pH < 5.5 should undergo DECT, while those with urinary pH > 5.5 should receive standard CT [22]. Recently, the radiation dose for DECT was reported to be comparable to standard CT (2.6 vs. 2.7 mSv). In fact, by further reducing the current in the scanner, DECT can still produce compositional stone analysis at 40% lower radiation dose, equivalent to that of low-dose CT [16]. Currently, ultra-low-dose DECT has managed to produce excellent differentiation between uric acid (sensitivity and specificity 100%) and non-uric acid stones (sensitivity 100%, and specificity 79%) [16].

The limitations of DECT include (a) higher costs of the scanner, (b) challenges in clinical workflow if prospective patient selection becomes necessary, (c) variability in reporting radiation dose and (d) indeterminate best energy levels for imaging as well as post-processing algorithms [4, 22].

In addition, a high-resolution CT scan producing thin (<5 mm) slices, viewed in the bone window, can be used to assess the internal architecture of urolithiasis. Using magnification, stones that appear homogeneous in architecture are less likely to fragment during ESWL compared to stones with heterogeneous profile [11]. However, studies on urinary stone fragility are still limited.

2.8 Differential Renal Function

Urolithiasis can have an impact on renal function. Differential renal function should be ascertained in situations where treatment decisions can be made more accurately, particularly when standard anatomical imaging reveals potential loss of renal parenchyma [5, 31]. The functional information will help to prioritise the treatment side in situations of bilateral urolithiasis and assist in deciding if kidney preservation or removal is indicated in chronic stone disease [31]. Also, baseline kidney function can be ascertained in the following treatment outcomes of upper urinary tract stone disease [5].

Although parenchymal thickness, measured by US or CT scan, can estimate renal function, there are situations such as chronic kidney disease or staghorn/complex stones, where the renal function cannot be properly determined (Fig. 2.3). Furthermore, in the past, the demonstration of contrast excretion on X-ray films, such as in IVU or excretory phase in contrast-enhanced CT or MR urography, are relied upon to provide functional information of the kidneys. However, this has now been brought into question [31].

Nuclear renal scan is regarded as the gold standard for evaluating differential renal function. This study can also evaluate for obstruction. Commonly used radio-isotope tracers include the purely glomerular-filtered 99m-technitium-

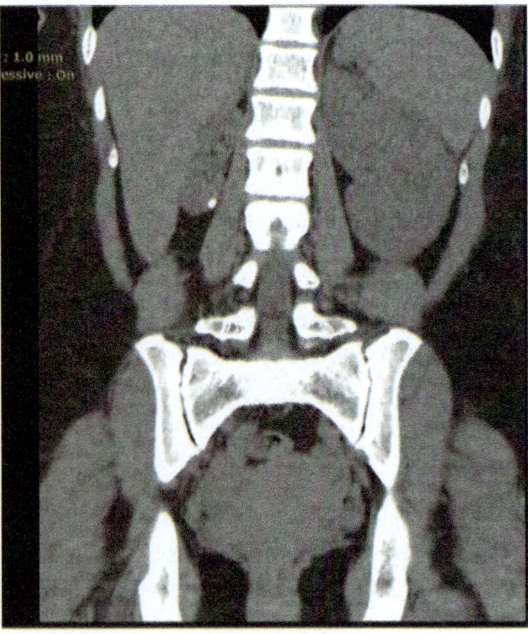

Fig. 2.3 NCCT showing right atrophic kidney due to an underlying urolithiasis

diethylene-triamine-pentaacetic acid (DTPA) and tubular-secreted, more efficient, 99m-technitium-mercapto-acetyl-triglycerine (MAG3) [32]. The value of differential renal function was proposed by Sreenevasan in 1974. In bilateral renal calculi, renography provided differential renal function information whereby the better kidney was operated on first, with positive post-operative outcomes [33]. However, renal isotope scans are not widely available, are costly, involves radiation exposure, are operator dependent and has a prolonged acquisition time, and in stone surgery, it does not contribute any anatomical information. The ability to assess obstruction via nuclear renography is compromised in cases of moderate-to-severe chronic kidney disease. Similarly, the assessment of renal function is limited in the setting of obstruction; thus, any obstruction needs to be alleviated first [5].

In view of those limitations, various derivatives of CT scans have been used to estimate renal function. Feder et al. studied the ratio of the parenchymal area of both kidneys and compared them with the MAG3 renal scan. Both showed a very high correlation between predicted and observed renal function, with an average difference of 4.7% between the two [34]. Samar et al. investigated 21 patients with unilateral obstructive uropathy and derived the percentage total renal volume of both normal and obstructed kidneys from helical CT scans. This was compared with percentage renal function determined from DTPA. Again, they demonstrated strong agreement between the two parameters, for both normal and obstructed kidneys [35]. In conclusion, CT-derived parameters seemed promising in predicting split renal function, although its utility needs to be tested in well-designed studies.

2.9 Conclusions

Imaging technology has improved over the years to improve accuracy in the detection of urinary calculi, and this helps with treatment planning. NCCT in adults and US scan in paediatric and pregnant patient groups have proven to be useful in detecting a majority of stones in the emergent and elective settings. The different iterations of NCCT with lower doses of ionising radiation have proven to be increasingly accurate compared to conventional imaging. Similarly for US scan, additional information on urolithiasis can be obtained via B-mode and Doppler features such as twinkling artefact, ureteral jets and resistive indices measurements. Using readily available scans, stone composition and hardness can now be deduced from advanced CT features such as double-energy CT. Furthermore, differential renal function can now be inferred from CT parameters, although this requires further validation.

References

1. Raheem IA, Khandwala YS, Sur RL, Ghani KR, Denstedt JD. Burden of urolithiasis: trends in prevalence, treatments, and costs. Eur Urol Focus. 2017;3:18–26.
2. Geraghty RM, Proietti S, Traxer O, Archer M, Somani BK. Worldwide impact of warmer seasons on the incidence of renal colic and kidney stone disease: evidence from a systematic review of literature. J Endourol. 2017;31(8):729–35.
3. Fulgam PF, Assimos DG, Pearle MS, Preminger GM. Clinical effectiveness protocols for imaging in the management of ureteral calculous disease: AUA technology assessment. J Urol. 2013;189:1230.
4. Moreno CC, Beland MD, Goldfarb S, et al. Acute onset flank pain—suspicion of stone disease (urolithiasis). ACR appropriateness criteria. Reston, VA: American College of Radiology; 2015.
5. Assimos D, Krambeck A, Miller NL, Monga M, Murad MH, Nelson CP, et al. Surgical management of stones: American Urological Association/Endourological Society guideline, part 1. J Urol. 2016;196:1153–60.
6. Türk C, Skolarikos A, Neisius A, et al. EAU Guidelines on Urolithiasis. In: EAoUG Office, Editor. EAU Guidelines. Edn published as the 35th EAU Annual Meeting, Amsterdam. Arnhem, The Netherlands: European Association of Urology Guidelines Office; 2020.
7. Jung H, Andonian S, Assimos D, Averch T, Geavlete P, Kohjimoto Y, et al. Urolithiasis: evaluation, dietary factors, and medical management: an update of the 2014 SIU-ICUD international consultation on stone disease. World J Urol. 2017;35:1331–40.
8. Riccabona M, Avni FE, Blickman JG, Dacher J-N, Darge K, Lobo ML, Willi U. Imaging recommendations in paediatric uroradiology. Minutes of the ESPR uroradiology task force session on childhood obstruc-

tive uropathy, high-grade fetal hydronephrosis, childhood haematuria, and urolithiasis in childhood. ESPR Annual Congress, Edinburgh, UK, June 2008. Pediatr Radiol. 2009;39:891–8.
9. Brisbane W, Bailey MR, Sorensen MD. An overview of kidney stone imaging techniques. Nat Rev Urol. 2016;13(11):654–62.
10. Villa L, Giusti G, Knoll T, Traxer O. Imaging for urinary stones: update in 2015. Eur Urol Focus. 2016;2(2):122–9. https://doi.org/10.1016/j.euf.2015.10.007.
11. Masch WR, Cronin KC, Sahani DV, Kambadakone A. Imaging in urolithiasis. Radiol Clin North Am. 2016; https://doi.org/10.1016/j.rcl.2016.10.002.
12. Mitterberger M, Pinggera GM, Pallwein L, et al. Plain abdominal radiography with transabdominal native tissue harmonic imaging ultrasonography vs unenhanced computed tomography in renal colic. BJU Int. 2007;100:887–90.
13. Ripolles T, Agramunt M, Errando J, Martinez MJ, Coronel B, Morales M. Suspected ureteral colic: plain film and sonography vs unenhanced helical CT. A prospective study in 66 patients. Eur Radiol. 2014;14:129–36.
14. Lipkin M, Ackerman A. Imaging for urolithiasis: standards, trends, and radiation exposure. Curr Opin Urol. 2016;26:56–62.
15. Lamb AD, Wines MD, Mousa S, Tolley DA. Plain radiography still is required in the planning of treatment for urolithiasis. J Endourol. 2008;22:2201–5.
16. Koo K, Matlaga BR. New imaging techniques in the management of stone disease. Urol Clin North Am. 2019;46(2):257–63. https://doi.org/10.1016/j.ucl.2018.12.007.
17. Wells ITP, Raju VM, Rowberry BK, et al. Digital tomosynthesis—a new lease of life for the intravenous urogram? Br J Radiol. 2011;84:464–8.
18. Smith-Bindman R, Aubin C, Bailitz J, Bengiamin RN, Camargo CA Jr, Corbo J, et al. Ultrasonography versus computed tomography for suspected nephrolithiasis. N Engl J Med. 2014;371:1100–10.
19. Mills L, Morley EJ, Soucy Z, Vilke GM, Lam SHF. Ultrasound for the diagnosis and management of suspected urolithiasis in the emergency department. J Emerg Med. 2018;54(2):215–20.
20. Gottlieb M, Long B, Koyfman A. The evaluation and management of urolithiasis in the emergency department: a review of the literature. Am J Emerg Med. 2018;36(4):699–706.
21. Smith RC, Rosenfield AT, Choe KA, et al. Acute flank pain: comparison of non-contrast-enhanced CT and intravenous urography. Radiology. 1995;194:789–94.
22. Nestler T, Haneder S, Hikamp NG. Modern imaging techniques in urinary stone disease. Curr Opin Urol. 2019;29:81–8.
23. El-Wahab OA, El-Tabey MA, El-Barky E, El-Baky SA, El-Falah A, Refaat M. Multislice computed tomography vs intravenous urography for planning supine percutaneous nephrolithotomy: a randomised clinical trial. Arab J Urol. 2014;12(2):1627.
24. Xiang H, et al. Systematic review and meta-analysis of the diagnostic accuracy of low-dose computed tomography of the kidneys, ureters and bladder for urolithiasis. J Med Imaging Radiat Oncol. 2017;61:582.
25. Rob S, Bryant T, Wilson I, Somani BK. Ultra-low-dose, low-dose, and standard dose CT of the kidneys, ureters, and bladder: is there a difference? Results from a systematic review of the literature. Clin Radiol. 2017;72:11–5.
26. Meher S, Gibbons N, DasGupta R. Renal stones in pregnancy. Obstet Med. 2014;7:103–10.
27. Kanal E, Greenberg T, Hoff MN, et al. ACR manual on MR safety. Reston, VA: American College of Radiology; 2020. p. 15–6.
28. Bowen DK, Tasian GE. Pediatric stone disease. Urol Clin North Am. 2018;45:539–50.
29. Bres-Niewada E, Dybowski B, Radziszeskiw P. Predicting stone composition before treatment—can it really drive clinical decisions? Cent European J Urol. 2014;67:392–6.
30. Celik S, Sefik E, Basmaci I, Bozkurt IH, Aydin ME, Yonguc T, Degirmenci T. A novel method for prediction of stone composition: the average and difference of Hounsfield units and their cut-off values. Int Urol Nephrol. 2018;50(8):1397–405. https://doi.org/10.1007/s11255-018-1929-3.
31. Nayyar R, Khattar N, Sood R. Functional evaluation before stone surgery: is it mandatory? Indian J Urol. 2012;28:256–62.
32. Taylor AT. Radionuclides in nephrourology, part 1: radiopharmaceuticals, quality control, and quantitative indices. J Nucl Med. 2014;55:608–15.
33. Sreenevasan G. Bilateral renal calculi. Ann R Coll Surg Engl. 1974;55:9–12.
34. Feder MT, Blitstein J, Mason B, Hoenig DM. Predicting differential renal function using computerized tomography measurements of renal parenchymal area. J Urol. 2008;180(5):2110–5.
35. Sarma D, Barua SK, Rajeev TP, Baruah SJ. Correlation between differential renal function estimation using CT-based functional renal parenchymal volume and ^{99m}Tc-DTPA renal scan. Indian J Urol. 2012;28:414–7.

Part II

Instrument for Endourological Treatment of Urinary Calculi

3 Understanding the Instruments: Endoscope

Shuji Isotani

Abstract

The purpose of this chapter is principally to provide the equipment information, knowledge, and tips while using the ureteroscope (URS); it may familiarize urologists with using the URS in their clinical practice. We begin with the brief history of URS, followed by the URS mechanical futures such as the differences with "rigid vs. flexible" and "fiber-optic scope vs. digital scope" in optics. "Durability and single-use ureteroscope" and "tips to prevent flexible ureteroscope damages" are also discussed.

3.1 Introduction

The continuous development of surgical devices and the advancement of endoscopic techniques have improved the treatment outcomes of retrograde ureteroscopic surgery [1]. In this chapter, we present an overview of emerging technologies of current endoscopy in the light of the recent versatility of endoscopes and current limitations. As ureteroscopy is the most common endoscopy we use, we used the development of ureteroscopy as the main example for the discussion of endoscopic development. The same principles also applied to other endoscopies, including cystoscopy and nephoscopy. Understanding the principles of the ureteroscopes that define current ureteroscopy is one of the important keys to establish an efficient and safe procedure with endoscopic treatment.

Two types of ureteroscopes exist in shape and handling: rigid ureteroscopy (r-URS) and flexible ureteroscopy (f-URS). Recently, significant advancements include new endoscopy design, especially in the flexible ureteroscopy (f-URS), and it made f-URS more effective auxiliary tools, with improvement in treatment protocols and in laser lithotripsy technology. We use the term retrograde intrarenal surgery (RIRS) as almost the same meaning as f-URS because retrograde intrarenal surgery is performed by flexible ureteroscopy. The f-URS can be used for all locations of the ureter. Thus, strictly speaking, the term f-URS covers a wider area of the treatment location of the ureter than RIRS. Now, the f-URS seems to be one of the major treatment modalities for upper urinary tract calculi all over the world [2–5]. We have much literature that confirmed the effectiveness and safety of URS in the treatment of renal stone [4, 6–8, 9, 10]. Studies have demonstrated that the feasibility of URS in stones less than 2 cm and illustrated the versatility and possibility of this technique [11–17]. The f-URS is considered the most beneficial therapeutic

S. Isotani (✉)
Department of Urology, Juntendo University, Tokyo, Japan
e-mail: s-isotani@juntendo.ac.jp

A. C.F. Ng et al. (eds.), *Practical Management of Urinary Stone*,
https://doi.org/10.1007/978-981-16-4193-0_3

option for most of the stones with the size and location of kidney stones except the staghorn stone, and the urologist should consider this new treatment.

Ureteroscopy is known as the name of the endoscope, which is designed to visualize within the upper urinary system (ureter and kidney) and work as an instrument to treat calicles, tumors, or strictures in the upper urinary system, and it is commonly used by urologists and endourologists. In the following sections, we will first provide the equipment information, knowledge, and tips while using the ureteroscope. We hope the information may help urologists to familiarize themselves with URS in their clinical practice.

3.2 Brief History of URS

The first rigid ureteroscopy (r-URS) was done in 1912 when Dr. Young introduced a pediatric cystoscope into a severe dilated right ureter of a child who had posterior urethral valves and he was pleasantly astonished by the renal pelvis. The following century has seen continued development and evolution of ureteroscopy to the smaller and better image in use. Then, the first flexible ureteroscope (f-URS) was reported in 1964 by Dr. Marshall, who used a 9F pediatric flexible cystoscope for the adult ureter; there was no working channel or active deflection at that time, and this is used for only for the diagnostic use [18]. In 1989, Dore et al. first reported his preliminary 15 cases of upper urinary stones treated by an evolutionally flexible ureteroscope [19]. Since then, much improvement has been made in f-URS technology in terms of smaller outer diameters, larger working channels, active deflection (maneuverability), and better visualization of the scope to facilitating the operator to increase the effectiveness of this treatment.

In the 1980s, f-URS was continuously improved, with both the development of fibrotic light sources and the scope deflection ability in passive or active direction, and in 1994, the evolutionally technological advancement brought a miniaturized flexible ureteroscope, with a tip diameter of 7.5 Fr and an adequate working-channel of 3.6 Fr. In 2001, a flexible ureteroscopy with active two-way exaggerated deflection (up to 270 degree) was introduced, and these scopes could provide the ability to reach the entire intrarenal collecting system in the surgery. In addition, about the imaging technique, the advancements in the endourological evolution of ureteroscopes are moving from fiber-optic imaging to digital imaging technology [10, 20]. The first digital flexible ureteroscopes have been reported by Zilberman et al. in 2011. The digital flexible ureteroscopes improved resolution and color representation, as well as 5.3 times larger image size compared with the standard fiber-optic flexible ureteroscope [20]. With combining new digital ureteroscopy and high-definition television, the image quality has dramatically improved. Moreover, accessory equipment such as baskets and laser lithotripsy technology have also improved the efficacy of the procedures [8]. Because the technology regarding the URS has improved, the f-URS has been accepted as the optimal treatment for renal calculi with very low morbidity; recently, there has been a huge surge in the number of ureterorenoscopic procedures being performed. URS has been rapidly diffusing worldwide, and it led to the expansion of indications in the USA, Europe, and Asia [1, 2, 4–6, 10, 12, 14].

The development of the flexible ureteroscopy overcomes the limitation of rigid scope and allows the urologist to inspect nearly the entirety of the inner kidney to find stones, treat them, and remove them using a variety of techniques. To achieve a safe and effective surgical procedure in the URS, ureteroscopy should have a good visual image of the operation field by imaging technology development, efficient irrigation flow with low intrarenal pressure, and good defluxion capability to achieve the access to all renal calyx. The ideal URS in the future may overcome such conflicting ideas both of the easy access to all renal cavities by better deflection capability with small shaft and excellent visuality by advanced imaging technology [9, 21].

3.3 Rigid vs. Flexible

3.3.1 Rigid Ureteroscope (Semirigid Ureteroscope)

Comparing the flexible ureteroscope (f-URS), the rigid ureteroscope (r-URS) can provide multiple entries and exits during fragment retrieval under better visualization of operation field with better irrigation efficiency. On the other hand, with r-URS, it is difficult to access the stone located in the upper ureter or renal collecting system. When urinary stone moving to the upper ureter or kidney by stone retropulsion, flexible ureteroscopy is required to pursuit the stone to the upper ureter and renal pelvis. Also, for the patient with an elevated bladder neck, huge prostates, narrow ureters, and very developed psoas muscles, it becomes a complex case by only the rigid URS. For these cases, it is better to prepare f-URS. Although the f-URS has been rapidly spreading in the world, the r-URS still has been one of the best treatment modalities for ureteral urolithiasis. For example, the r-URS could be performed before f-URS. The advantage of using r-URS before f-URS is that the ureter becomes passively dilated under direct vision by r-URS, and surgeons can identify the real compliance of the ureter by advancing the scope to know the ideal ureteral access sheath (UAS) size according to the patient's anatomy. An additional benefit is that in the limited case of second-look procedures, missed fragments that migrated down into the lower ureter can be easily removed by r-URS without UAS placement [22–24]. From the result of the Clinical Research Office of the Endourological Society (CROES) URS global study including 9681 patients, the rigid URS was the most used procedure for ureteral stones in all locations. The stone-free rates with r-URS were 94.2%, 84.5%, and 76.6% for distal, middle, and proximal ureteral stones, respectively. For stones located in proximal ureter, failure and retreatment rates were significantly higher for r-URS than for f-URS [17]. The reported incidence of complications was low: 3.8% to 7.7% as intraoperative complications and 2.5% to 4.6% as postoperative complications [17]. In Table 3.1, the futures of rigid URS and flexible URS are summarized.

Table 3.1 Comparison of rigid URS and flexible URS

	Rigid scope	Flexibe scope
Working channel	Large	Small
Vision with blood	Better	Poorer
Irrigation	Better	Poorer
Durability	Long	Short
Maneuverability	Limited	Great

3.3.2 Flexible Endoscope

The flexible ureteroscope was developed to reach intrarenal structures by the deflection of the tip of the ureteroscope. The basic design of f-URS manipulation is the combination of deflection and rotation of the scope. Because the f-URS is deflected in only one plane by the scope handle, the surgeon needs to rotate the scope to reach the aimed place where the surgeon wants to observe. For example, the right-handed operator can visualize the calyces in the right kidney located posteriorly and anteriorly by supination and extra-supination of the ureteroscope, respectively.

The first flexible URS was developed by Marshall in 1964 [18]; the continual improvement with technological innovations has noticed in f-URS technology afterward pursuing smaller diameters, larger working channels, more maneuverability by active deflection, and better visualization of the scope to facilitating the effectiveness of RIRS [10, 25].

About the optimal target of f-URS (as the same meaning as RIRS here), in 2017, Sanguedolce et al. reviewed the literature regarding "RIRS: retrograde intrarenal surgery" and found that the main target of RIRS is renal stones of 1–2 cm in size, and the surgical outcomes were considered safe and effective, even in patients with specific conditions such as bleeding diathesis, anatomical malformation, or pregnancy. They concluded that RIRS is a well-established procedure under constant evolution with advances in technique and technology [1].

Today, most of the new generation f-URSs (both fiber-optic and digital scopes) are equipped with acceptable optical quality, a 270-degree deflection capability in both directions, and a standard 3.6 Fr working channel. Now, the f-URS has gained worldwide popularity due to its minimal invasiveness and satisfactory outcomes [1] (Table 3.2).

However, there are still some issues regarding the use of the flexible ureteroscope. One of the biggest concerns is the durability of the scope. The flexible ureteroscope is fragile and requires its usage with caution as well during the surgery as sterilization. One randomized comparative trial, which evaluated the lifespan of different new generation ureteroscopes, including Wolf Viper, Olympus URF-P5, Gyrus-ACMI DUR-8 Elite, and Stryker FlexVision U-500, showed that the mean device durability was ranged from 5.3 to 18 cases before major repairs because of poor visibility (42%), a decrease of maneuverability (25%), and damage of working channel due to laser misfiring (8%) [26]. There were other several papers that have been published about the durability of the flexible ureteroscope. In 1998 White and Moran, in 2000 Afane [27], and more recently in 2006 Monga demonstrated longevity ranging from 6 to 25 procedures in use [28]. To increase the durability of the flexible ureteroscope, in 2002, Pietrow reported that they increased the durability up to an average of 27.5 uses (range 19–34) before repairs [29]. In 2006, Traxer demonstrated that there is an increase in the performance of the instruments if they are used by an experienced endourologist [30]. They reported that it was reaching 50 procedures to first repair with a digital flexible ureteroscope. Even in these reports, in general, the need for repair frequently occurs with the ureterorenoscope, and the endourologist needs to take careful consideration not to damage the scope by the surgical procedure, and further improvements in scope durability would be needed. Actually, an initial purchasing cost of f-URS is around USD 25,000 plus costs for the video processor and viewing monitor [31]. The use of flexible ureteroscopes is associated with a high financial burden. Thus, the durability of f-URS became one of the most important issues about f-URS.

Also, there are many kinds of f-URS available in the market right now, such as fiber-optic, digital, disposable, or reusable ureteroscopes. There is some difference between each other in terms of durability, image quality, maneuverability, shaft diameter, and also working channel arrangement. These factors usually conflict with each other. For example, the smallest currently available ure-

Table 3.2 Currently available flexible URS with its features

Company/model	Type	Tip caliber (Fr)	Shaft caliber (Fr)	Working channel (Fr)	Deflection
Olympus URF-P5	Fiber-optic	5.3	8.4	3.6	180/275
Olympus URF-P6	Fiber-optic	4.9	7.95	3.6	275/275
Olympus URF-P7	Fiber-optic	4.9	7.95	3.6	275/275
Olympus URF-V	Digital	8.3	9.9	3.6	180/275
Olympus URF-V2	Digital	8.5	8.4	3.6	275/275
Olympus URF-V3	Digital	8.5	8.4	3.6	275/275
Storz Flex-X2/X2s	Fiber-optic	7.5	7.5	3.6	270/270
Storz Flex-XC	Digital	8.5	8.4	3.6	270/270
Wolf Viper	Fiber-optic	6	8.8	3.6	270/270
Wolf Boa	Digital	6.6	8.7	3.6	270/270
Wolf Cobra	Fiber-optic	6.0	9.9	3.6	270/270
Wolf Cobra vision	Digital	5.2	9.9	3.3 × 2	270/270
Boston Scientific–Lithovue	Digital	7.7	9.5	2.4 and 3.3	270/270
Pussen	Digital	9.0	9.5	3.6	270/270
PolyScope	Fiber-optic	8.0	8.0	3.6	>250

teroscope is based on the fiber-optic ureteroscope rather than the digital ureteroscope, although the best image quality is provided by the digital ureteroscope rather than the fiber-optic ureteroscope. These conflicting factors make it difficult to compare these scopes.

3.4 Fiber-Optic vs. Digital Imaging System

Apart from maneuverability proprieties, image quality is a key factor affecting efficacy, safety, and versatility of ureteroscopy. There are two types of image systems existing in the flexible ureteroscopy: fiber-optic and digital imaging systems. In Table 3.3, the futures of fiber-optic and digital imaging are summarized.

Table 3.3 Comparison of fiber-optic and digital scopes

	Fiber-optic	Digital
Principle	Rod-lens	Chip-on-tip
Image	Moiré, smaller	Clearer, bigger
Camera head	Add-on	Inbuild
Setup	Longer	Easyer
Durability	Shorter	Better
Cost	Less	High
Diameter	Smaller	Larger

3.4.1 Fiber-Optic Endoscope

Historically, the first f-URS was started with a fiber-optic imaging system bundling flexible optical fibers between the distal tip and the proximal eyepiece [18]. Before introducing the digital flexible ureteroscopes, flexible fiber-optic ureteroscopes helped to develop the endourological surgical treatment options for the management of urolithiasis in the upper ureter and intrarenal collecting system. The thin flexible glass fibers that were covered by a cladding with a low refraction index allow the light transmission over a long distance with minimal losses. The bundle of glass fibers is orchestrated coherently in order to produce one big image at the end of instruments. The visualization capability is variable between the manufacturers according to the difference of number and quality in the optic fibers for the image transmission. The number and quality of the optic fibers reflect the durability and maneuverability of the scopes.

With fiber-scope, a honeycomb effect, in other words, the Moire effect, and the fuzzy image can be seen on the screen (Fig. 3.1a) [31]. An increasing number of fiber-optic bundles may decrease the honeycomb effect, but these thinner fibers would be more easily broken in the scope.

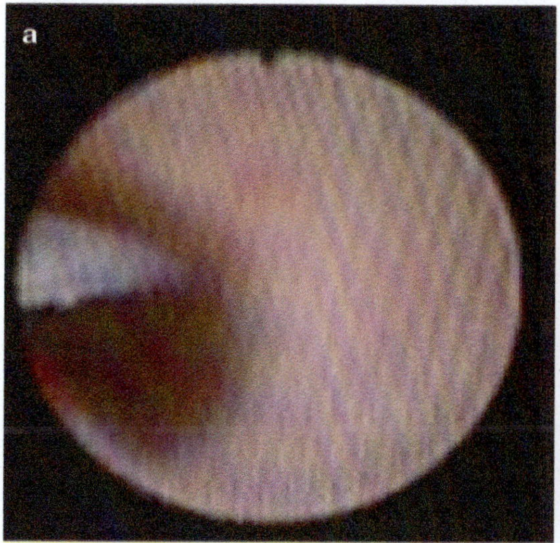

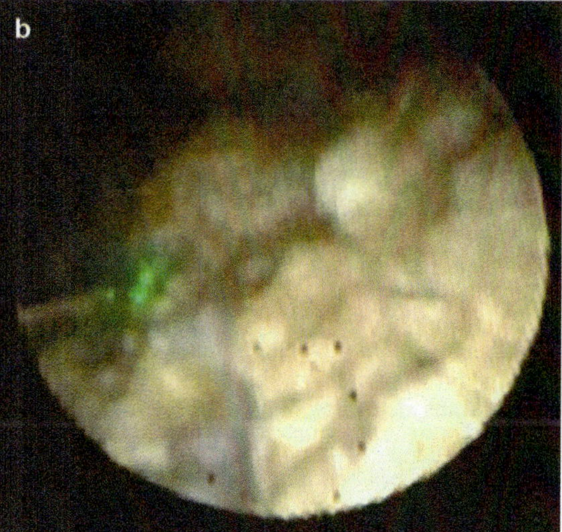

Fig. 3.1 (**a**) Moire effect; (**b**) broken fibers in endoscope

The fiber-optic fibers are easily broken when passed through the ureter, and during times of extreme deflection, such as entry into the lower pole, the broken fiber is presented as a black dot on the screen (Fig. 3.1b). As the additional fibers continue to break, visualization continues to deteriorate until the repair is ultimately required. In addition, the leakage of the ureteroscope, which was usually developed by a small scar or hole in the jacket of the ureteroscope, leads to progressive fogging of the image to require repair. Pietrow et al. showed in 2002 that with an average of 15.3 passes, 20 or more optical fibers were broken using Olympus 7.5 Fr flexible ureteroscopes [29].

Although the image quality is not good as the digital ureteroscope, one of the benefits of the fiber-optic ureteroscopes is better accessibility in the whole renal pelvis. All of the fiber-optics had better end-tip deflection compared with the digital f-URS because the fiber-optic scope does not have the bulky and rigid configuration of the digital camera unit at the tip of ureteroscopes. Thus, to approach a difficult lower pole calyx, it might be better to use a fiber-optic f-URS with the risk of breaking fibers [21]. It appears to be the strong benefit from our daily practice that in certain cases, some additional degrees of deflection would have been key for treatment success by the fiber-optic ureteroscope. Another benefit of the fiber-optic ureteroscope is that it has smaller distal tip diameter than the digital scope [21]. The small size of ureteroscopes is the fundamental key point to achieve successful ureteroscopy by acquiring better insertion and irrigation flow, and it may provide higher single-session success rates.

3.4.2 Digital Endoscope

Digital imaging technology has been used in the area of gastrointestinal and lower urinary tract endoscopy; it has been introduced to flexible ureteroscopes in 2006 as the world's first digital f-URS DUR-D (Gyrus-ACMI). The traditional fiber-optic bundles were replaced by nine wires that transmit the digital signal from the image system located at the tip of the scope to the camera control unit. The tip of the endoscope uses a complementary metal-oxide semiconductor (CMOS) imager system [26, 31]. This imaging system eliminates the fragile flexible low-resolution fiber-optics and provided excellent imaging quality. The second-generation digital ureteroscope that came into the market in August 2008 utilized a CCD chip as the image capture device URF-V (Olympus). The URF-V had an 8.5F tapered tip and a working channel of 3.6F. It has a 180–275 degrees up-down deflection ability. This digital ureteroscope provided better visualization in the upper collecting system, good maneuverability, and deflection ability when applying either a laser fiber or a basket through the working channel; however, it had a larger diameter than a standard 4.9 F fiber-optic ureteroscope.

There are two types of imaging sensors that exist in the market right now. The digital ureteroscope by Karl Storz and the complementary metal oxide semiconductor (CMOS) imaging sensor by Richard Wolf. The CMOS is a generic term for the process used to produce these image sensors, along with a multitude of other semiconductor items such as computer RAM and processors like those from Intel and other manufacturers. Thus, CMOS image sensors can be made in the same fabs as these other items, with the same equipment at a lower cost than CCD image sensors. The other imaging sensor is a charge-coupled device sensor (CCD) equipped with a digital ureteroscope made by Olympus. CCD achieved higher-quality imaging than CMOS but required a manufacturing process that is different from that used for manufacturing other computer chips such as processors and RAM. This means that specialized CCD fabs have to be constructed, and they cannot be used for making other components, thereby making CCD more expensive than CMOS [32]. The next-generation digital ureteroscopes are likely to integrate ultra-miniaturized digital image sensors with increasing image resolution catching up with current display resolution standards such as "Full HD" or "4 k."

The benefit of digital ureteroscopes is that it achieves better image quality than fiber-optic f-URS. By this superiority, the digital ureteroscopes achieved significantly shorter operative time in several clinical studies. In the literature, some studies showed that better image quality provides higher precision for diagnosis and treatment and a shorter procedure time [10, 21, 33]. Somani and coworkers demonstrated that the advantage of the digital ureteroscope in cases of stone treatment was the decreased operative time by 20% [32]. Also, for detection of upper urinary tract urothelial carcinoma, most authors stated that digital ureteroscopes seem to achieve better tumor detection rates. The other benefit of digital ureteroscopes is their durability. The digital f-URS has been reported to have superior durability than fiber-optic models at first. However, the initial enthusiasm for improved durability of the digital f-URS has not been well established. In 2018, Legemate demonstrated significant variability in the durability of both the digital and fiber-optic scopes from 10 to 79 uses prior to repair [34, 35]. In 2019, Temiz et al. also concluded that the digital f-URS was associated with a higher initial cost but offered no additional benefit with regard to scope durability or surgical outcomes compared to standard fiber-optic scopes [33]. There appears to be little difference between fiber-optic and digital ureteroscopes in durability.

3.5 Reusable vs Single-Use Endoscope

Despite the technological development of flexible ureteroscopes, including fiber-optic and digital scopes, durability remains a major concern. Due to the high cost and limited durability, the cost–benefit of the ureteroscopes has become an important factor for initiating and maintaining f-URS programs worldwide, especially in developing countries. To solve this problem, LithoVue (Boston Scientific) became available as the first complete disposable digital flexible ureteroscope in 2016 [36]. Now, there are some single-use ureteroscopes available or under development, such as Uscope (Zhuhai Pusen Medical Technology), NeoFlex (Neoscope Inc.), and Shaogang or YC-FR-A (YouCare Tech), and most of them were provided with a CMOS digital image [37]. The initial series of studies about single-use ureteroscope suggested that these single-use ureteroscopes may be viable and cost-effective alternatives to reusable flexible ureteroscopes [38]. However, there were some discrepancies observed between these studies when the same characteristics were compared with digital flexible ureteroscopes [39]. This variability suggests that further research must be carried out to concretely determine the comparability of single-use ureteroscope image quality and performance. Also, in 2017, Martin et al. demonstrated that single-use URS might be cost-beneficial at centers with a lower case volume per year, but institutions with a high volume of cases may find the reusable URS cost-beneficial based on their cost-benefit analysis [40]. The environmental impact of a single-use ureteroscope is another factor that needs greater attention. McGrath Shannon examined a comparative study about the carbon footprint of single-use and reusable ureteroscopes in 2018 [41]. They concluded that the environmental impacts of the reusable flexible ureteroscope and the single-use flexible ureteroscope are comparable, even it is challenging to predict the potential environmental implications. More studies are needed to demonstrate the efficiency, cost-effectiveness, and the other factors of these devices that are more difficult to use than the usual reusable flexible ureterorenoscopes. Also, currently, available models continue to undergo rapid innovation with several new models that may be promised. Continued innovation and healthy competition in this field will lead to improved devices that are more cost-effective. In this rapidly changing field, more research is needed to validate the clinical performance and efficacy of these single-use flexible ureteroscopes.

3.6 Tips to Prevent Flexible Endoscope Damages

As we know, the flexible ureteroscope is fragile. The approach to minimizing the cost of flexible ureteroscope damage is improving the technique to maximize the longevity of the flexible scope. There are some reports published to identify the factors to enhance the longevity of a ureteroscope. The factors such as the lower pole stone, multiple passes of the scope during the operation, and the scope cleaning methods have been suggested [29]. Also, recently, multiple accessories have been created to facilitate the expanded applications of flexible ureteroscopy. Hosny et al. summarized the current techniques that can be immediately adopted to maximize f-URS use and reduce the need for repairs in 2019 [42]. They recommend using a semirigid ureteroscope prior to f-URS to calibrate and dilate the lower ureter, keeping f-URS as straight as possible, confirming the adequate lubrication on the f-URS and a well-lubricated hydrophilic guidewire during insertion. Also, at the operation, the gentle manipulation of the handpiece deflection lever and avoiding the maximum deflection for prolonged periods reduce the deflection-related injury. The surgeon should hold the f-URS by the handpiece and always maintain the f-URS in a neutral/loosely coiled position. To have easier access to the stone prior to lithotripsy, repositioning lower pole stones to the upper pole is recommended. Also, they emphasize that confirming the ureteral access sheath (UAS) is not restricting f-URS deflection (ideally, the UAS should be in the proximal ureter below the uretero-pelvic junction) and removal of the f-URS with UAS together when finished. About the laser fiber, smaller diameter laser fibers should be used if possible, being aware of keeping f-URS in a straight position during the insertion of laser fiber, avoiding the laser firing when the fiber is not clearly visible (1/4 of the screen) and at extreme f-URS deflection. After the surgery, it was recommended to perform the pressure leak test for every case (immediate repair if leak identified), and cleaning and sterilization should be done according to the manufacturer's guidelines. Finally, the scope should be stored carefully in dedicated cases to avoid trapping.

References

1. Sanguedolce F, Bozzini G, Chew B, Kallidonis P, De La Rosette J. The evolving role of retrograde intrarenal surgery in the treatment of urolithiasis. Eur Urol Focus. 2017;3(1):1–10.
2. Isotani S, Noma Y, Wakumoto Y, Muto S, Horie S. Endurological treatment trend of upper urinary urolithiasis in Japan from the Japanese Diagnosis Procedure Combination Database. Int J Urol. 2019;25:373.
3. Ordon M, Urbach D, Mamdani M, Saskin R, Honey RJD, Pace KT. The surgical management of kidney stone disease: a population based time series analysis. J Urol. 2014;192(5):1450–6.
4. Geraghty RM, Jones P, Somani BK. Worldwide trends of urinary stone disease treatment over the last two decades: a systematic review. J Endourol. 2017;31(6):547–56.
5. Pietropaolo A, Proietti S, Geraghty R, Skolarikos A, Papatsoris A, Liatsikos E, et al. Trends of "urolithiasis: interventions, simulation, and laser technology" over the last 16 years (2000–2015) as published in the literature (PubMed): a systematic review from European section of Uro-technology (ESUT). World J Urol. 2017;35(11):1651–8.
6. Li JK, Teoh JY, Ng C-F. Updates in endourological management of urolithiasis. Int J Urol. 2019;26(2):172–83.
7. Rukin NJ, Siddiqui ZA, Chedgy ECP, Somani BK. Trends in upper tract stone disease in England: evidence from the hospital episodes statistics database. Urol Int. 2017;98(4):391–6.
8. Proietti S, Knoll T, Giusti G. Contemporary ureteroscopic management of renal stones. Int J Surg. 2016;36(Pt D):681–7.
9. Giusti G, Proietti S, Villa L, Cloutier J, Rosso M, Gadda GM, et al. Current standard technique for modern flexible ureteroscopy: tips and tricks. Eur Urol. 2016;70(1):188–94.
10. Alenezi H, Denstedt JD. Flexible ureteroscopy: technological advancements, current indications and outcomes in the treatment of urolithiasis. Asian J Urol. 2015;2(3):133–41.
11. Kumar A, Kumar N, Vasudeva P, Jha SK, Kumar R, Singh H. A prospective, randomized comparison of shock wave lithotripsy, retrograde intrarenal surgery and Miniperc for treatment of 1 to 2 cm radiolucent lower calyceal renal calculi: a single Center experience. J Urol. 2015;193(1):160–4.
12. Zumstein V, Betschart P, Abt D, Schmid H-P, Panje CM, Putora PM. Surgical management of urolithiasis—a systematic analysis of available guidelines. BMC Urol. 2018;18(1):1–8.
13. Drake T, Grivas N, Dabestani S, Knoll T, Lam T, MacLennan S, et al. What are the benefits and harms of ureteroscopy compared with shock-wave lithotripsy in the treatment of upper ureteral stones? A systematic review. Eur Urol. 2017;72(5):1–15.
14. Assimos D, Krambeck A, Miller NL, Monga M, Murad MH, Nelson CP, et al. Surgical management of stones: American Urological Association/Endourological Society guideline, part II. J Urol. 2016;196(4):1161–9.
15. Ordon M, Andonian S, Blew B, Schuler T, Chew B, Pace KT. CUA Guideline: Management of ureteral calculi. Can Urol Assoc J. 2015;9(11–12):E837–51.

16. Donaldson JF, Lardas M, Scrimgeour D, Stewart F, MacLennan S, Lam TBL, et al. Systematic review and meta-analysis of the clinical effectiveness of shock wave lithotripsy, retrograde intrarenal surgery, and percutaneous nephrolithotomy for lower-pole renal stones. Eur Urol. 2015;67(4):612–6.
17. Castro EP, Osther PJS, Jinga V, Razvi H, Stravodimos KG, Parikh K, et al. Differences in ureteroscopic stone treatment and outcomes for distal, mid-, proximal, or multiple ureteral locations: the Clinical Research Office of the Endourological Society ureteroscopy global study. Eur Urol. 2014;66(1):102–9.
18. Marshall VF. Fiber optics in urology. J Urol. 1964;91(1):110–4.
19. Dore B, Orget J, Grange P, Aubert J. [Flexible ureteroscopy. Diagnostic and therapeutic significance. Apropos of 15 cases]. Annales d'urologie. Ann Urol (Paris); 1989;23(5):377–382.
20. Zilberman DE, Lipkin ME, Ferrandino MN, Simmons WN, Mancini JG, Raymundo ME, et al. The digital flexible ureteroscope: in vitro assessment of optical characteristics. J Endourol. 2011;25(3):519–22.
21. Dragos LB, Somani BK, Sener ET, Buttice S, Proietti S, Ploumidis A, et al. Which flexible ureteroscopes (digital vs. fiber-optic) can easily reach the difficult lower pole calices and have better end-tip deflection: in vitro study on K-Box. A PETRA evaluation. J Endourol. 2017;31(7):630–7.
22. Giusti G, Proietti S, Rodríguez-Socarrás ME, Saitta G, Bellinzoni P, Gaboardi F. Semirigid ureteroscopy: step by step. J Endourol. 2020 May;34(S1):S13–6.
23. Mursi K, Elsheemy MS, Morsi HA, Ghaleb A-KA, Abdel-Razzak OM. Semi-rigid ureteroscopy for ureteric and renal pelvic calculi: Predictive factors for complications and success. Arab J Urol. 2013;11(2):136–41.
24. Rana AM, Aquil S, Khawaja AM. Semirigid ureteroscopy and pneumatic lithotripsy as definitive management of obstructive ureteral calculi during pregnancy. Urology. 2009;73(5):964–7.
25. Wright AE, Rukin NJ, Somani BK. Ureteroscopy and stones: current status and future expectations. World J Nephrol. 2014;3(4):243–8.
26. Knudsen B, Miyaoka R, Shah K, Holden T, Turk TMT, Pedro RN, et al. Durability of the next-generation flexible fiberoptic ureteroscopes: a randomized prospective multi-institutional clinical trial. Urology. 2010;75(3):534–8.
27. Afane JS, Olweny EO, Bercowsky E, Sundaram CP, Dunn MD, Shalhav AL, et al. Flexible ureteroscopes: a single center evaluation of the durability and function of the new endoscopes smaller than 9Fr. J Urol. 2000;164(4):1164–8.
28. Monga M, Best S, Venkatesh R, Ames C, Lee C, Kuskowski M, et al. Durability of flexible ureteroscopes: a randomized, prospective study. J Urol. 2006;176(1):137–41.
29. Pietrow PK, Auge BK, Delvecchio FC, Silverstein AD, Weizer AZ, ALBALA DM, et al. Techniques to maximize flexible ureteroscope longevity. Urology. 2002;60(5):784–8.
30. Traxer O, Dubosq F, Jamali K, Gattegno B, Thibault P. New-generation flexible ureterorenoscopes are more durable than previous ones. Urology. 2006;68(2):276–9.
31. Gridley CM, Knudsen BE. Digital ureteroscopes: technology update. Res Rep Urol. 2017;9:19–25.
32. Somani BK, Al-Qahtani SM, de Medina SDG, Traxer O. Outcomes of flexible ureterorenoscopy and laser fragmentation for renal stones: comparison between digital and conventional ureteroscope. Urology. 2013;82(5):1017–9.
33. Temiz MZ, Colakerol A, Ertas K, Tuken M, Yuruk E. Fiberoptic versus digital: a comparison of durability and cost effectiveness of the two flexible ureteroscopes. Urol Int. 2019;102(2):181–6.
34. Legemate JD, Kamphuis GM, Freund JE, Baard J, Zanetti SP, Catellani M, et al. Durability of flexible ureteroscopes: a prospective evaluation of longevity, the factors that affect it, and damage mechanisms. Eur Urol Focus. 2018 Mar 10:1–7.
35. Lin C-C, Wu LS-H, Huang S-S, Lin C-F, Chen W-H, Wu C-T. Surgical technique to achieve high durability of flexible ureteroscopes: a single hospital experience. Biomed J. 2018;41(6):385–90.
36. Proietti S, Dragos L, Molina W, Doizi S, Giusti G, Traxer O. Comparison of new single-use digital flexible ureteroscope versus nondisposable Fiber optic and digital ureteroscope in a cadaveric model. J Endourol. 2016;30(6):655–9.
37. Scotland KB, Chan JYH, Chew BH. Single-use flexible ureteroscopes: how do they compare with reusable ureteroscopes? J Endourol. 2019;33(2):71–8.
38. Taguchi K, Usawachintachit M, Tzou DT, Sherer BA, Metzler I, Isaacson D, et al. Micro-costing analysis demonstrates comparable costs for LithoVue compared to reusable flexible fiberoptic ureteroscopes. J Endourol. 2018;32(4):267–73.
39. Cho SY, Lee JY, Shin DG, Seo IY, Yoo S, Park HK. Evaluation of performance parameters of the disposable flexible ureterorenoscope (LITHOVUE) in patients with renal stones: a prospective, observational, single-arm, multicenter study. Sci Rep. 2018;8(1):9795–6.
40. Martin CJ, McAdams SB, Abdul-Muhsin H, Lim VM, Nunez-Nateras R, Tyson MD, et al. The economic implications of a reusable flexible digital ureteroscope: a cost-benefit analysis. J Urol. 2017;197(Pt 1):730–5.
41. Davis NF, McGrath S, Quinlan M, Jack G, Lawrentschuk N, Bolton DM. Carbon footprint in flexible ureteroscopy: a comparative study on the environmental impact of reusable and single-use ureteroscopes. J Endourol. 2018;32(3):214–7.
42. Defidio L, De Dominicis M, Di Gianfrancesco L, Fuchs G, Patel A. Improving flexible ureterorenoscope durability up to 100 procedures. J Endourol. 2012 Oct;26(10):1329–34.

Understanding the Instruments: Endourology Accessory

4

Kantima Jongjitaree and Ekkarin Chotikawanich

4.1 Introduction

Endourology has become an advanced surgery nowadays, especially the intraluminal procedure. Advanced technology provides a smaller ureteroscope, a wider range degree of deflection, and higher image quality. The new generation of the scope allows urologists access into the ureter and kidney without limitation. Both diagnostic and therapeutic procedures have been popular and rising with this endoscopy. Many instruments have been developed to facilitate intraluminal surgery. Guidewire, stone basket, ureteral access sheath (UAS), and anti-retropulsion device are the instruments commonly used while performing ureteroscopy. There are many designs of these instruments in the market. Understanding them is an important issue. This chapter will present the details of these common instruments.

4.2 Basket

Basket is a common stone retrieval device. The properties of the basket are the ability to open with enough radial force in the ureter, capture, and disengage the stone. The ideal basket has been designed in an atraumatic shape with a higher linear penetration force in order not to damage the endoscope and collecting system by the basket tip. As the flexible ureteroscopes are getting smaller day by day, the basket should be small and fit in the narrow space, flexible and easy for deflection. Baskets in a urologic procedure generally come in 1.3–2.2Fr in size for using through flexible and semirigid ureteroscope working channels. The size of the basket also matters. The flow of irrigant fluid is significantly decreased when the working channel is occupied by a large instrument. The smaller diameter basket has less strength and allows greater scope deflection when it has been in the flexible ureteroscope. The smaller size of the basket, 1.5Fr Sacred heart Halo® (Sacred heart medical®) and 1.9Fr Escape® nitinol basket (Boston Scientific®), allows passage of laser fiber along with it for simultaneous lithotripsy while capturing the stone (side by side approach). On the other hand, the smaller tip tends to kink and bend after repetitive insertion, so it decreases durability in complex procedures comparing with the larger one [1]. In a study, Korman et al. compared three small baskets with a size less than 1.5Fr [2]. They were 1.5Fr Halo® (Sacred Heart Medical), 1.5Fr N-Circle® Nitinol Tipless Stone Extractor (Cook Urological®), and 1.3Fr OptiFlex ® (Boston Scientific®). The results were not significantly different in extraction times in the caliceal model, but the OptiFlex® had the slowest extraction times in the ureteral model.

K. Jongjitaree · E. Chotikawanich (✉)
Division of Urology, Department of Surgery, Siriraj Hospital, Mahidol University, Bangkok, Thailand

A. C.F. Ng et al. (eds.), *Practical Management of Urinary Stone*,
https://doi.org/10.1007/978-981-16-4193-0_4

Designs of the basket are in various configurations. They differ in size, wire material, stiffness, opening dynamic, and the ability to capture and engage the stone.

4.2.1 Tip Designs

4.2.1.1 Tipped Basket

Knowing as older generation stainless steel-tipped at the end of the basket, the example is Segura® basket (Boston Scientific) and the Bard Dimention® (Bard Urology). They have more radial strength and rigidity. High radial dilatation force is useful for the stone that hugged in edematous ureteral mucosa but tipped end of basket causing more ureteric and renal papilla injury. Bleeding from mucosa frequency obscures the visualization and causes a problem in diagnostic ureteroscopy.

4.2.1.2 Tipless Basket

A newer-generation basket that is developed by removing stainless tip (Fig. 4.1b) but still provides good dilatation force, kink resistance, and memory properties of a new material is nitinol. Tipless nitinol baskets have been known to increase the efficacy and reduce trauma to the ureter and the renal papilla compared to older generation stainless steel-tipped baskets. The nitinol tipless baskets in the market include the N Circle® (Cook Urological), 1.9Fr Zero Tip® (Boston Scientific), Optiflex® (Boston Scientific), 2.2Fr Dormia® No-Tip (Coloplast), 1.9Fr Skylite® tipless nitinol (Bard Urology), and 1.5Fr Halo® (Sacred Heart Medical). Nishant Patel et al. [3] compared five tipless nitinol baskets and reported that the 1.5 Fr Halo® (Sacred Heart Medical) provided the highest resistive force to penetration, highest radial dilatation force, and least impediment in scope deflection.

4.2.1.3 Configurations

(a) Helical Design (Fig. 4.1a)

The mechanism of this type of basket is a rotation to engage the stone. This provides the advantage in less ureteral mucosa entrapment but has more difficulty in engaging the small stone. This basket is not suitable to capture the stone in the kidney as its shape causes more difficulty for capturing and may cause damage to a renal papilla.

(b) Spherical Design (Fig. 4.1b)

This type of basket provides an overall less dilatational force than the helical basket. It is easy to capture the stone in the kidney. The disadvantage of this basket is the difficulty of extracting multiple stones in one capture.

(c) End-Cage Design (Fig. 4.1c)

This holds like a regular basket and releases like a three-prong grasper. The design provides 50% better retention strength than grasper and better release ability than a regular basket. The open end allows more directing in line with the scope visualization and targeting ahead to capture the stone, while regular baskets capture the stone from a side of the basket. This ability facilitates capturing the stone that impacted urothelial mucosa. In stuck too large stone to remove, it

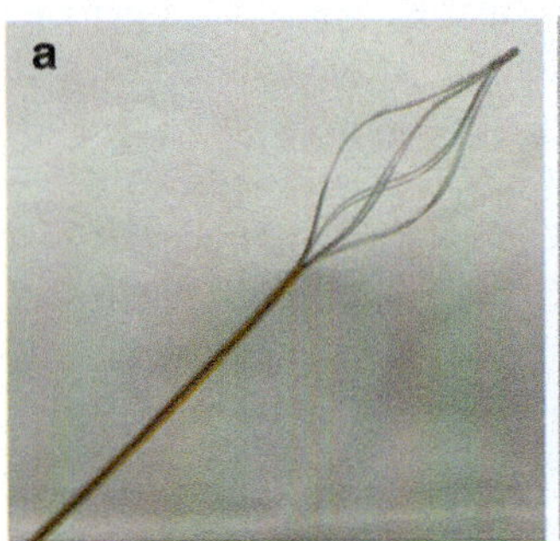

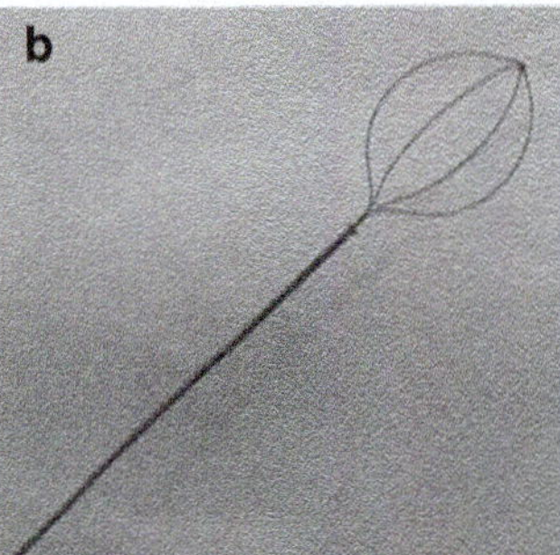

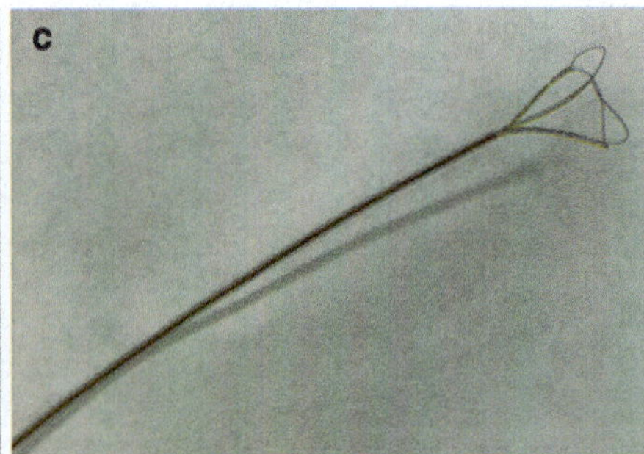

Fig. 4.1 Tip of a basket in various configurations. (**a**) Helical stainless steel tip basket (Gemini® 4 wire basket, Boston Scientific). (**b**) Spherical nitinol tipless basket (Zero tip® nitinol stone retrieval basket, Boston Scientific). (**c**) End-gage basket (Ngage® nitinol stone extractor, Cook Urological)

also permits easier release of stone than a tipless basket. The examples of this type of basket are 1.7Fr and 2.2Fr NGage® (Cook Urological) and 1.9Fr Dakota® nitinol stone retrieval device with Opensure handle (Boston Scientific). Both NGage and Dakota have similar durability, but Dakota has demonstrated versatility in releasing a larger stone (more than 8 mm) [4].

The baskets that have a more linear opening dynamic provide greater control, the opening sequence of the basket, entrapping a stone without over-excursion of the basket, and easier keeping basket tip in the field of view. This mechanism facilitates capturing mobile stones, especially in the renal calyx. The basket that has a true linear opening dynamic is the Ncircle® (Cook Urological). The others mostly had combined linear opening dynamic when small size opening and then exponential opening dynamic at the greater degree of opening. Comparing to the basket that has exponential opening dynamics, it has greater radial dilatation force but more difficult to control. As a result, most of the baskets increase the difficulty in stone capture when they are fully opened. Many studies showed that the 2.2Fr Ncircle® (Cook Urological) was the most rapid targeting basket width and best facilitated efficient stone capturing from the ureteral and calyceal model [5–7]. The 2.2Fr Ncompass® (Cook Urological) has a webbed configuration that best facilitates capturing stones as small as 1 mm in size.

A common complication of the basket was the ureteric injury. The cause of injury was entrapping too large stones during extraction. In this situation, releasing the stone from the basket was difficult. Some baskets have been designed to solve this problem. The 1.9Fr Escape® stone basket (Boston Scientific) can transform four wires into two wires at its base to free the entrapped stone. The Dimension® stone basket (Bard Urology) has a turning wheel at the handle to increase the basket size. The 1.5Fr Halo® (Sacred Heart Medical) has a rotatory wheel on the handle that allows rotation of the engaged stone.

After the innovation and development of a newer model of baskets, the incident of major urethral injury, ureteral avulsion decreases from 0.5% in 1982–1986 to 0% in 1992–1998 [8]. On the other hand, to prevent complications from stone basketing, avoidance of forceful manipulation is mandatory. Stone extraction should be reserved for stone less than 6 mm; in stones larger than 6 mm, fragmentation or ureteral dilatation may be necessary.

4.3 Guidewire

Numerous guidewires are now commercially available. The purpose of the guidewire is to provide safe access to the renal calyx and to be an inner portion of a coaxial system for passage of other instruments. Ideal guidewires have the property that can successfully pass through narrow ureters without causing any damage. The physical properties of guidewires included strength, bending force, and surface friction. Optimal strength of guidewires facilitates passage through tortuous ureter or coaxial passage stably guided the UAS compared with the floppy; Amplatz® (Boston Scientific) (Fig. 4.2b) is the most suitable for this purpose. A slippery surface with the optimum floppy tip of the guidewire can decrease ureteric injury; Glidewire® (Terumo) has the best property for this. The new model of guidewire developed in various sizes, tips, surface coatings, and strengths depends on the purpose of the operation.

1. Strength

The basic construction of a guidewire has two different layers: the inner layer determines the rigidity of the guidewire composed of a solid wire core, and the outer layer determines lubricity of the guidewire and is the layer that covers the inner layer by a tightly coiled steel wire that may be round or flat. The flat one makes the guidewire have a smoother surface. The stiffer guidewire provides strength that can straighten a tortuous ureter. Older generation guidewire is made of stainless steel. It is cheap but causes organ injury due to its strength and lack of deformability. The kinking usually occurred and becomes permanent. An example of this type of wire is Amplatz Super Stiff® wire (Boston Scientific). A newer generation of the guidewire

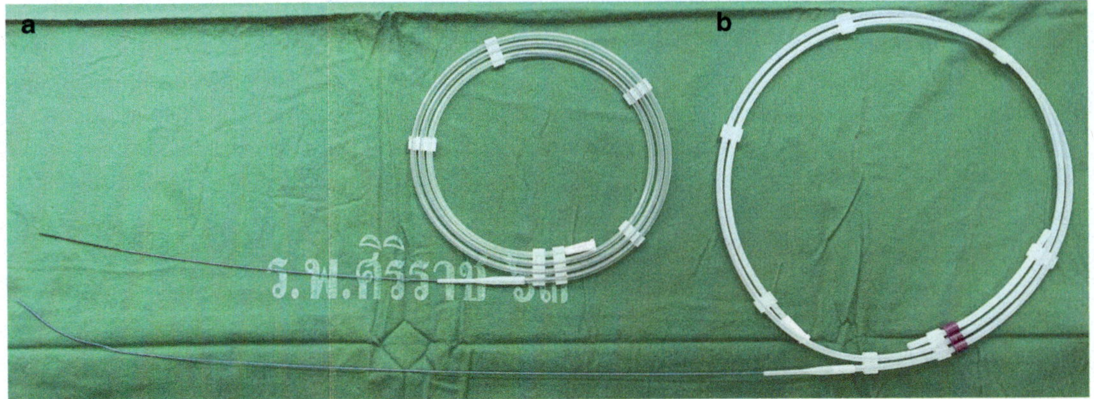

Fig. 4.2 (a) 0.035 inch × 150 cm hybrid guidewire with 5 cm hydrophilic floppy distal tip and rigid proximal shaft (Sensor® guidewire, Boston Scientific). (b) 0.038 inch × 145 cm stiff guidewire with 6 cm floppy distal tip and rigid proximal shaft (Amplatz® Super Stiff, Boston Scientific)

is made of nitinol. It is a metal alloy of nickel and titanium that has unique properties that have shape memory, kink resistance, and superelasticity with 10–30 times that of ordinary metal. The examples of this type of wire are Glidewire® (Terumo), Zebra® wire (Boston Scientific), Roadrunner® (Cook Urological), and U-nite® (Bard Urology).

2. Size

The size varies from 0.018 inch to 0.038 inch in diameter and 145–150 cm in length. The common size in the general endoscopic procedure is 0.038 inch with 150 cm in length.

3. Tips

Three types of tips were developed: straight, angle, and J type. The curve tip has better angulation for lateral displaced ureteric orifice. The flexible tip has benefits in the backloading of flexible ureteroscope and prevents instrument damage.

4. Surface Coating

The outer layer of the guidewire had the following surface coating substances: PTFE (Teflon) and various hydrophilic polymers for low friction characteristics. PTFE coating reduced the coefficient of friction to half the uncoated value. The example of this type of wire is roadrunner® (Cook Urological), Glidewire® (Terumo), and PTFE Bard® guidewire (Bard Urology). The slippery manner makes the guidewire easy to access the ureter or even bypass the stone but not suitable to use as a safety guidewire due to its instability.

The newer model of the guidewire, the hybrid guidewire (Fig. 4.2a), has a hydrophilic tip at 3 cm of the distal end and stiff proximal part. Examples of this model are Sensor® wire (Boston Scientific), Soloplus® (Bard Urology), Ultratrack® (Olympus), Motion® (Cook Urological), and Rio tracer® (Rocamed). Three properties of the smooth hydrophilic distal tip, kink resistance, and backloading were developed to solve the instability problem while the floppy tip is safe to ureters.

Many functions of the guidewire in the endoscopic procedure included instrument insertion (over the guidewire) in the ureteroscope and ureteral access sheath insertion as a safety guidewire, use in retrograde pyelography, and dilating ureteric orifice or ureteric stricture. There was controversy about whether a safety guidewire is mandatory. EAU guidelines recommend a safety guidewire to assist endoscope passage. The safety guidewire has benefited in the prompt placement of a ureteral stent in the case of ureteric injury. There is also a disadvantage of guidewire usage during the procedure. The insertion of a guidewire parallel to the ureteroscope and UAS will decrease the luminal size. A guidewire can damage the ureter and pelvis by the tip, and the bleeding may interfere with visualization in diagnosis ureteroscopy. Recent studies [9, 10] have suggested that there was no increase in intraoperative complications without the use of a safety guidewire. They concluded that the safety guidewire may not be mandatory unless it is a difficult procedure or complicated case.

4.4 Ureteral Access Sheath (UAS)

This instrument design straightens ureters and facilitates the insertion of flexible ureteroscope without ureter disturbance. UAS includes two parts: the inner obturator and the outer sheath (Fig. 4.3). The inner taper dilator tip can also be used as a ureteric dilator.

The outer surface of UAS is coated with a hydrophilic substance to facilitate entry. UAS is produced in various characteristics including length, diameter, tip design, and material. The size of UAS varies from 9.5 to 13Fr in inner diameter and 11–18Fr in outer diameter. The length of UAS is from 13 to 55 cm. The common sizes of UAS in endoscopy are 11/13 to 12/14Fr. The length of UAS in a female is 36 cm and in a male is 36–48 cm upon the location of the disease. Additional advantages of UAS are decreasing intrapelvic pressure and maintaining it below 20 cmH_2O with an irrigant fluid pressure of 200 cmH_2O [11], improving irrigation flow and visibility, decreasing the need to empty the bladder, decreasing operative time, facilitating ureteral reentry, and protecting the ureteroscope. Ideally, UAS should have a property that resists bucking and kinking, hydrophilic coating with minimal friction to the ureter for safety insertion, and an adequate inner diameter that allows passing of ureteroscope and irrigant fluid. The larger diameter provides better irrigation flow, superior instrument passage, and larger stone extraction. On the other hand, the larger UAS has more failure rate of insertion and causes more injury to the ureter. Although it has a slippery outer sheath surface, device insertion failure was reported as 44% in 12/15Fr UAS [12]. The success rate of UAS insertion increased in a pre-stented patient with a failure rate at 0–12%. Also, preoperative stenting could help to decrease ureteric injury by UAS [13]. The optimum duration of pre-stenting was still under-investigated, but most of the literature recommends at least 5 days of ureteric stent insertion [14]. Other factors that increase the success rate of UAS insertion include older age, former endoscopic ureteral surgery, and small stone burden [15, 16]. Alpha-blocker was proposed to facilitate UAS insertion and decrease ureteric injury [17], but further study is required to confirm the observation.

To pass UAS safely, semirigid URS 6Fr was used to complete the inspection of the ureter and to make sure that no ureteric stone will be trapped between the ureter and UAS. A safety guidewire and a stiff guidewire should be passed under direct vision. UAS placement is required insertion over a stiff guidewire and under fluoroscopy. High insertion force should be avoided in UAS placement. Some centers do not routinely do ureteroscopy before UAS insertion but using dual lumen ureteral catheter (Fig. 4.4) instead. The placement of a stiff guidewire is required only

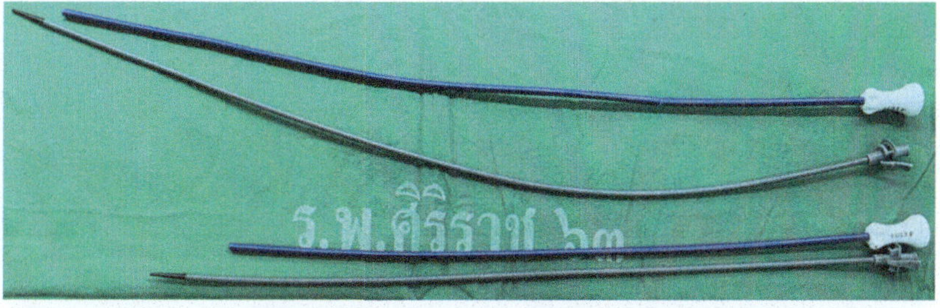

Fig. 4.3 Ureteral access sheath in 11/13Fr × 36 cm (above) and 46 cm (below) (Navigator® HD, Boston Scientific)

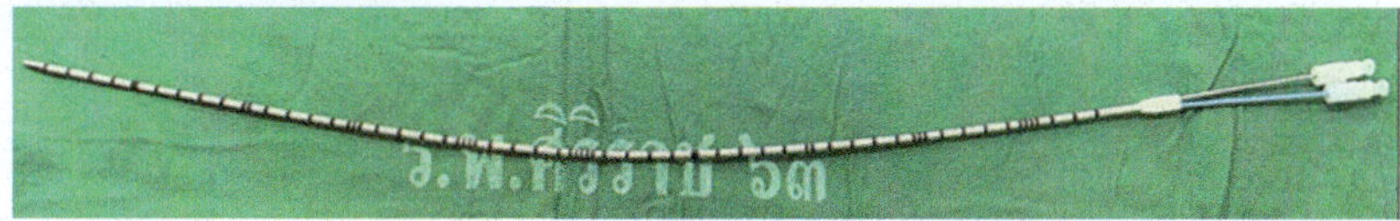

Fig. 4.4 Dual lumen ureteral catheter (Cook Urological)

coaxial insertion along the dual lumen ureteral catheter under fluoroscopy. Traxer also recommended a thorough inspection of the ureter during UAS removal during the end of surgery for the assessment of any ureteric injury [13].

The complications from UAS insertion included ureteric ischemia and an increased risk of ureteric stricture. The incidence of complication increases with the inappropriate size of UAS usage that causes ureteric wall tension and compresses submucosal capillaries. In 10/12Fr UAS, 75% of the blood supply of the ureter was maintained compared with 35% in the larger diameter of UAS.

A postoperative ureteric stent is still controversial. Many studies [18, 19] recommend ureteric stent insertion after UAS usage to reduce the risk of symptomatic ureteric obstruction. The study showed ureteric stent associated with lower overall pain score and decreased hospital readmission rate due to ureteric obstruction. On the other hand, in the study of Sirithanaphol et al. [20] that randomly compared postoperative stenting and no-stenting in uncomplicated flexible ureterorenoscopy with UAS, the result showed that there was no significant difference in postoperative pain, analgesic requirement, postoperative fever, urinary tract infection, irritative voiding symptom scores, and length of hospital stay between the two groups. Moreover, there was an increased operative time in the stenting group. The decision of stenting after UAS usage is upon the surgeon's preference and patient conditioning.

There are controversies in the benefit of UAS. Some studies report that UAS usage decreases operative time and saves the operating room cost [21], but other studies found that operation time was higher in the UAS usage group [22]. The stone-free rate is a concerning issue; L'esperance et al. [23] found that UAS usage significantly improved the stone-free rate from 67% to 79%, but some recent studies disagree with this report by concluding that no significant difference between the two groups [21, 22, 24]. AUA guidelines in the surgical management of stones (2016) recommend the use of UAS when performing flexible URS for complex, high volume renal stone, but EAU guidelines (2016) state that the use of UAS depends on the surgeon's preference.

In the newer model of UAS design, the UAS can be inserted without second wire usage. It has a slit and a notch at the tip of the dilator (Fig. 4.5) that allows a guidewire to be backloaded over the coaxial guidewire through the apex and exit through the side hole to become an extraluminal safety guidewire. This type of UAS has a lower buckling force and requires more force to remove the dilator. The examples of this design are Flexor parallel Rapid release® ureteral access sheath (Cook Urological) and Re-Trace® (Coloplast). The study of De et al. [25] found that the Navigator® HD was the most slippery and rigid while Cook sheaths were least traumatic.

Bi-flex® ureteral access sheath (Rocamed) (Fig. 4.6) has two working channels with 3Fr in diameter that allow safety guidewire insertion and contrast media injection within UAS.

Another model, a balloon-based UAS utilized the UAS insertion into both dilatation and UAS insertion in single-step, causing less trauma to the ureter by reducing axial force [24]. A new UAS with suction port and UAS with deflection tip is under-investigated.

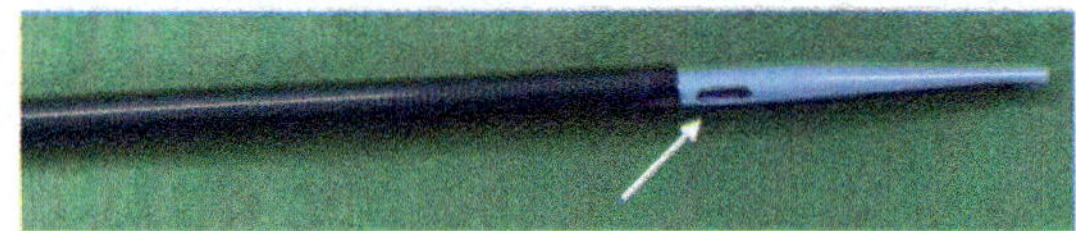

Fig. 4.5 Flexor parallel Rapid Release® ureteral access sheath (Cook Urological) had a slit and a notch at the tip of the dilator (arrow)

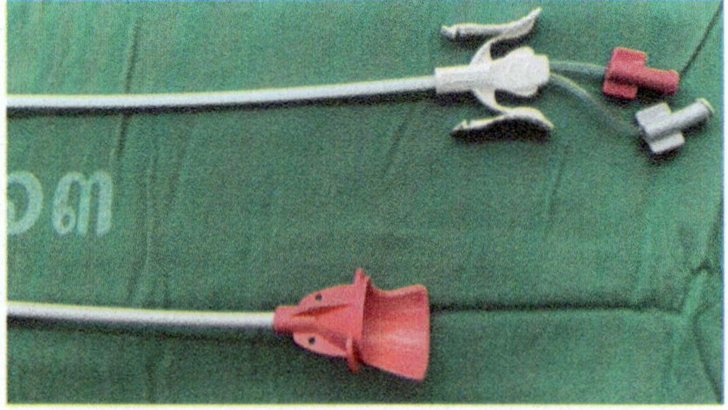

Fig. 4.6 Bi-flex® ureteral access sheath (Rocamed), which has two working channels at the proximal end

4.5 Anti-retropulsion Device

Stone migration is always a challenge during ureteroscopy and stone manipulation. The incidence of stone migration occurs from 5% to 40% of ureteroscopy. The risk of stone migration depends on many factors, including the location of the stone, type and the setting of lithotripter, degree of hydronephrosis, and pressure of irrigation flow. The stone migration reduces the stone-free rate, increases operative time, and may require conversion of semirigid ureteroscopy to flexible ureteroscopy. Many devices have been invented to solve this problem.

1. Mechanical Wire Basket

The examples of this type of basket include Stone cone® (Boston Scientific), Accordion® (Accordion Medical), Escape® (Boston Scientific), and Ntrap® (Cook Urological). These anti-retropulsive devices provided an advantage, and they can be used as stone retrieval devices.

- Escape® nitinol stone retrieval basket (Boston Scientific) is a 1.9Fr, 4-wire nitinol basket. The diameter in the standard position is 11 and 15 mm in fully opened. It has been designed for use with holmium laser fiber in the most semirigid and flexible ureteroscopy. The stone is captured while simultaneous laser lithotripsy is performed. However, the simultaneous usage of both basket and laser occupies most of the working channel lumens, causing laser fiber position restriction, poor irrigation flow, and limited visualization.
- The Stone Cone® (Boston Scientific) (Fig. 4.7b) is 0.43 mm nitinol wire with PTFE cover forming in expandable taper cone at the distal end available in 7 and 10 mm in size. Only fragments less than 2.5 mm are uncapturable and retropulsive to the proximal ureter. Studies had reported 100% no stone migration during both laser and pneumatic lithotripter [26, 27]. Minor complications of Stone Cone® included ureteral abrasion and submucosal cone wire placement. However, at a 3-year follow-up, there was also no stricture or hydronephrosis in patients used with Stone Cone® [28]. These studies concluded that Stone Cone® is effective in preventing stone retropulsion, with no long-term adverse effects on ureters [29].
- The Ntrap® (Cook Urological) (Fig. 4.7a) is a 2.6Fr device with 7 mm tightly woven nitinol mesh in the umbrella shape basket at the end. It can prevent stone migration up to 1.5 mm of the fragment. With the stiff tip, there are reports of the risk of ureteral perforation with Ntrap [30]. Faharat et al. reported that the rate of secondary procedure in ureteroscopy with Ntrap (Cook Urological) was 17%, which was lower than the control group (28%) [31]. However, there was a higher rate than Stone Cone® that had a rate of secondary procedure at 5%.
- The Accordion® (Accordion Medical) is a tool with a film occlusion that expands behind the stone. It is more resistant to laser damage than the Stone Cone and Ntrap.

XenX® (Rocamed) was introduced in 2012; it has a function as a normal hydrophilic guidewire when closed and as a nitinol ureteral mesh when open.

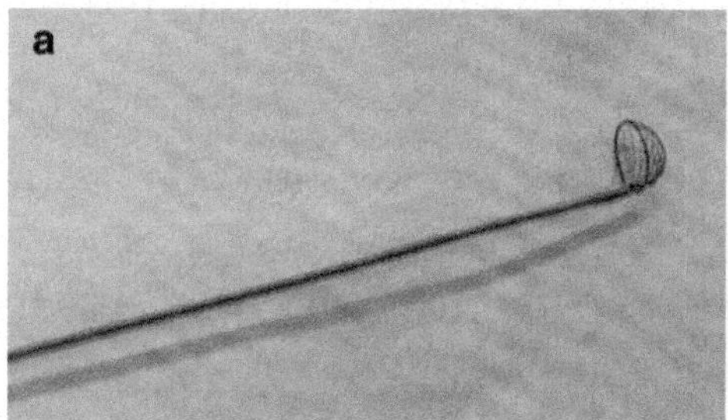

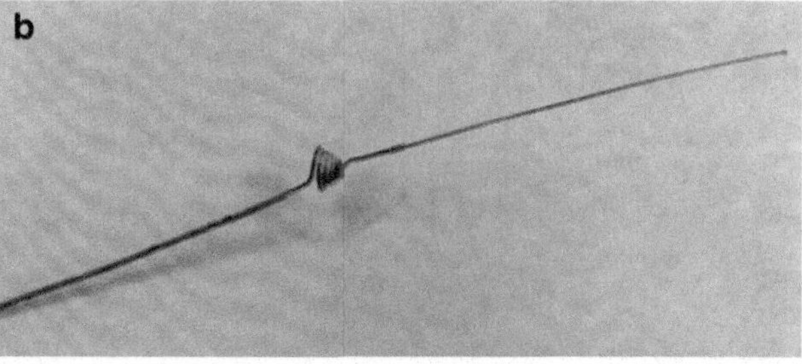

Fig. 4.7 Tip of anti-retropulsion device. (**a**) The Ntrap® (Cook Urological). (**b**) The Stone Cone® (Boston Scientific)

2. Mechanical Balloon Basket

The Passport® (Boston Scientific) is a 3Fr wire with an inflatable balloon in the middle. Originally it was designed as a ureteric dilatation device, but it can be used as an anti-retropulsion device. The common problem occurring 31% was the failure to advance the device proximal to the stone.

3. A Gel-Based Plug

- Backstop® (Boston Scientific) is a reverse-thermosensitive dissolvable polymer that forms a plug in the ureter to prevent stone migration. The gel will form at body temperature, and after completing the procedure, cold saline was used to irrigate the Backstop to turn the gel into solute again or it will be dissolved in 45 min at body temperature.

There was a report [32] of off-label use of lidocaine or lubricant jelly injected through a 6Fr ureteral catheter at the level proximal to the stone. The stone-free rate was significantly higher in the lidocaine group than in the control (96% vs. 28%). Stone retropulsion occurred in 1 out of 25 patients (4%). The disadvantage of this method was obscuring visualization caused by jelly.

The cost-effectiveness of an anti-retropulsion device for ureteroscopy and lithotripsy has been considered. Ursiny et al. reported that an average additional cost of operation with an anti-retropulsive device was $384 compared with $952 in non-use groups [33]. The cost-effectiveness will be achieved if the retropulsion rate is greater than 6.3%.

4.6 Conclusion

The endourologic procedure nowadays has been facilitated by modern technology and advanced equipment. Understanding the devices and accessories as well as updating the knowledge is mandatory for the maximum benefits and safety of the patient.

References

1. Chotikawanich E, Korman E, Monga M. Complications of stone baskets: 14-year review of the manufacturer and user facility device experience database. J Urol. 2011;185(1):179–83.
2. Korman E, Hendlin K, Chotikawanich E, Monga M. Comparison of small diameter stone baskets in an in vitro caliceal and ureteral model. J Endourol. 2011;25(1):123–7.
3. Patel N, Akhavein A, Hinck B, Jain R, Monga M. Tipless nitinol stone baskets: comparison of penetration force, radial dilation force, opening dynamics, and deflection. Urology. 2017;103:256–60.
4. Bechis SK, Abbott JE, Sur RL. In vitro head-to-head comparison of the durability, versatility and efficacy of the NGage and novel Dakota stone retrieval baskets. Transl Androl Urol. 2017;6(6):1144–9.
5. Monga M, Hendlin K, Lee C, Anderson JK. Systematic evaluation of stone basket dimensions. Urology. 2004;63(6):1042–4.
6. Lukasewycz S, Skenazy J, Hoffman N, Kuskowski M, Hendlin K, Monga M. Comparison of nitinol tipless stone baskets in an in vitro caliceal model. J Urol. 2004;172(2):562–4.
7. Hendlin K, Lee C, Anderson JK, Monga M. Radial dilation force of tipless and helical stone baskets. J Endourol. 2004;18(10):946–7.
8. de la Rosette JJ, Skrekas T, Segura JW. Handling and prevention of complications in stone basketing. Eur Urol. 2006;50(5):991–8. discussion 8-9
9. Dickstein RJ, Kreshover JE, Babayan RK, Wang DS. Is a safety wire necessary during routine flexible ureteroscopy? J Endourol. 2010;24(10):1589–92.
10. Ulvik O, Rennesund K, Gjengsto P, Wentzel-Larsen T, Ulvik NM. Ureteroscopy with and without safety guide wire: should the safety wire still be mandatory? J Endourol. 2013;27(10):1197–202.
11. Rehman J, Monga M, Landman J, Lee DI, Felfela T, Conradie MC, et al. Characterization of intrapelvic pressure during ureteropyeloscopy with ureteral access sheaths. Urology. 2003;61(4):713–8.
12. Monga M, Gawlik A, Durfee W. Systematic evaluation of ureteral access sheaths. Urology. 2004;63(5):834–6.
13. Traxer O, Thomas A. Prospective evaluation and classification of ureteral wall injuries resulting from insertion of a ureteral access sheath during retrograde intrarenal surgery. J Urol. 2013;189(2):580–4.
14. De Coninck V, Keller EX, Rodriguez-Monsalve M, Audouin M, Doizi S, Traxer O. Systematic review of ureteral access sheaths: facts and myths. BJU Int. 2018;122(6):959–69.
15. Mogilevkin Y, Sofer M, Margel D, Greenstein A, Lifshitz D. Predicting an effective ureteral access sheath insertion: a bicenter prospective study. J Endourol. 2014;28(12):1414–7.
16. Shields JM, Bird VG, Graves R, Gomez-Marin O. Impact of preoperative ureteral stenting on out-

come of ureteroscopic treatment for urinary lithiasis. J Urol. 2009;182(6):2768–74.
17. Koo KC, Yoon JH, Park NC, Lee HS, Ahn HK, Lee KS, Kim DK, Cho KS, Chung BH, Hong CH. The impact of preoperative α-adrenergic antagonists on ureteral access sheath insertion force and the upper limit of force required to avoid ureteral mucosal injury: a randomized controlled study. J Urol. 2018;199(6):1622–30.
18. Torricelli FC, De S, Hinck B, Noble M, Monga M. Flexible ureteroscopy with a ureteral access sheath: when to stent? Urology. 2014;83(2):278–81.
19. Rapoport D, Perks AE, Teichman JM. Ureteral access sheath use and stenting in ureteroscopy: effect on unplanned emergency room visits and cost. J Endourol. 2007;21(9):993–7.
20. Sirithanaphol W, Jitpraphai S, Taweemonkongsap T, Nuanyong C, Chotikawanich E. Ureteral stenting after flexible ureterorenoscopy with ureteral access sheath; is it really needed?: a prospective randomized study. J Med Assoc Thai. 2017;100:174.
21. Kourambas J, Byrne RR, Preminger GM. Does a ureteral access sheath facilitate ureteroscopy? J Urol. 2001;165(3):789–93.
22. Traxer O, Wendt-Nordahl G, Sodha H, Rassweiler J, Meretyk S, Tefekli A, et al. Differences in renal stone treatment and outcomes for patients treated either with or without the support of a ureteral access sheath: the clinical research Office of the Endourological Society Ureteroscopy Global Study. World J Urol. 2015;33(12):2137–44.
23. L'Esperance JO, Ekeruo WO, Scales CD Jr, Marguet CG, Springhart WP, Maloney ME, et al. Effect of ureteral access sheath on stone-free rates in patients undergoing ureteroscopic management of renal calculi. Urology. 2005;66(2):252–5.
24. Berquet G, Prunel P, Verhoest G, Mathieu R, Bensalah K. The use of a ureteral access sheath does not improve stone-free rate after ureteroscopy for upper urinary tract stones. World J Urol. 2014;32(1):229–32.
25. De S, Sarkissian C, Torricelli FC, Brown R, Monga M. New ureteral access sheaths: a double standard. Urology. 2015;85(4):757–63.
26. Gonen M, Cenker A, Istanbulluoglu O, Ozkardes H. Efficacy of Dretler stone cone in the treatment of ureteral stones with pneumatic lithotripsy. Urol Int. 2006;76(2):159–62.
27. Maislos SD, Volpe M, Albert PS, Raboy A. Efficacy of the stone cone for treatment of proximal ureteral stones. J Endourol. 2004;18(9):862–4.
28. Eisner BH, Dretler SP. Use of the stone cone for prevention of calculus retropulsion during holmium:YAG laser lithotripsy: case series and review of the literature. Urol Int. 2009;82(3):356–60.
29. Shabana W, Teleb M, Dawod T. Safety and efficacy of using the stone cone and an entrapment and extraction device in ureteroscopic lithotripsy for ureteric stones. Arab J Urol. 2015;13(2):75–9.
30. Ahmed M, Pedro RN, Kieley S, Akornor JW, Durfee WK, Monga M. Systematic evaluation of ureteral occlusion devices: insertion, deployment, stone migration, and extraction. Urology. 2009;73(5):976–80.
31. Farahat YA, Elbahnasy AE, Elashry OM. A randomized prospective controlled study for assessment of different ureteral occlusion devices in prevention of stone migration during pneumatic lithotripsy. Urology. 2011;77(1):30–5.
32. Zehri AA, Ather MH, Siddiqui KM, Sulaiman MN. A randomized clinical trial of lidocaine jelly for prevention of inadvertent retrograde stone migration during pneumatic lithotripsy of ureteral stone. J Urol. 2008;180(3):966–8.
33. Ursiny M, Eisner BH. Cost-effectiveness of anti-retropulsion devices for ureteroscopic lithotripsy. J Urol. 2013;189(5):1762–6.

5 Understanding the Instruments: Intra-corporeal Lithotripsy—Non-laser Types

Ritesh Goel, Prabhjot Singh, and Rajeev Kumar

Abstract

Intra-corporeal lithotripters can be broadly divided into laser- and non-laser-based devices. With the advent of laser technology, the use of mechanical lithotripters has declined considerably. However, for certain procedures like percutaneous nephrolithotomy and semi-rigid ureteroscopy, mechanical lithotripters still have a role. Newer advanced combined lithotripters are well suited for miniature access and providing comparable outcomes to laser lithotripters at an affordable price.

Keywords

Intra-corporeal · Lithotripters · Electro-hydraulic · Pneumatic · Ultrasonic

5.1 Introduction

The ability to break stones using energy devices has been the cornerstone of miniaturization of access for urolithiasis. Both percutaneous nephrolithotomy (PCNL) and flexible or semi-rigid ureterorenoscopy (URS) require intra-corporeal lithotripsy (ICL). The high stone-free rates provided by both these techniques make them the procedures of choice for the majority of stones, particularly those where extra-corporeal shock wave lithotripsy (SWL) may not be the best choice. Since their inception in the 1960s as a rigid mechanical jackhammer type of instrument, ICLs have evolved to their present thinner and more agile working elements with varied mechanisms of action. ICLs have been the backbone of success of PCNL, and, with recent modifications, they also provide good ergonomics for URS. The type of access, PCNL versus URS, and calibre of instrument used are the main limiting factors for any endourological procedure. Broadly, ICLs can be classified into laser and non-laser lithotripters. With the advent of laser lithotripters that have extremely fine fibre delivery systems, high power options and versatility in all access devices, the use of non-laser ICLs has declined. However, they continue to be the workhorse for PCNLs, particularly when regular or mini-tracts are used and also in resource-poor settings where the cost of a non-ICL device is far lower than a laser.

In this chapter, we will review different types of non-laser ICLs. Non-laser ICLs differ from each other based on their working principle, compatible instruments, hybrid technology and costs. There are three main types of non-laser ICLs: electrohydraulic, electrokinetic (ballistic) and ultrasonic systems.

R. Goel · P. Singh · R. Kumar (✉)
Department of Urology, All India Institute of Medical Sciences, New Delhi, India
e-mail: rajeev.urology@aiims.edu

A. C.F. Ng et al. (eds.), *Practical Management of Urinary Stone*,
https://doi.org/10.1007/978-981-16-4193-0_5

5.2 Classification of Lithotripters

5.2.1 Electrohydraulic Lithotripters (EHLs)

EHL was one of the oldest techniques of ICL, first reported by Yutkin et al. in the late 1950s for clinical use in stone fragmentation [1]. Prior to its use in PCNL and semi-rigid URS, it was primarily used for fragmentation of bladder calculi. EHL uses a coaxial probe that generates electrohydraulic shock waves upon application of an electric current. Fragmentation is a result of electric discharge produced through a fluidic medium. In the presence of electric discharge, heat is generated, and fluid gets vaporized. This vaporization results in the formation of a cavitation bubble, which expands rapidly and then collapses. This results in the formation of hydraulic shock waves that travel to the probe in contact with the stone. Three different shock waves are generated within each cavitation bubble: expansion of bubble, collapse and then rebound of bubble.

URAT-1 (Medexport) was the first commercially available EHL. It consisted of a 10Fr rigid probe with a pulse generator and could be used in a 24Fr cystoscope [2]. The energy was stored within the capacitors that allowed variations in power, rate and duration of EHL. The probe used for EHL for URS ranges from 1.4Fr to 5Fr diameter. Initial usage of EHL probes was under fluoroscopic control without endoscopic control (direct insertion of the probe without ureteroscopy). This led to an increased risk of stone migration, ureteral injury and strictures [3].

One of the major drawbacks of the EHL probe is that cavitation bubble expansion was not under the operator's control. As the size of the bubble expands, the ureteral wall may be distended beyond the safety window. Even when the probe was not in direct contact with the mucosa, it led to mucosal injury and rarely caused ureteral perforation. To counter the threat of ureteral perforation, the aim should be to create low-energy pulses with higher fragmentation capability. Studies have shown [4] that using higher voltages and overall low capacity creates a small but steep 'laser-like' pulse. These pulses have high mechanical energy and are safer than traditional probes.

5.2.1.1 Data on EHL

In a study of 89 patients [5], EHL was used in the management of ureteral calculi using semi-rigid ureteroscopes. The mean calculus size was 8.2 mm (3–19 mm), mean operating time was 29 min (10–120 min), and complete fragmentation was seen in 91.5% of patients. Following complications were observed: haematuria in 2.2% of patients, urinary tract infection in 3.4% of patients and post-procedure ureteric colic in 2.2% of patients. Four patients suffered minor ureteric perforation (4.5%) and were managed conservatively. In another study of 43 patients with solitary ureteral calculi [6], 36 patients (84%) required single sitting with EHL probes; in 6 patients (14%), calculus were pushed back to the kidney and later required SWL. Overall success rate of endoscopic intervention was 98%. The mean operating time was 26.4 min, and the duration of post-operative hospital stay was a mean of 2.5 days. Four (9%) patients suffered minor ureteral perforations and were managed with double-J stenting.

5.2.2 Pneumatic Lithotripters (PLs)

PLs have been one of the oldest and most widely used ICLs in urology. In simple terms, PLs work like a hammer as pressurized air fires a projectile onto a metal rod that hits the stone. Clean pressurized air at 0.35–0.5 MPa pushes a metallic projectile on the plate at the end of the metal rod; this transfers the kinetic energy to the stone particle in contact with the probe (Fig. 5.1).

This modality was first introduced after the development of Swiss LithoClast System (Fig. 5.2) (Microvasive-Boston Scientific Corp., Boston, Massachusetts) in 1996. Its benefits include compatibility with existing pressurized air channels available in most operating rooms and the availability of reusable probes of varying sizes. These advantages allow for a reduction in operating costs. Probes are available from 1.8Fr

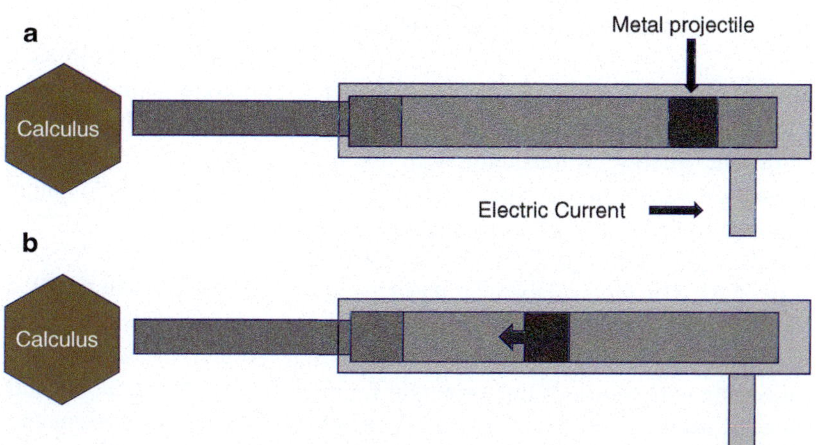

Fig. 5.1 (**a**) Pneumatic lithotripter with inner channel comprising a metal projectile and probe in contact with calculus. (**b**) On application of electric current clean pressurized air pushes metal projectile towards the metal plate of the probe in contact with calculus, delivering mechanical energy

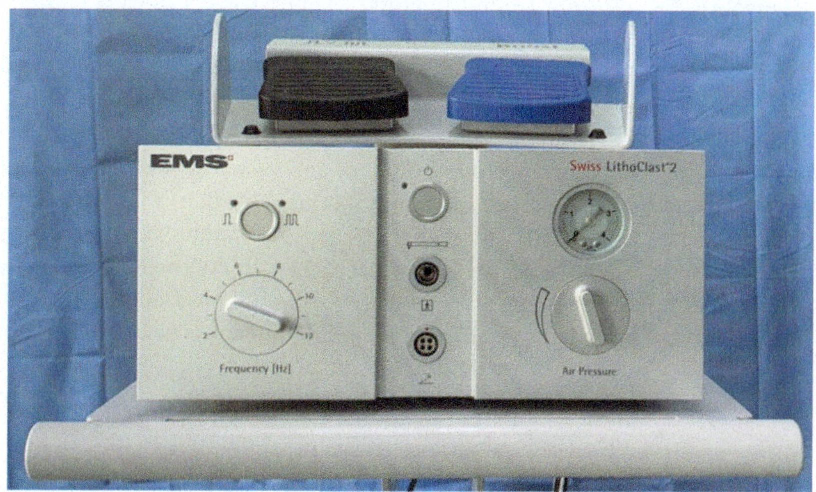

Fig. 5.2 Swiss LithoClast 2 apparatus™ (EMS) with foot pedal

to 8Fr for different sheaths and can be used using the same console.

The biggest advantage of PL is the low cost of device, reusable probes, flexibility for use in both URS and PCNL, and high effectiveness in stone fragmentation with low complications. PL devices are often available for less than US$700 and require only electricity to function. This makes them the first choice in many institutions with limited resources.

PL suffers from several limitations as well. The probe of the LithoClast can reach a velocity of 12.1–33.3 m/s and a probe displacement of maximum of 2.53 mm. This is directly related to the diameter of the probe and the pressure of the air. Earlier, only rigid probes were available, which provided good stone fragmentations but did not offer any manoeuvrability. Presently, flexible probes have been developed, but this has come at the cost of probe displacement and reduction in energy delivered for stone fragmentation. This is directly related to the deflection angle of the probe; when the flexible probe is bent, the energy delivered decreases [7]. Another limitation is the proximal migration of the stone fragments, which was seen in up to 18% of the patients [8].

Lithovac (Microvasive-Boston Scientific, Boston, Massachusetts) was developed as a modification to the Swiss LithoClast probe to address the problem with proximal migration. It allows continuous suction of small fragments of the stone and prevents proximal migration, resulting in up to 95% stone-free rates and complete fragmentation without the need for a secondary procedure [9].

5.2.3 Ultrasonic Lithotripsy (USL)

Application of alternating electric current to plates on opposite sides of a crystal produces ultrasonic energy. Ultrasound, with its high-frequency waves, causes compression and rarefaction on the particles alternately, which results in cavitation in the transmission media (Fig. 5.3). On the collapse of these cavities, there is a development of a pressure gradient that can destroy solid objects [10]. After initial failed attempts of use of this principle for fragmenting urinary and biliary stones, the development of ultrasonic lithotrite in the 1970s established the efficacy of this method. This lithotrite, with the help of an ultrasound transducer, vibrates a hollow probe transmitting energy to the stone, resulting in fragmentation. Simultaneous suction and irrigation by the USL probe help in removing the stone fragment and keeping the probe cool, preventing thermal injuries to adjacent tissues [11].

Apart from PCNLs, USL has been used for bladder and renal stones [12, 13]. In the ureter, blind fluoroscopy-guided USL had better results than EHL and PL with fewer complications [12]. With advances in technology, USL under direct ureteroscopic vision with 4.5–6Fr probes is possible. Another development is the 2.5Fr solid wire probe, which transmits energy transversally compared to the longitudinal energy by a hollow probe [12].

5.2.3.1 Data on PL and USL

Chaussey et al. treated 118 ureteral stones and found a success rate of 96.6% [14]. USL is particularly useful in conditions like steinstrasse and large ureteral stone [15]. Combination of PL and USL led to the introduction of the LithoClast Ultra$^{(R)}$ device, combining the speed of PL and fragment evacuation property of USL. Though the earlier in vitro results were promising [7], a later randomized trial found no difference in stone-free rates with PL versus USL alone [16].

The CyberWand Dual Ultrasonic Lithotriptor System™ (Olympus) (Fig. 5.4) uses a dual probe assembly combining an ultrasonic probe and an intermittent impact action probe. This dual probe allows fragmentation of hard stones and simultaneous suction of fragmented stones. The

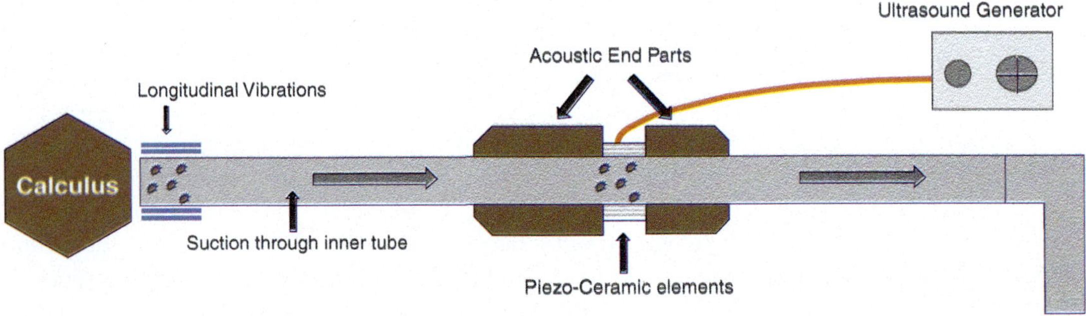

Fig. 5.3 Ultrasonic probe with ultrasound generator in contact with stone and simultaneous suction of fragmented particles

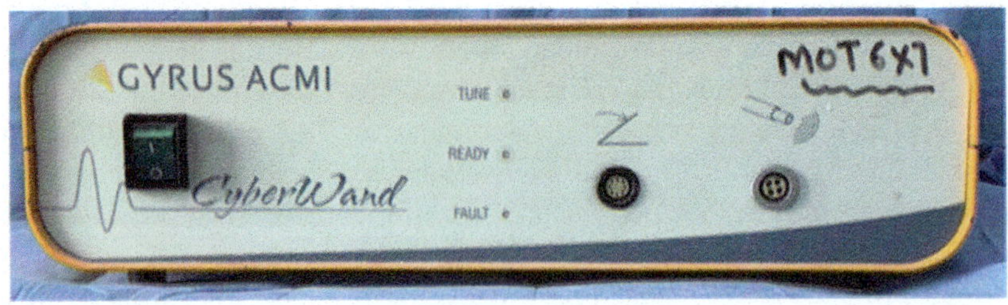

Fig. 5.4 CyberWand™ (Olympus) apparatus with foot control pedal

CyberWand has a 0.375 cm or 11.25Fr wide and 40 cm long probe, which is single-use only. The large diameter and single-use probe limit its use to large-sized nephroscopes.

5.3 Combination of Ultrasonic and Pneumatic Lithotripters

Combination probes utilize benefits of both pneumatic and ultrasonic probes. Pneumatic component provides greater mechanical force to fragment larger and harder stones, whereas the ultrasonic probe provides finer fragmentation. It incorporates the active suction elements of ultrasonic probes, which is not seen with pneumatic probes. The options include Swiss Master LithoClast™, Swiss LithoClast™ Trilogy and Shock Pulse™ (Olympus). The Swiss Master LithoClast (Fig. 5.5) uses Swiss LithoClast™ probes varying from 2.4Fr to 6Fr.

5.3.1 Swiss LithoClast™ Master

This device involves the simultaneous use of a pneumatic effect for coarse fragmentation and USL for finer fragmentation. It also has a controlled suction for evacuations of stone fragmentation. In a study of 27 patients with bladder calculi treated using the Swiss LithoClast™ Master [17], complete stone clearance was seen in 26 patients (96%). Mean stone size was 20 mm (5–40 mm), and median lithotripsy duration was 60 min (20–144 min). Auxiliary procedures like transurethral resection of the prostate (TURP) were done in 2 patients. All patients were discharged the next day after surgery.

In another prospective study [18], 60 patients with renal calculi planned for PCNL were included. They were randomized into two groups: standard pneumatic lithotripters (Group 1) and Swiss LithoClast™ Master (Group 2). Group 2 had a significantly lower average duration of fragmentation and clearance at 58 min compared to 65 min in Group 1 ($p < 0.01$). Group 1 had a significantly higher incidence of residual fragments than Group 2 (53% vs. 4%, $P < 0.01$). Both the modalities were comparable in their rate of complications. Bleeding was seen in 1 patient (3.33%) in Group 1 and 3 patients in (10%) Group 2, whereas urine leak was seen in 3 patients (10%) in Group 1 and 5 patients (16.7%) in Group 2.

In a study comparing the CyberWand™ with the Swiss LithoClast™ Master [19], 138 patients with staghorn calculi undergoing PCNL were randomized to the CyberWand dual probe (Group A, $n = 71$) and Swiss LithoClast Master (Group B, $n = 67$). Both groups were comparable with respect to the age of the patients, size of the calculus and overall complications. Fragmentation time was significantly shorter in Group A (77.14 ± 21.39 min) than in Group B (84.25 ± 20.62 min) ($P = 0.049$). No difference was observed in the one-stage stone clearance rate and blood loss between the two groups ($P = 0.854$).

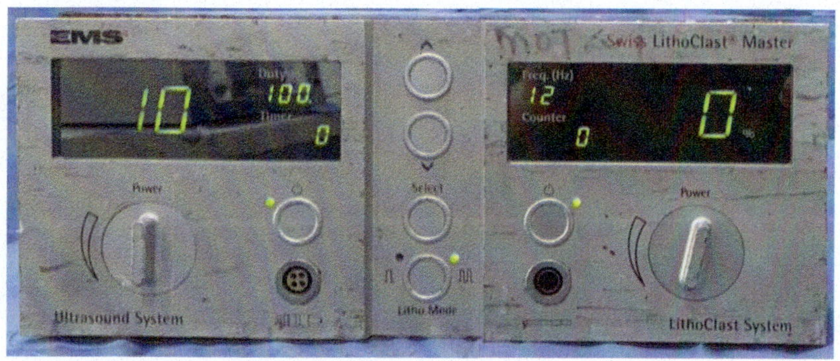

Fig. 5.5 Swiss LithoClast™ Master (EMS)

5.3.2 The ShockPulse-SE™ (Olympus)

The ShockPulse-SE™ (Olympus) (Fig. 5.6) is a dual-acting lithotripter that uses constant ultrasonic wave energy with regular intermittent ballistic shock-wave energy at a high-frequency rate of 300 Hz. Its inner lumen is larger, allowing for faster suction of fragments. It also has a single hand piece that allows simultaneous control of both the lithotripsy mechanism. It has also eliminated the need for a foot switch and helps better ergonomics. Both the single-use and reusable probes range from 2.91Fr to 11.3Fr. A prospective randomized trial compared ShockPulse (Group 1) with PL (Group 2). A total of 119 patients undergoing PCNL were randomized into two groups: Group 1 (61 patients) and Group 2 (58 patients). Both the groups were comparable in demographic and clinical characteristics. Stone-free rates were also comparable between the two groups: 78.69% versus 74.13% ($P = 0.66$). However, the duration of the procedure and mean fragmentation time were significantly lower in Group 1. The mean duration of the procedure was 43.23 ± 18.49 min in Group 1 and 51.53 ± 19.48 min in Group 2 ($P = 0.0188$). The mean calculus fragmentation time was 17.95 ± 15.25 min in Group 1 and 24.37 ± 11.12 min in Group 2 ($P = 0.0096$). Both groups were comparable in overall complications rates ($P = 0.58$) [20].

5.3.3 Swiss LithoClast™ Trilogy

The Swiss LithoClast™ Trilogy (Fig. 5.7) involves ballistic, ultrasonic and suction in a single probe. An automatic adaptive algorithm delivers constant ultrasonic energy for fine fragmentation and dusting of stones with the simultaneous electromagnetic current generated ballistic

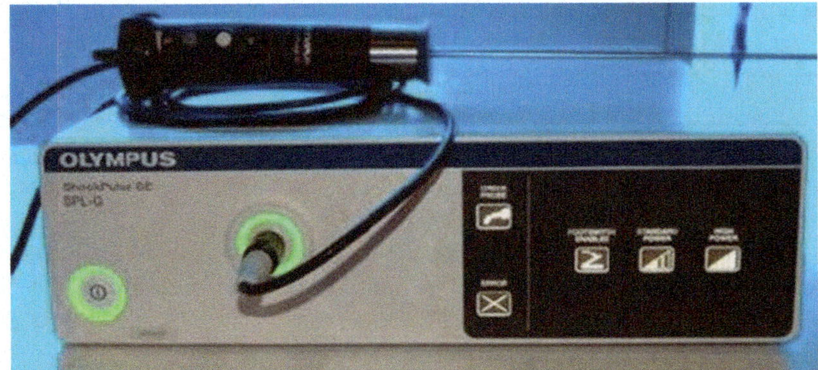

Fig. 5.6 ShockPulse-SE™ (Olympus)

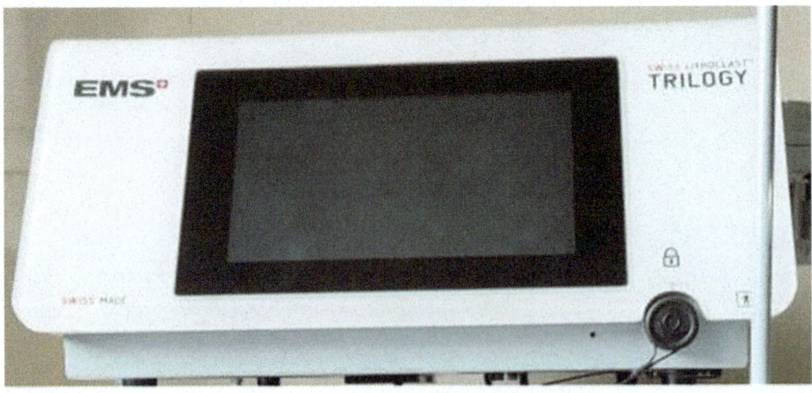

Fig. 5.7 Swiss LithoClast™ Trilogy (EMS)

energy for fragmentation of larger and harder stones. The probe size varies from smallest being 1.1 mm to largest being 3.9 mm with varying lengths.

In vitro studies with LithoClast Trilogy have shown superior results compared to available combination devices. This increased efficiency can be attributed to a larger probe diameter and greater tip displacement during both ultrasonic and impactor actions [21]. It has been effectively used as an alternative to laser cysto-lithotripsy for a large bladder calculus [22]. In a randomized trial, 31 patients with renal calculi were included. They were divided into two groups: standard PCNL ($n = 20$) and mini PCNL access ($n = 11$). The mean volume of renal calculus was 3776.1 + 2132 mm^3 for mini PCNL compared to 7096 ± 6441 mm^3 for standard PCNL. The mean haemoglobin drop was 1.24 ± 0.64 g/dL for mini PCNL and 1.23 ± 0.89 g/dL standard PCNL. The total duration of the procedure was 53.4 ± 23.8 min for mini PCNL and 65.2 ± 23.5 for standard PCNL. The total duration of lithotripsy use was 14.7 ± 12.4 min for mini PCNL and 12.0 ± 8.9 min for Standard PNL. Immediate and 1-month follow-up stone clearance rates were 93% and 96%, respectively. There were three Clavien-Dindo grade I and one grade II complications [23].

5.4 Safety Concerns

With the advent of newer techniques like SWL and laser lithotripsy, the flaws of the conventional techniques are frequently highlighted. In ex vivo studies, EHL was shown to have the highest rate of acute tissue damage [4, 24]. Studies in rabbits show abrasion and haemorrhage on direct application, which worsened with time on histological evaluation mostly attributed to rapid heat generation at the probe tip [25]. A plasma shield with a stainless-steel coil with a perforated end cap has been developed for the probe to reduce collateral damage [25]. Though economical for bladder stones, the role of EHL is limited in ureteric stones.

PL, on the other hand, does not cause serious tissue injury. In animal experiments, there was no macroscopic lesion seen with direct application of PL, even though microscopic changes were present, which resolved within weeks [24]. In a study by Teh et al. in human patients with bladder and ureteric stones, direct application of probe to soft tissue caused minimal trauma [26].

USL, when examined for safety, did better than EHL and PL [27, 28]. In a porcine study, even after direct application for 3.4 mm probe on urothelium did not lead to iatrogenic ureteral perforation. Backed by various other studies [29] [30] [31], USL has been found to be the safest technique. However, the USL probe tends to get heated during the procedure, resulting in frequent breakdowns [31].

5.5 Comparisons

USL may achieve a higher fragmentation rate than EHL. In a study of 100 patients undergoing URS, 67 patients received USL and 33 underwent EHL [32]. Both the groups were comparable with respect to stone size, location and composition. Among the USL group, complete fragmentation was observed in 92.5% of patients compared to 72.7% of patients in the EHL group.

In a prospective, randomized study [8], EHL was compared with PL for fragmentation rate and rate of complications in patients undergoing URS. In EHL group, 29 out of 34 patients (85.3%) had complete fragmentation, compared to 89.5% in the PL group ($p = 0.12$). Both groups had similar rates of proximal migration of stone fragments requiring SWL. The two groups differed significantly in their complication rates. The rate of ureteral perforations was significantly higher in patients treated with EHL (6/34) – 17.6% compared with 2.6% cases (1/38, $p < 0.01$) in PL. Results were consistent with multiple earlier reported studies reflecting the increased risk of ureteral perforation in cases treated with EHL [33].

In a study of 227 patients undergoing PCNL [31], 107 underwent USL, 83 had PL, and 37 required both PL and USL. The groups were comparable in their mean operative time and length of hospital stay. In the USL group, the absence of stone fragments on post-operative X-ray was seen in 96.9% patients and a final complete clearance after SWL in 97.2%. In the PL group, 81.9% of patients had the absence of stones on post-operative scans on the first day, and 18.1% required SWL, leading to a complete fragmentation rate of 91.5%. On follow-up at 3 months post-operatively, the stone-free rates were 97.2% in the USL group and 91.5% in the PL group. Hence, USL provided better stone-free rates than pneumatic lithotripters.

USL, when used through rigid endoscopes, can provide fragmentation rates reaching up to 100%, but when combined with pneumatic lithotripsy, stone-free rates are seen in the range of 80–90% [34].

5.6 Mechanical Lithotripters

Mechanical lithotrites are manually operated lithotripters such as stone crushing forceps that can fragment stones while passing through a 25Fr cystoscope sheath or a 26Fr resectoscope sheath. A 24Fr lithotrite with a curved coaxial jaw also exists for larger stones and is introduced into the bladder blindly. The Mauermayer stone crushing forceps [35] consist of a 25Fr lithotrite sheath and a working element with a channel to introduce 7Fr sized instruments like EHL probes or laser fibres. Stones up to a size of 2 cm in the largest dimension can be fragmented rapidly and easily removed. All devices applied in the bladder are used under visual control.

5.7 Conclusion

Intra-corporeal lithotripters are the most vital part of the armamentarium of endourological surgeries. Their use has declined in the past few years because of their safety concerns, advancement of laser modality and miniaturization of the techniques. However, modern combination probes provide excellent stone-free rates and good safety outcomes and are ever so commonly increasingly used in rigid nephroscopies. EHLs had the best fragmentation potential, but their use was limited because of the higher risk of ureteral injuries. Pneumatic and ultrasonic probes were better suited to ureteral surgeries, but they lack the flexibility of laser fibres. Despite these shortcomings, these instruments still have a place in endourological practice.

References

1. Mitchell ME, Kerr WS Jr. Experience with the electrohydraulic disintegrator. J Urol. 1977;117(2):159–60. https://doi.org/10.1016/s0022-5347(17)74598-3.
2. Eaton JM, Malin JM, Glenn JF. Electrohydraulic lithotripsy. J Urol. 1972;108:865–6.
3. Raney AM. Electrohydraulic ureterolithotripsy. Urology. 1978;13(3):284–5.
4. Vorreuther R, Corleis R, Klotz T, Bernards P, Engelmann U. Impact of shock wave pattern and cavitation bubble size on tissue damage during ureteroscopic electrohydraulic lithotripsy. J Urol. 1995;153(3 Pt 1):849–53.
5. See ACH, Ng FC, Ch'ng HC. Electrohydraulic lithotripsy: an effective and economical modality of endoscopic ureteric lithotripsy. Aust N Z J Surg. 1997;67:551–3.
6. Yang SS, Hong JS. Electrohydraulic lithotripsy of upper ureteral calculi with semirigidureteroscope. J Endourol. 1996;10(1):27–30. https://doi.org/10.1089/end.1996.10.27.
7. Auge BK, Sekula JJ, Springhart WP, Zhu S, Zhong P, Preminger GM. In vitro comparison of fragmentation efficiency of flexible pneumatic lithotripsy using 2 flexible uteroscopes. J Urol. 2004;172:967–70.
8. Hofbauer J, Höbarth K, Marberger M. Electrohydraulic versus pneumatic disintergration in the treatment of ureteral stones: a randomized, prospective trial. J Urol. 1995;153:623–5.
9. Delvecchio FC, Kuo RL, Preminger GM. Clinical efficacy of combined Lithoclast and Lithovac stone removal during ureteroscopy. J Urol. 2000;164:40–2.
10. Howards SS, Merrill E, Harris S, Cohn J. Ultrasonic lithotripsy. Investig Urol. 1974;11(4):273–7.
11. Fuchs GJ. Ultrasonic lithotripsy in the ureter. Urol Clin North Am. 1988 Aug;15(3):347–59.36.
12. Marberger M, Stackl W, Hruby W. Percutaneous lithalopaxy of renal calculi with ultrasound. Eur Urol. 1982;8:236–42.
13. Çetin S, Ozgür S, Yazicioglu A, Ünsal K, Ilker Y. Ultrasonic lithotripsy of bladder stones. Int Urol Nephrol. 1988;20(4):3615.

14. Chaussy C, Fuchs G, Kahn R, Hunter P, Goodfriend R. Transurethral ultrasonic ureterolithotripsy using a solid-wire probe. Urology. 1987;29(5):531–2.
15. Gur U, Lifshitz D, Lask D, Livne PM. Utereral ultrasonic lithotripsy revisited: a neglected tool? J Endourol. 2004;18(2):137–40.
16. Lehman DS, Hruby GW, Phillips C, Venkatesh R, Best S, Monga M, et al. Prospective randomized comparison of a combined ultrasonic and pneumatic lithotrite with a standard ultrasonic lithotrite for percutaneous nephrolithotomy. J Endourol. 2008;22(2):285–9.
17. Kingo PS, Ryhammer AM, Fuglsig S. Clinical experience with the Swiss lithoclast master in treatment of bladder calculi. J Endourol. 2014 Oct;28(10):1178–82.
18. Rai RS, Patrulu K, Rai R, Gupta E, Kayastha A, Sawhney S. Lithoclast(®) master in intracorporeal lithotripsy during percutaneous nephrolithotomy: our experience. Med J Armed Forces India. 2008;64(3):232–3.
19. Li Y, Zeng F, Yang Z, Chen H. Zhong Nan Da Xue Xue Bao. Yi Xue Ban. 2013;38(8):853–856. https://doi.org/10.3969/j.issn.1672-7347.2013.08.016
20. Yadav BK, Basnet RB, Shrestha A, Shrestha PM. Comparison between shockpulse and pneumatic lithotripsy in percutaneous nephrolithotomy. World J Urol. 2020; https://doi.org/10.1007/s00345-020-03239-3. Epub 2020 May 24.
21. Carlos EC, Wollin DA, Winship BB, et al. In vitro comparison of a novel single probe dual-energy lithotripter to current devices. J Endourol. 2018;32(6):534–40. https://doi.org/10.1089/end.2018.0143.
22. Sninsky BC, Flamiatos JF, Nakada SY. The end of "Cutting for Stone"? Using the lithoclast trilogy for cystolitholapaxy on a 4 cm bladder stone per urethra. Urol Case Rep. 2019;26:100964. https://doi.org/10.1016/j.eucr.2019.100964. Published 2019 Jul 10.
23. Sabnis RB, Balaji SS, Sonawane PL, et al. EMS Lithoclast Trilogy™: an effective single-probe dual-energy lithotripter for mini and standard PCNL. World J Urol. 2020;38(4):1043–50. https://doi.org/10.1007/s00345-019-02843-2.
24. Piergiovanni M, Desgrandchamps F, Cochand-Priollet B, Janssen T, Colomer S, Teillac P, et al. Ureteral and bladder lesions after ballistic, ultrasonic, electrohydraulic, or laser lithotripsy. J Endourol. 1994;8(4):293–9.
25. Bhatta KM, Rosen DI, Flotte TJ, Dretler SP, Nishioka NS. Effects of shielded or unshielded laser and electrohydraulic lithotripsy on rabbit bladder. J Urol. 1990;143(4):857–60.
26. Teh CL, Zhong P, Preminger GM. Laboratory and clinical assessment of pneumatically driven intracorporeal lithotripsy. J Endourol. 1998;12(2):163–9.
27. Begun FP. Modes of intracorporeal lithotripsy: ultrasound versus electrohydraulic lithotripsy versus laser lithotripsy. Semin Urol. 1994;12(1):39–50.
28. Zengin K, Sener NC, Bas O, Nalbant I, Alisir I, Zengin K, et al. Comparison of pneumatic, ultrasonic and combination lithotripters in percutaneous Nephrolithotripsy. Int Braz J Urol. 2014;40(5):650–5.
29. LeRoy AJ, Segura JW. Percutaneous ultrasonic lithotripsy. AJR Am J Roentgenol. 1984;143(4):785–8.
30. Radfar MH, Basiri A, Nouralizadeh A, Shemshaki H, Sarhangnejad R, Kashi AH, et al. Comparing the efficacy and safety of ultrasonic versus pneumatic lithotripsy in percutaneous nephrolithotomy: a randomized clinical trial. EurUrol Focus. 2017;3(1):82–8.
31. Karakan T, Diri A, Hascicek AM, Ozgur BC, Ozcan S, Eroglu M. Comparison of ultrasonic and pneumatic intracorporeal lithotripsy techniques during percutaneous nephrolithotomy. Scientific World Journal. 2013;2013:604361. https://doi.org/10.1155/2013/604361. Published 2013 Aug 18.
32. Vicente J, Caparrós J, Salvador J, Parra L, Rios G. Electrohydraulic and ultrasonic lithotripsy in 100 consecutive cases of primary ureteral stones. Urol Int. 1991;47:16–9.
33. Zheng W, Denstedt JD. Intracorporeal lithotripsy: update on technology. Urol Clin. 2000 May 1;27(2):301–13.
34. Leveillee RJ, Lobik L. Intracorporeal lithotripsy: which modality is best? Curr Opin Urol. 2003;13(3):249–53. https://doi.org/10.1097/00042307-200305000-00014.
35. Mauermayer W, Hartung R. The bladder-stone punch—a new principle of visual lithotripsy. Urologe A. 1976;15:164–6.

Understanding the Instruments: Intracorporeal Lithotripsy—Laser

6

Ji Won Kim and Sung Yong Cho

Abstract

Laser is an acronym for "Light Amplification by Stimulated Emission of Radiation." The main structure of a laser system includes a pumping source, an optical oscillator, and a laser amplifier. The optical oscillator generally consists of an optical resonator with mirrors and an amplifier. The laser beam is generated by stimulated emission. The Ho:YAG laser used in the urology field is a flash-lamped pumping Q-switched laser system, but a thulium fiber laser is a diode laser pumping master oscillator power amplifier (MOPA) system.

The lasers mainly used in the urology field are the neodymium-doped YAG (Nd:YAG) laser frequency-converted to 532 nm by potassium titanyl phosphate (KTP), the thulium- or holmium-doped YAG (Tm:YAG or Ho:YAG) laser at 2013 nm or 2120 nm, and the thulium-doped double-clad fiber (Tm fiber) laser around 2000 nm. All of these lasers are solid-state lasers different from gas, chemical, semiconductor, dye, and free-electron lasers. The Ho:YAG laser has been the first choice for treating urolithiasis, benign prostatic hyperplasia, urothelial and bladder tumors, and urinary tract strictures or polyps.

Commercially available Ho:YAG, Tm:YAG, and thulium fiber laser machines are introduced here. The mechanistic aspects of stone fragmentation and tissue destruction are related to photothermal, photoacoustic, and thermomechanical ablation; the stone absorption rate; and the laser fiber-to-stone distance with fluid absorption. Recently, the Tm fiber laser was introduced for the management of urologic diseases, and many probable advantages have been discussed. Different Tm fiber laser machines with different specifications from different companies will be available in the near future. Clinicians need to stay alert to perspectives from users in real practice, and the results of in vitro experiments can be different from those inside operating rooms.

Keywords

Urolithiasis · Urinary calculi · Nephrolithotomy · Percutaneous · Ureteroscopy · Minimally invasive surgical procedures · Laser

J. W. Kim
Department of Photonics and Nanoelectronics, Hanyang University ERICA, Ansan, Republic of Korea
e-mail: jwk7417@hanyang.ac.kr

S. Y. Cho (✉)
Department of Urology, Seoul National University, College of Medicine, Seoul National University Hospital, Seoul, South Korea
e-mail: moretry@snuh.org

A. C.F. Ng et al. (eds.), *Practical Management of Urinary Stone*,
https://doi.org/10.1007/978-981-16-4193-0_6

Notes on Transcription

2 mm	2 millimeters
2 μm	2 micrometers
OR	Operating room
Ho:YAG	Holmium:YAG
TFL	Thulium fiber laser
2 W	2 Watts
2 Hz	2 Hertz
2 mm/s	2 millimeters per second
2 kg	2 kilograms
2×	2 times

6.1 Introduction

Many kinds of lasers have been used in the urology field, such as neodymium-doped YAG (Nd:YAG) lasers with KTP (potassium titanyl phosphate; green light), holmium-doped YAG (Ho:YAG) lasers, and thulium-doped YAG (Tm:YAG) lasers. They are mainly solid-state lasers that use rare earth–doped materials such as Nd, Ho, and Tm. Since the Ho:YAG laser was introduced 20 years ago, it has been the first choice for treating urolithiasis and benign prostatic hyperplasia in the urology field. Recently, its application has been extended to urothelial tumors, urinary tract strictures, and polyps, indicating its versatility.

In this chapter, we will review the definition and mechanisms of lasers, how they create and transmit energy, and future perspectives. Additionally, we will compare holmium and thulium fiber lasers (TFL), a newly introduced laser.

6.2 Definition of Laser and How Lasers Work

Light is a type of electromagnetic wave that transmits energy in space. Electromagnetic waves include radio waves, microwaves, infrared, visible light, ultraviolet, X-rays, and gamma rays, which are classified by frequency. Typically, light refers to the electromagnetic waves detectable by human eyes, which are in the range of ultraviolet and infrared, as shown in Fig. 6.1.

Laser is an acronym for "Light Amplification by Stimulated Emission of Radiation," which was conceptually suggested by Albert Einstein in 1916. The first laser, that is, a ruby laser, was demonstrated by T. H. Mainman in 1960, and it has shown remarkable progress in output power and energy, becoming the essential tool in numer-

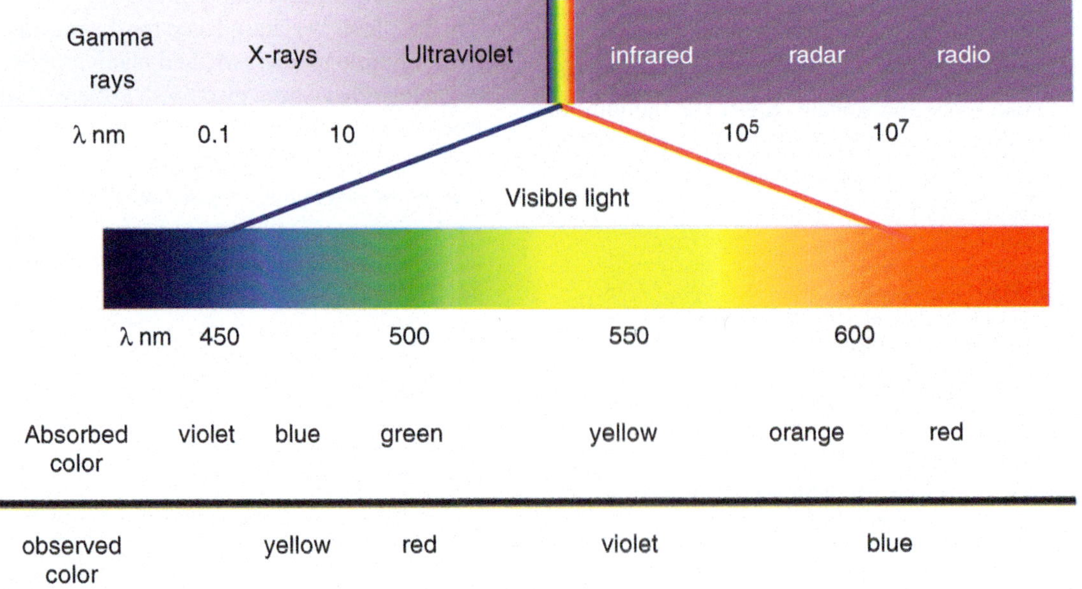

Fig. 6.1 The spectrum of electromagnetic waves

ous areas of application, including industry, communication, defense, spectroscopy, and medicine. This can be attributed to its excellent properties, such as coherence, directionality, monochromaticity, and high intensity.

One of the advantages of lasers is that they can emit light in a very short time interval from tens of femtoseconds to hundreds of nanoseconds in the so-called pulsed mode of operation, allowing the application of very high energy light to a very localized area in a very short time, which cannot be accomplished by another way. That is, only lasers can emit the same energy light with an adjustable pulse width, leading to a very high peak power (typically calculated as the pulse energy divided by the pulse duration for an ideal pulse shape), as seen in Fig. 6.2. For example, if the laser in the continuous-wave (CW) mode of operation has 1 mW of output, it cannot hurt tissues or skin at all and may not even be felt. However, when a single pulse with a 10-ns pulse width is applied with the same energy, i.e., 1 mJ pulse energy and 100 kW peak power, it can not only damage tissue and skin but also is strong enough to cut or drill a hole in a metal sheet.

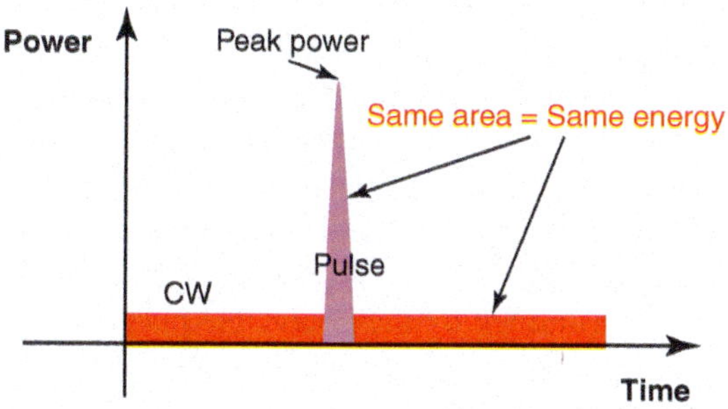

Fig. 6.2 Comparison between CW and pulsed modes of operation in lasers

The pulse width (or pulse duration), pulse energy, repetition rates, peak power, and average power are shown in Fig. 6.3. The laser pulses do not have a rectangular pulse shape like those shown on the left side of this figure, but are theoretically Gaussian-like, as shown on the right side of this figure. For the Gaussian-like pulse shape, the pulse duration is defined by full width at half maximum (FWHM). The average power is the rate of energy transfer per second, and 1 W is defined as a derived unit of 1 joule per second. Thus, the average power becomes the pulse energy multiplied by the number of pulses per second, that is, the repetition rate (Hz), which is the inverse of the pulse period.

6.3 Structure to Generate Lasers

The main structure of a laser system includes a pumping source, an optical oscillator, and a laser amplifier, as shown in Fig. 6.4. The optical oscillator consists of an optical resonator with mirrors and an amplifier. The optical resonator basically comprises two opposing plane-parallel or curved mirrors at right angles to the axis of the laser

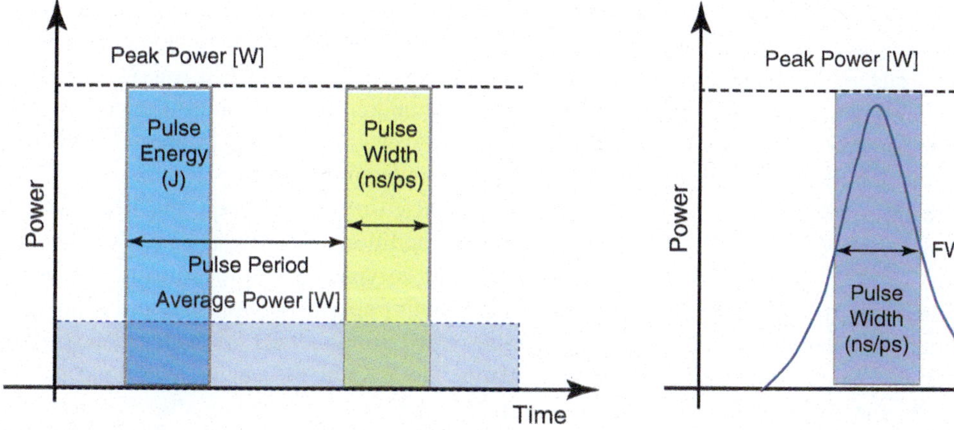

Fig. 6.3 The shape of laser pulses

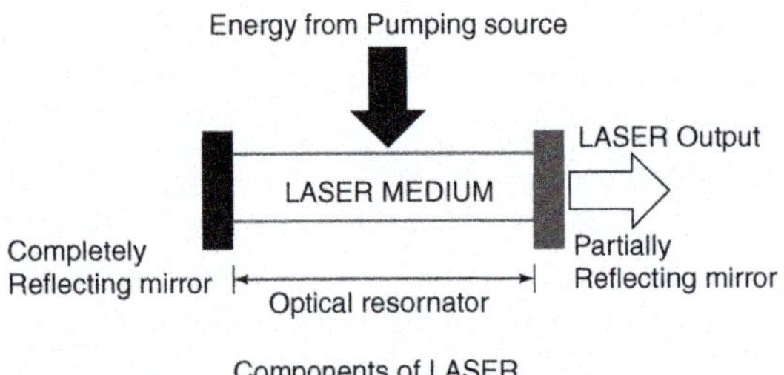

Fig. 6.4 Main structure of a laser system

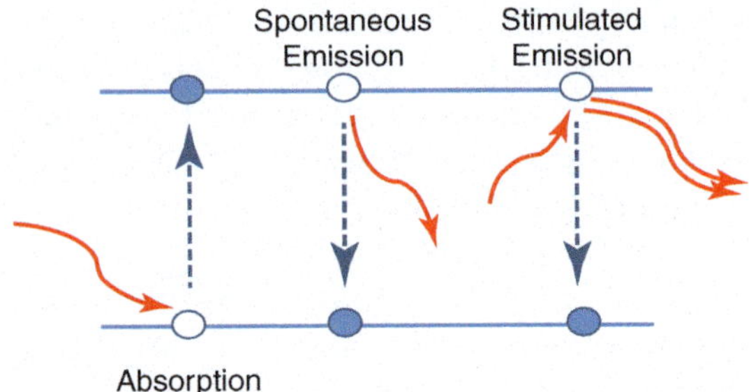

Fig. 6.5 The mechanism of stimulated emission of the laser

material and provides a highly selective feedback signal, inducing the stimulated emission in the laser amplifier. The laser amplifier includes a laser medium and acts as an energy source. These two mirrors in the two ends of the cavity, a highly reflecting mirror and a partially reflective mirror as the output coupler.

Figure 6.4 shows the basic configuration of the laser oscillator. The action providing energy to a laser medium is called pumping and can be achieved in various ways, such as absorbing other light energy, electrical discharge, and chemical reactions. In an optical pumping system, the pumping source is located parallel to the laser medium surrounded by the oscillator cavity.

Electrons in the active atoms of the laser medium are excited to a higher energy level by pumping and emit light when they drop to a lower energy level. The energy of the emitted light equals the difference in the two energy levels. Generally, the excited electrons in most materials drop immediately to a lower energy level, emitting light with no constraint, called spontaneous emission. In contrast, electrons in laser materials can stay much longer at the higher energy level than other materials so that they can drop to the lower energy level stimulated by the incident light signal, emitting the light of the same characteristics with the incident light signal, such as frequency, direction, and phase. This process is called stimulated emission and is the mechanism by which lasers work. A specific wavelength can add additional energy to each single pulse as a constructive method. When the signal gain by the stimulated emission exceeds the loss in the laser resonator under the condition of population inversion, the laser action is initiated (Fig. 6.5).

Pumping in most solid-state lasers is realized using a radiation source with a spectral output that closely matches the absorption bands of the gain medium. An arc discharge lamp is the popular radiation pump source for lasers, called flash-lamp pumping, with high energy and a low repetition rate. But they suffer from a low electrical-optical efficiency and short lifetime despite their low cost. Flash lamp pumping is used for Ho:YAG and Tm:YAG lasers.

Diode pumping utilizes a laser diode as the pump source (DPSSL typically means diode-pumped solid-state laser). Diode pumping has the advantage of high electrical-optic efficiency, long lifetime, robust operation, and compactness but has been limited by the obtainable pulse energy and high cost. Therefore, a laser pumping system should be selected by considering the physical configuration of a laser medium and the target specifications. For example, if a laser system with high energy over tens of millijoules at repetition rates less than 100 Hz is needed, the flash-lamp-pumped laser is the best choice. However, if the treatment is better with low energy laser beams (<hundreds of microjoules) at high repetition rates over a few hundred kilohertz, it is better to use a diode pumping laser system.

For pulsed-mode operation, the laser system requires additional elements. The Q-switching technique is typically employed to obtain high-energy laser pulses with a pulse width from sub-nanosecond to hundreds of nanoseconds. The quality factor Q of the cavity is defined as the ratio of the energy stored in the cavity to the energy loss per cycle. A high-energy Q-switched pulse is generated when a cavity Q is restored from a low Q value in a short time by a Q-switch device in the optical oscillator. The other way is to amplify the temporally modulated signal from the master oscillator in the power amplifier. This method is heavily used in a fiber-based MOPA configuration. For example, the Ho:YAG laser with energy over tens of millijoules (mJ) at tens of hertz has a flash-lamp-pumped Q-switched laser configuration, but the Tm fiber laser with less than 1 mJ operated over tens of kilohertz has a diode-laser-pumped MOPA configuration employing Tm fibers.

6.4 Why Can the Lasers with the Same Power Show Different Results?

Many parameters, such as wavelength, pulse energy, pulse duration, repetition rate, and beam quality, should be considered when laser light is applied to a target.

1. The first is the laser wavelength, which determines the absorption ratio of the light energy incident upon the target. For example, it is much more efficient to use Tm- or Ho-doped lasers emitting ~2.1 μm for tissues high in moisture since the water absorption at ~2.1 μm is hundreds of times stronger than that at ~1.0 μm.
2. The next factor is pulse energy. After all, lasers transmit energy in the form of light, generating heat in the target. Thus, the higher the pulse energy, the higher the instantaneous temperature the target reaches.
3. Although the pulsed laser has the same pulse energy in the same wavelength, the laser–material interaction can be greatly dependent on the pulse duration. It is generally known that laser pulses with a shorter pulse width can induce a higher instantaneous temperature on the hitting point of the target, but less thermal damage around it. This relationship is similar to nailing with a hammer. The sharpness of the nail tip and the applied force from the hammer correspond to the pulse width and the pulse energy, respectively. However, the obtainable pulse energy is limited by the pulse duration due to damage in the laser system, so a pulse energy and pulse duration optimized for the application should be chosen.

The lasers mainly used in the urology field are the neodymium-doped YAG (Nd:YAG) laser frequency-converted to 532 nm by potassium titanyl phosphate (KTP), the thulium- or holmium-doped YAG (Tm:YAG or Ho:YAG) laser at 2010 nm or 2120 nm, and the thulium-doped double-clad fiber (Tm fiber) laser around 2000 nm. All of these lasers are solid-state lasers different from gas, chemical, semiconductor, dye, and free-electron lasers.

Ho:YAG lasers from different companies can show different clinical performances due to differences in the specifications, including pulse shape, repetition rates, peak energy, and beam quality. The way the pulsed operation is achieved also limits the laser performance obtainable. Some engineering differences may not show clinically significant differences.

YAG (yttrium–aluminum–garnet) is a synthetic crystalline material and is commonly used as a medium material in various solid-state lasers. The intentional introduction of impurities into this crystal lattice is called doping, and holmium or thulium ions can be doped into this crystal to produce holmium or thulium lasers, respectively.

All of the Ho:YAG, Tm:YAG, and Tm fiber laser outputs can be coupled to a silica fiber delivery cable, allowing the laser beam to deliver to the target with minimal energy loss. The fiber delivery cable is thin enough to be easily bent, so it is very useful in flexible ureteroscopy.

6.5 What Lasers Does Urology Currently Have Available

Ho:YAG has been the first choice to treat urolithiasis, benign prostatic hyperplasia, urethral strictures, and urothelial tumors in the urology field. That is because holmium lasers can be completely absorbed within 0.4 mm safely, ablate all kinds of stones, and act as a knife for cutting, ablating, and enucleating tissue with thin and flexible laser fibers.

6.6 Holmium Laser

The emission wavelength of holmium lasers is about 2120 nm in the near-infrared range, which is highly absorbable in water. The optical penetration depth in water is about 400 μm at 2140 nm, so the Ho laser beam thermally expands and vaporizes water. Because most of the energy from the flash-lamp heats the resonator, a large-volume cooling system is necessary to preserve the original energy and frequency. The setting of a single oscillator is confined to 30 W or less, and high-power holmium laser machines contain several oscillator systems with a large cooling system.

There are many commercially available holmium laser machines with different specifications. The 120 W laser was released by Lumenis in 2014, and MOSES technology of the fourth generation was added to this 120 W laser machine in 2017. The thinnest diameter of laser delivery fibers is still 200 μm due to the coupling limitation of the spatially multimodal laser output. The noise during laser firing ranges from 50 to 80 decibels, namely the level of light traffic to busy crossroads, and the difference in noise levels depends upon the size of the machine and the capacity of the cooling system. The next generation of Ho:YAG laser is expected to deliver a sequence of pulse trains, resulting in a higher ablation rate of urinary calculi and tissues. The absorption rate is higher than that of other lasers such as Tm:YAG and thulium fiber lasers.

6.7 Thulium Laser

Tm lasers can be used in the continuous wave mode or the pulsed mode. Typically, the laser emission wavelengths used in the urology field are about 2010 nm for Tm:YAG lasers and 1940 nm for Tm fiber lasers. Because the Tm:YAG laser cannot be used for stone fragmentation, its application is decreasing, and no further information will be discussed in this chapter.

Different from other solid-state lasers, the fiber laser is ideally immune to the heat generated during laser operation due to the waveguide structure with an extremely large ratio of surface area to volume. Thus, TFL can adopt an air-cooling system up to hundreds of watts in output and does not require a huge cooling system like the Ho:YAG laser. Also, since all of the free-space laser components used in other solid-state lasers, such as mirrors, polarizers, and Q-switches, can be replaced by the equivalent fiber-based components in fiber lasers, the fiber laser can be very compact, connected in a series from start to end, and highly robust in operation. Moreover, TFL has high flexibility in operating laser wavelengths from 1700 nm to 2100 nm, which can be optimized for an applied target. For example, TFL at 1940 nm has a four times higher absorption coefficient (14 mm^{-1}) than the Ho:YAG laser at 2120 nm (3 mm^{-1}). In addition, TFL has excellent spatial beam quality, and its output can be easily coupled to a delivery fiber cable with a diameter of 50 to 100 μm, which is impossible to realize with multimode Ho:YAG lasers. The achievable peak power per pulse in TFL is much lower than that of the Ho:YAG laser, but this disadvantage can be compensated by operating at high repetition rates up to several 100 kHz accompanied by long pulse duration owing to operating flexibility in the fiber MOPA configuration. Because of these excellent characteristics, some commercially available TFLs are being introduced in the urology field.

Since the first study on the applicability of TFL for renal stone fragmentation was performed in 2005, there have been limited in vivo studies utilizing TFL. The results look promising for laser lithotripsy and tissue ablation. Clinical trials should be conducted to show the full applicability of TLF considering the promising results reported in the existing literature.

6.8 Mechanistic Aspects of Stone Fragmentation and Tissue Destruction

Lasers have been used for stone fragmentation and incision, ablation, or vaporization for prostate, stricture tissue of the urinary tract, and urothelial tumors. The pulse duration with peak power of the laser, the stone absorption rate of the absorption coefficient, and the laser fiber-to-target distance with fluid absorption are key factors for stone fragmentation tissue destruction in terms of laser characteristics.

Several major mechanistic processes have been suggested for stone fragmentation, such as photothermal, photoacoustic, and thermomechanical ablation.

1. The first is photothermal ablation, which maximizes the transmission of energy through contact lithotripsy with a longer pulse duration for dusting and stone fragmentation.
2. Photoacoustic ablation is dependent upon pulse duration and energy. Short pulse and high peak powers may result in photoacoustic ablation.
3. Thermomechanical ablation is known as explosive vaporization to maximize the transmission of energy to the water and is related to water absorption. A short pulse causes stone fragmentation induced by the collapse of the shockwave-generated bubbles. If the energy of the laser gets into spaces filled by water in the stone or tissue, so-called inter-crystalline spaces or pores, vaporization, and thermal expansion of the water occur, causing cracks and thus fragmenting stones and ablating tissues.

In terms of the fiber-to-stone distance, Moses contact and distance modes from the Lumenis® company provide different sequenced multi-pulses of the Ho:YAG laser compared to the single, spherical short pulse, and long pulse profiles. The Moses distance mode makes a big vapor bubble first with low energy and a short duration pulse followed by a longer, higher energy pulse, allowing less stone retropulsion and increased ablation rates. And the Moses distance mode showed 100% more fragmentation than a short pulse at a 1-mm distance. Therefore, this technique was useful, especially for stone dusting techniques for smaller fragments and better vision. Other pulse modulation techniques, such as the “Virtual Basket” from Quanta and lasers with less retropulsion function from Jena Surgical®, were released onto the market.

6.9 Potential Advantages of Thulium Fiber Laser Compared to Holmium Laser from Clinical Perspectives

In in vitro experiments, due to the possibility of achieving lower pulse energy and higher frequency, TFL showed increased fragmentation and dusting efficiency with much smaller dusts than the Ho:YAG laser. It may mean that the operating time of flexible ureteroscopy can be decreased with TFL compared to using the Ho:YAG laser.

The small volume and low weight of TFL machines occupy less operating space. However, the height of this machine should be close to that of the operating tables for easy handling. It may mean that we have to remember that the TFL machine system includes the machine and its table unless it is located inside the shelf of an endoscopy cart. Even considering that the actual size of the TFL machine includes the complexity of the machine and its table, the weight of the TFL machine is much lighter than all Ho:YAG laser machines.

Since the Ho:YAG laser has to consume much energy, it needs a dedicated 250-W high-power electrical outlet, and the operating rooms where the machine can be used are limited. In contrast, TFL machines use only 110–220-W standard power outlets. Thus, they can be used in all operating rooms.

Due to the excessive heat produced, a more powerful cooling system is therefore needed for the Ho:YAG laser system. Hence, the Ho:YAG laser machine can make noises up to 50 to 80 decibels and interferes with communication in the operating room. Stop-and-go techniques for shooting lasers are basically necessary to get clear vision, check the status of the tips of the laser fibers, and decrease intrarenal pressure and temperature. However, the noise produced by a TFL machine is significantly less than that of Ho:YAG lasers.

6.10 Controversial Points of the So-Called Advantages of Thulium Fiber Lasers: Are They Exaggerated?

In terms of retropulsion, stone ablation rates are increased when there is less retropulsion during stone fragmentation, dusting, or pop-dusting. However, stone fragments can float and move inside the renal calyces not only by the laser but also by the irrigation fluid in real practice. Less retropulsion and increased number of fragments and dust may mean that surgeons have to increase the irrigation speed to obtain clear vision and increase the number of fragments floating inside the calyces. Small fragments may hide inside the dust and correspond to longer navigation time and dusting time.

Another interesting minor point is that surgeons sometimes try to actively utilize retropulsion when the stones are difficult to reach because of the anatomical features. For example, the stones in the upper pole can be difficult to reach when the miniaturized nephroscope advances through a lower pole tract during percutaneous nephrolithotomy. Otherwise, the stones can be located in the calyces with no favorable approach location during flexible ureteroscopic surgery. In these situations, surgeons may utilize the retropulsion of stones and the irrigation fluid. Thus, floating stones can be fragmented by this whirlpool effect ("popcorn" effect). All of these points may mean that further investigation on the roles of lasers, irrigation fluid, and other factors in retropulsion in real practice is necessary to clarify their clinical significance.

Very low pulse energies, very high pulse frequencies, and very long pulse durations may increase dusting effects and also surgical efficiency. However, the upper and lower limits of these parameters should be tested to get clinical significance in terms of safety in real practice. It may mean that we have to ask ourselves how much energy and frequency are actually needed for effective fragmentation. These parameters may reduce the use of stone baskets during flexible ureteroscopic surgery. However, it may mean increased intrarenal temperature of the irrigation fluid and damage from improper handling of flexible ureteroscopy. Additionally, excessive long pulse duration may lead to collateral photothermal damage and carbonization. Excessive heat absorption by fluid may lead to a suboptimal fiber-to-stone distance, and this means increased power output and heat generation. Another point is that the parameters of retropulsion, pulse energy, frequency, and pulse durations would not be considered for performing percutaneous nephrolithotomy.

The vulnerability to external shock and the durability of laser fibers should be tested in real practice, and these positive attributes can attract attention to the utility of TFL machines.

6.11 Summary

This chapter reviewed the definition of a laser, how the laser is generated, and how it works. Ho:YAG has been the first choice for the management of urologic diseases, and TFL is showing promising results in experiments. Although there is much promotion-related information, clinicians need to stay alert to the perspectives from users in real practice and that the results of in vitro experiments can be different from those inside operating rooms.

Acknowledgments This work was supported by a grant (No. 2019R1C1C1008339) from the National Research Foundation (NRF) funded by the Korean government (MSIT).

7 Understanding the Instruments: Ureteric Stent

Kantima Jongjitaree and Ekkarin Chotikawanich

The ureteric stent is a tubed catheter placed within a ureteral lumen to maintain its patency. Traditional double J stent has a J shape of each end of the stent (Fig. 7.1). This design provides the anchoring function and keeps the stent in place.

7.1 Size

Stent size varies from 3Fr to 8Fr. A common size of the stent in general urologic practice is 4.7Fr and 6Fr. The larger stent size improves urinary flow compared with the smaller one. Moreover, the larger stent size has less migration rate. Stent size does not relate to a stent-related symptom, but the oversized ureteric stent can cause damage on ureter.

7.2 Material

The materials that use for making ureteric stent are mainly made of polymer and metallic.

1. Polymer

Historically ureteric stents are made of polyethylene, but due to its limitation in rigidity and causing stone encrustation, they were substituted with the newly developed material. Silicone appears the best performance in long-term stone encrustation. They had 30% less stone encrustation at 10 weeks compared with other five different polymeric materials [1]. However, the softness and less of the rigidity of a silicone stent is an obstacle for stent insertion. Polyethylene with polyurethane mixture is another popular material for the ureteric stent. It has resistance against stone encrustation while providing designable rigidity.

2. Metallic

The purpose of this type of stent is to increase the ability to resist high compression force to stent lumen. They are now made of nitinol (nickel with titanium alloy mixture). The property of this material provides a specific memory that can retrieve their shape. These stents expand in high temperatures (55 °C) and recoil at low temperatures (below 10 °C). Metallic stents provide greater patency rate, longer indwelling time, and better management of ureteric stricture. The major disadvantages of the metallic stent are stone encrustation, ingrowth of the tumor, epithelial hyperplasia, and difficult to change. However, they have a long time to maintain good efficacy in urinary drainage (41% over 37 months) [2] and do not need to change frequently.

K. Jongjitaree · E. Chotikawanich (✉)
Division of Urology, Department of Surgery, Siriraj Hospital, Mahidol University, Bangkok, Thailand

A. C.F. Ng et al. (eds.), *Practical Management of Urinary Stone*,
https://doi.org/10.1007/978-981-16-4193-0_7

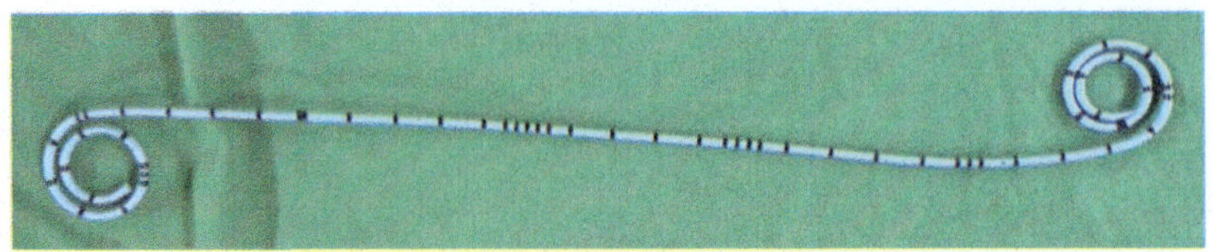

Fig. 7.1 Standard double J stent has a pigtail to each end of the stent

7.3 Design

1. Resonance Metallic Stent
This type of reinforced stent has greater resistance to radial compression force. It can use in malignant obstruction which usually has a high compression force without a significant reduction of inner luminal diameter. This stent has been lasting up to 12 months or longer. In the study of Wah et al. [3], resonance metallic stent improved urinary drainage comparing with traditional double J stent over 1 year.

2. Grooved Stent
This stent has external grooves along the stent lumen. This design aimed to improve urinary drainage by providing more pathways via the grooves. The example of this type of stent was LithoStent® (Olympus).

3. Spiral Stent
This stent has metallic wire within it to maintain spiral shape. The advantage of this shape is superiority to conform to the ureteric shape. The example of this type of stent is Percuflex Helical® (Boston Scientific).

4. Self-Expanding Meshed
This stent has been developed to improve urinary flow while causing less stent-related symptoms. This stent causes less irritation to the ureterovesical junction and bladder trigone. The mesh design also has the benefits of decreasing luminal obstruction. The problems of this type of stent are difficult for changing and higher cost compared to a normal stent.

5. Tail Stent
This stent has a loop of the polymer at the distal end instead of a classical pigtail (Fig. 7.2b). This design was aimed to decrease bladder irritation and stent symptoms. The study of Yew et al. [4] demonstrated that this type of stent caused minimal pain during stent insertion, but another study [5] reported there was no reduction of the incident of flank pain that resulted from urinary reflux. The example of these stents is Inlay® (Bard) and Polaris® loop ureteral stent (Boston Scientific) (Fig. 7.2a).

6. Dual Durometer
This type of stent is also developed for patient acceptability and comfort by having different rigidity in each part of the stent. The proximal part placed in the kidney has harder rigidity and softer at the distal part which is placed in the bladder. The example of these stents are Percuflex Plus® (Boston Scientific), Bard Inlay® (Bard), and Polaris® (Boston Scientific).

7. Magnetic Tipped
It was developed for decreasing the cost of cystoscopy to remove the stent. The benefit is obviously in the pediatric patient. With magnet at the distal end, it can be successfully removed in 29 out of 30 patients in one study [6].

8. Novel Stent Design
The new developing stent is biodegradable stent that provides the advantage of self-degradation and does not require removal. They are composed of Uriprene, poly-L-lactic acid, polyglycolic acid, and caprolactone that can dissolve in urine over time. Further studies are required for this type of stent.

7.4 Indications

1. For Treatment
The placement of ureteric stent that directly on treatment purpose is drainage of ureteral

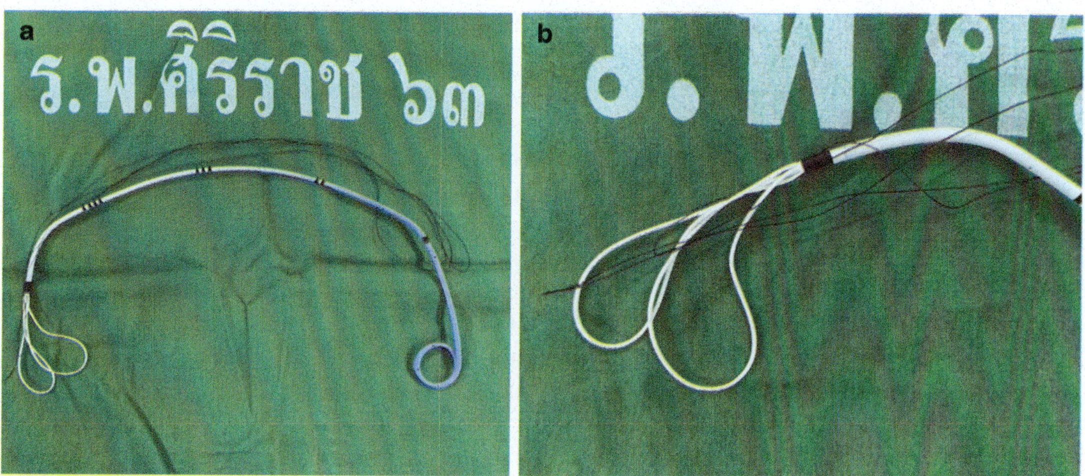

Fig. 7.2 (**a**) Polaris® loop ureteral stent (Boston Scientific) and (**b**) loop at distal end instead of a pigtail

obstruction, inner core stent for anastomosis in urologic organ, and conservative treatment in ureteric injury.

2. For Post-Procedure Prophylaxis

The imperative indications of post-procedure ureteric stent insertion are a solitary kidney or in kidney transplant. For uncomplicated ureteroscopy, other indications are to be discussed in the needful of stent insertion.

Stent symptoms interfere quality of life of patients. There were more postoperative pain and lower urinary tract symptoms in patients in the ureteric stent group compared with the non-stent group after semirigid ureteroscopy for distal ureteric calculi [7]. Routine stenting following uncomplicated ureteroscopy does not lower the complication rate and unplanned hospital readmission and increase treatment cost [8]. Moreover, routine stenting after ureteroscopy did not increase the stone-free rate. In the study of Prasanchaimontri et al. [9] compared stenting in post-ureteroscopy stone removal and found that there was no difference in stone-free rates. According to the literature [10], the indications for post-ureteroscopy ureteral stent insertion have been controversial. The relative indications include significant ureteral edema, impacted stone, incomplete procedure, preoperative ureteric stricture, intraoperative ureteric injury, prolong operative time more than 90 min, stone burden more than 2 cm, and recent history of urinary tract infection. Ureteric stenting after ureteral access sheath insertion has been controversial. Many literatures [11, 12] recommended placement of ureteric stent after insertion of UAS due to a high prevalence of significant transient pain for 24 hours. The study showed ureteric stent associated with lower overall pain score and decreasing hospital readmission rate due to ureteric obstruction. On the other hand, in the study of Sirithanaphol et al. [13] that randomized the comparison of postoperative stenting in uncomplicated flexible ureterorenoscopy with UAS, the results were no significant difference in postoperative pain, analgesic requirement, postoperative fever, urinary tract infection, irritative voiding symptom scores, and length of hospital stay between the two groups. Moreover, there was an increased operative time in the stenting group. The decision of stenting after UAS usage is upon the surgeon's preference and patient conditioning.

7.5 Complications

7.5.1 Stent-Related Symptoms

Placement of ureteral catheter does not only relieve urinary obstruction, but the stent itself can cause localized inflammation of the ureter and bladder and produce the related symptoms. Stent-related symptoms occur over 80% of patients with ureteric stent insertion [14]. Symptoms include voiding symptoms, frequency (50–60%), urgency (57–60%), incomplete emptying (76%), hematuria (25%), suprapubic pain (30%), flank pain (19–32%), nocturia (60%), incontinence, and sexual dysfunction (32%). The symptoms affect daily life activity and reduce working capacity [15]. There were 32% of patients needed to remove a ureteric stent sooner than planning [16].

The suspected mechanism of voiding dysfunction is probably from the distal coil of the stent that interferes with bladder mucosa especially during urination. Physical activities aggravate symptoms by increasing the movement of the coiled bladder explaining that the symptoms often occur during the day more than at night [17]. Stent length associates with the intravesical position of the distal coil of the stent. Longer stents are associated with the frequency of urination, and the symptoms worsen when the distal coil crossed the midline [18]. Longer stents tended to make trigonal irritation or form an incomplete distal loop [19]. Stent size does not correlate with the stent symptoms [20] [21]. The study of Candela et al. [21] compared three different ureteric stents (6Fr Percuflex, 4.8Fr, and 6Fr HydroPlus); they reported there was no difference in stent symptoms among groups. Moreover, voiding dysfunction may be the result of infection and stone encrustation of the stent.

The mechanism of flank pain is supposed to be from refluxing urine from the bladder to the renal pelvis. It does not associate with the location of the upper coil of the stent [18, 22].

The correlation between stent material and rigidity has been controversial. Many studies [15, 23, 24] concluded that there was no association between QOL and stent material composition. On the other hand, a randomized control trial of 155 patients reported that there was a higher incidence of bladder's irritating symptoms in those patients who have a firm pigtail stent compared with a soft pigtail stent [25].

7.6 Prevention and Management of the Stent-Related Symptoms

Stent-related complications can prevented with lessened ureteric stent insertion. It is important to evaluate the indications of ureteric stent insertion individually. Considering this morbidity, routine stenting should be avoided. If ureteric stent insertion is mandatory, there are many strategies to decrease ureteric stent side effects and complications.

1. Stent Length and Positioning

The position of the upper coil does not affect the symptoms, while many studies confirm that lower coil crosses the midline [26] and incomplete distal coils [19] are the factors that associate with increasing voiding dysfunction. The length of the stent correlates directly with the position of the lower coil, and the overlong length of the ureteric stent should be avoided. The literature proposed the formula to calculate the appropriate stent length. The example from the study of Hao P et al. [27] calculated ureteral stent from the length = 0.125 × body height + 0.5 cm or using the vertical distance from the second lumbar vertebra to pubic symphysis −2 cm. In pediatric population the formula is length = patient age (year) + 10 [28]. However, in a recent randomized study [29] comparing multi-length 22–30 cm to 24 cm ureteric stent, they did not show a significant difference in stent-related symptoms or health-related quality of life.

2. Stent Distal Loop Modifications

The distal loop is the key point of bladder irritation. Modifications of the distal tail of the ureteric stent were proposed. Tail stent (Boston Scientific) was designed to minimize bladder irritation by tapering their size from 7 Fr at proximal to 3 Fr at the distal end and changing the distal end to loop polymer instead of coil shape (Fig. 7.2b). This stent provides significantly lower irritating symptoms but does not decrease in flank pain [5]. Improving the stent consistency has been considered, dual durometer® has different rigidity in the same stent, and the distal end has softer material for decreasing bladder irritation.

3. Stent Coating

There were several drugs developed for eluting the stent to improve stent discomfort. Ketorolac (NSAIDs) was first proposed by Krambeck et al. [30], and the result of comparative study with normal stent showed ketorolac-loaded stents appeared to cause less pain. Ketorolac coating stent provided a high concentration of ketorolac in the bladder and ureter while decreasing systemic side effects of NSAIDs [31]. This stent can decrease stent-related discomfort especially in young adults [32]. Antimicrobial was another drug that developed for coating the stent. Biofilm formation and stone encrustation can aggravate the inflammatory pathway and cause stent-related pain. With antibacterial property, povidone-iodine coated stent had fewer bacterial adhesions and stone encrustations. Moreover, it showed to improve lubricity [33] of the stent. Mendez-Probst et al. [34] investigated triclosan coating stent and reported the triumph triclosan-eluting stent had significantly decreased in stent-related symptoms. The antimicrobial mechanism of the triclosan is interfering in the stability of the bacterial cell wall. However, triclosan itself cannot reduce the infection; therefore, combination therapy with standard antibiotics should be considered.

The newer model of the drug-eluting stent was a drug with anti-tumor activity such as paclitaxel [35] and zotarolimus [36]. The mechanisms of anti-tumor drugs are reducing tissue hyperplasia reaction and anti-inflammatory. Further in human-study is required before concluding the benefit of this type of stent.

4. Pharmacologic

(a) *Alpha-Blocker*

Alpha 1A and 1D adrenoreceptors are commonly found in the bladder and ureter and inhibit the alpha adrenoreceptor causing smooth muscle relaxation in the prostate, bladder neck, and distal ureter. The use of alpha adrenoreceptor blockers is proposed to improve voiding dysfunction from ureteric stent insertion. The mechanisms of action are dilatation of the ureter, reduce basal tone, and decrease peristalsis frequency causing a reduction in flank pain. Local trigone smooth muscle relaxation decreases irritating symptoms. Alfuzosin 10 mg once daily for 4 weeks can decrease pain and urinary symptoms and improve in general health index score [37]. Other studies [38, 39] with alfuzosin 10 mg once daily for 10 days or 6 weeks show the same result with improving stent-related morbidity. Efficacy of alfuzosin and terazosin is superior compared to tamsulosin. However, a study [40] shows that significant improvement in pain was found in tamsulosin oral 2 weeks after double J stent insertion in ureteroscopic stone removal compared with the placebo group. Tamsulosin improves urinary symptoms, pain, and general health in all domains except sexual index [41]. The side effects of alpha-blockers are hypotension and retrograde ejaculation. There was a report of retrograde ejaculation that worsens sexual dysfunction in ureteric stent insertion patients, but this side effect is reversible.

(b) *Anticholinergic*

Anticholinergic drugs act directly to the muscarinic receptor in the bladder. These drugs can lower the symptoms of bladder irritation and urgency. A randomized control study [42] reported that using solifenacin in patients who underwent ureteroscopy with ureteric stent insertion significantly lowered the total symptom score including sexual index. Moreover, the later literature found the solifenacin was able to improve urinary symptoms, pain, and general health [43]. Tolterodine 4 mg extended-release once daily for 6 weeks showed to improve pain and urinary symptom index score [39]. However, neither extended-release oxybutynin nor phenazopyridine provided benefit over placebo [44]. Common side effects of anticholinergic are dementia, blurred vision, headache, dry mouth, and urinary retention. Consider the use of these anticholinergic drugs in the elderly with caution because the drugs can cross the blood-brain barrier to cause cognitive impairment.

(c) *Combined Alpha-Blockers with Anticholinergic*

Theoretically, the synergistic effect of anticholinergic and alpha-blockers will improve stent symptoms. The combination of tamsulosin and oxybutynin [45] or pregabalin and solifenacin [46] showed improvement of pain and general health in many studies. However, Wang et al. [43] studied comparing solifenacin and tamsulosin or placebo; the result showed that a combination of solifenacin and tamsulosin did not gain benefits over solifenacin monotherapy.

(d) *Other Medications*

NSAIDs and opioids are widely used in the postoperative period of ureteroscopy with stone removal. They decrease postoperative pain but do not have any impact on voiding symptoms. Beiko et al. [47] reported that ketorolac intravesical installation immediately after stent placement after ESWL showed decrease in irritating symptoms at 1 hour after the intervention. Other pain-relieving methods were also proposed. Periureteric injection of botulinum toxin can decrease postoperative pain but does not effect on irritating symptoms [48].

Mirabegron is a beta-3 agonist. The study of Tae et al. [49] observed that patients who received mirabegron 50 mg once daily after the ureteroscopic procedure with ureteric stent insertion had successfully reduced the discomfort.

7.7 Other Complications

A ureteral stent is a foreign body to the urinary system. The bacterial colonization can produce the biofilm layer with adhesive property to the stent. This makes bacterial eradication rarely successful by antibiotic alone. Stent colonization reported 42–90% of ureteric stent insertion [50]. Persistent bacteriuria or complicated urinary infection from ureteric stent insertion can cause removing or changing the ureteric stents too early from treatment planning. Urine culture in a patient with ureteric stent shows having both gram-negative and gram-positive bacteria, while only gram-negative bacteria are commonly found in the normal population [51]. The antibiotic therapy should be adjusted according to change in bacteriology. Moreover, the persistence of urea-splitting organisms can cause stone encrustation from the changing environment to facilitate stone growth.

Stone encrustation is another common complication of ureteric stent insertion. Leaving the ureteric stent in the urine can promote stone encrustation up to 76% in 12 weeks [52]. The incidence of stone encrustation is increasing and occurs rapidly in the occasional population such as those stone former and pregnancy. Stone encrustation associates directly with bacterial adhesion by enhancing a favorable environment for bacteria and biofilm formation. Bacteria can enhance stone growth especially urea-splitting organisms. Proposing the different stent materials aim to decrease stone encrustation, bacterial adhesion, and biofilm formation. Compared to a metallic stent, silicon and polyurethane stents have a higher resistance to stone encrustation [1]. Special stent coatings were developed to lessen the problems. Glycosaminoglycan (CAG) is a natural stone inhibitor in human urine; it was used to coat on the surface of the ureteric stent. The studies reported the decrease in stone encrustation in a ureteric stent with CAGs coated [53]. Heparin, one of the CAGs, also showed delaying time to stone encrustation up to 12 months [54]. Other coating substances that were proposed to reduce stone encrustation and biofilm formations were hydrogel [55] and phosphorylcholine (PC) [56]. They provided a hydrophilic environment on the surface and provided an unsuitable environment for biofilm formation. PTFE was used to coat the stent surface and made the stent slippery by low friction coefficient and resistance to van der Waals force. Moreover, they also decreased tissue growth and bacterial colonization [57, 58]. Antibiotic and antimicrobial coated stents were also investigated to form mechanisms that decrease bacterial growth and eradicate them directly [59]. Daptomycin, linezolid, tigecycline, rifampicin, cefotaxime, vancomycin, silver, triclosan, chitosan, and povidone-iodine coated [60, 61] were tested and demonstrated inhibiting bacterial growth.

Other complications of ureteric stent insertion were stent migration, stent fracture, forgotten stent, and knotting of the stent. Stent migration was found higher in softer material and hydrophilic coated stent. The knotting of ureteric stent had been reported in many studies [62–65]. The cause of the knotted stent was unknown, but the incidence was higher in a multi-length ureteric stent [65]. Excessive length of the ureteral stent may be the risk factor of knotting. Various removal techniques were proposed including gentle traction, retrograde ureteroscopy with laser ablation, percutaneous antegrade removal, and open ureterotomy.

7.8 Conclusion

The ureteric stent is a common endourologic accessory. The benefits of the ureteric stent have been involved in benign and malignant disease management. Apart from the benefits, the stent itself can cause complications. Understanding the indications for insertion and stent-related complications is mandatory. The special ureteric stent should be considered in a selected case to lessen the side effects and complications.

References

1. Tunney MM, Keane PF, Jones DS, Gorman SP. Comparative assessment of ureteral stent biomaterial encrustation. Biomaterials. 1996;17(15):1541–6.
2. Campschroer T, Lock MT, Lo RT, Bosch JL. The Wallstent: long-term follow-up of metal stent placement for the treatment of benign ureteroileal anastomotic strictures after Bricker urinary diversion. BJU Int. 2014;114(6):910–5.
3. Wah TM, Irving HC, Cartledge J. Initial experience with the resonance metallic stent for antegrade ureteric stenting. Cardiovasc Intervent Radiol. 2007;30(4):705–10.
4. Yew J, Bellman G. Modified "tubeless" percutaneous nephrolithotomy using a tail-stent. Urology. 2003;62(2):346–9.
5. Dunn MD, Portis AJ, Kahn SA, Yan Y, Shalhav AL, Elbahnasy AM, et al. Clinical effectiveness of new stent design: randomized single-blind comparison of tail and double-pigtail stents. J Endourol. 2000;14(2):195–202.
6. Taylor WN, McDougall IT. Minimally invasive ureteral stent retrieval. J Urol. 2002;168(5):2020–3.
7. Borboroglu PG, Amling CL, Schenkman NS, Monga M, Ward JF, Piper NY, et al. Ureteral stenting after ureteroscopy for distal ureteral calculi: a multi-institutional prospective randomized controlled study assessing pain, outcomes and complications. J Urol. 2001;166(5):1651–7.
8. Haleblian G, Kijvikai K, de la Rosette J, Preminger G. Ureteral stenting and urinary stone management: a systematic review. J Urol. 2008;179(2):424–30.
9. Prasanchaimontri P, Nualyong C, Taweemonkongsap T, Chotikawanich E. Impact of ureteral stent size on stone-free rates in ureteroscopic lithotripsy for ureteral stones: randomized controlled trial. J Med Assoc Thail. 2017;100:162.
10. Knudsen BE, Beiko DT, Denstedt JD. Stenting after ureteroscopy: pros and cons. Urol Clin North Am. 2004;31(1):173–80.
11. Torricelli FC, De S, Hinck B, Noble M, Monga M. Flexible ureteroscopy with a ureteral access sheath: when to stent? Urology. 2014;83(2):278–81.
12. Rapoport D, Perks AE, Teichman JM. Ureteral access sheath use and stenting in ureteroscopy: effect on unplanned emergency room visits and cost. J Endourol. 2007;21(9):993–7.
13. Sirithanaphol W, Jitpraphai S, Taweemonkongsap T, Nuanyong C, Chotikawanich E. Ureteral stenting after flexible ureterorenoscopy with ureteral access sheath; is it really needed?: A prospective randomized study. J Med Assoc Thail. 2017;100:174.
14. Joshi HB, Okeke A, Newns N, Keeley FX Jr, Timoney AG. Characterization of urinary symptoms in patients with ureteral stents. Urology. 2002;59(4):511–6.
15. Joshi HB, Newns N, Stainthorpe A, MacDonagh RP, Keeley FX Jr, Timoney AG. Ureteral stent symptom questionnaire: development and validation of a multidimensional quality of life measure. J Urol. 2003;169(3):1060–4.
16. Ringel A, Richter S, Shalev M, Nissenkorn I. Late complications of ureteral stents. Eur Urol. 2000;38(1):41–4.
17. Chew BH, Knudsen BE, Nott L, Pautler SE, Razvi H, Amann J, et al. Pilot study of ureteral movement in stented patients: first step in understanding dynamic ureteral anatomy to improve stent comfort. J Endourol. 2007;21(9):1069–75.
18. Al-Kandari AM, Al-Shaiji TF, Shaaban H, Ibrahim HM, Elshebiny YH, Shokeir AA. Effects of proximal and distal ends of double-J ureteral stent position on postprocedural symptoms and quality of life: a randomized clinical trial. J Endourol. 2007;21(7):698–702.
19. Rane A, Saleemi A, Cahill D, Sriprasad S, Shrotri N, Tiptaft R. Have stent-related symptoms anything to do with placement technique? J Endourol. 2001;15(7):741–5.
20. Erturk E, Sessions A, Joseph JV. Impact of ureteral stent diameter on symptoms and tolerability. J Endourol. 2003;17(2):59–62.

21. Candela JV, Bellman GC. Ureteral stents: impact of diameter and composition on patient symptoms. J Endourol. 1997;11(1):45–7.
22. Ho CH, Tai HC, Chang HC, Hu FC, Chen SC, Lee YJ, et al. Predictive factors for ureteral double-J-stent-related symptoms: a prospective, multivariate analysis. J Formos Med Assoc. 2010;109(11):848–56.
23. Bregg K, Riehle RA Jr. Morbidity associated with indwelling internal ureteral stents after shock wave lithotripsy. J Urol. 1989;141(3):510–2.
24. Pryor JL, Langley MJ, Jenkins AD. Comparison of symptom characteristics of indwelling ureteral catheters. J Urol. 1991;145(4):719–22.
25. Lennon GM, Thornhill JA, Sweeney PA, Grainger R, McDermott TE, Butler MR. 'Firm' versus 'soft' double pigtail ureteric stents: a randomised blind comparative trial. Eur Urol. 1995;28(1):1–5.
26. El-Nahas AR, El-Assmy AM, Shoma AM, Eraky I, El-Kenawy MR, El-Kappany HA. Self-retaining ureteral stents: analysis of factors responsible for patients' discomfort. J Endourol. 2006;20(1):33–7.
27. Hao P, Li W, Song C, Yan J, Song B, Li L. Clinical evaluation of double-pigtail stent in patients with upper urinary tract diseases: report of 2685 cases. J Endourol. 2008;22(1):65–70.
28. Palmer JS, Palmer LS. Determining the proper stent length to use in children: age plus 10. J Urol. 2007;178(4 Pt 2):1566–9.
29. Calvert RC, Wong KY, Chitale SV, Irving SO, Nagarajan M, Biyani CS, et al. Multi-length or 24 cm ureteric stent? A multicentre randomised comparison of stent-related symptoms using a validated questionnaire. BJU Int. 2013;111(7):1099–104.
30. Krambeck AE, Walsh RS, Denstedt JD, Preminger GM, Li J, Evans JC, et al. A novel drug eluting ureteral stent: a prospective, randomized, multicenter clinical trial to evaluate the safety and effectiveness of a ketorolac loaded ureteral stent. J Urol. 2010;183(3):1037–42.
31. Chew BH, Davoudi H, Li J, Denstedt JD. An in vivo porcine evaluation of the safety, bioavailability, and tissue penetration of a ketorolac drug-eluting ureteral stent designed to improve comfort. J Endourol. 2010;24(6):1023–9.
32. Lingeman JE, Preminger GM, Goldfischer ER, Krambeck AE, Comfort ST. Assessing the impact of ureteral stent design on patient comfort. J Urol. 2009;181(6):2581–7.
33. Khandwekar AP, Doble M. Physicochemical characterisation and biological evaluation of polyvinylpyrrolidone-iodine engineered polyurethane (Tecoflex(®)). J Mater Sci Mater Med. 2011;22(5):1231–46.
34. Mendez-Probst CE, Fernandez A, Denstedt JD. Current status of ureteral stent technologies: comfort and antimicrobial resistance. Curr Urol Rep. 2010;11(2):67–73.
35. Liatsikos EN, Karnabatidis D, Kagadis GC, Rokkas K, Constantinides C, Christeas N, et al. Application of paclitaxel-eluting metal mesh stents within the pig ureter: an experimental study. Eur Urol. 2007;51(1):217–23.
36. Kallidonis P, Kitrou P, Karnabatidis D, Kyriazis I, Kalogeropoulou C, Tsamandas A, et al. Evaluation of zotarolimus-eluting metal stent in animal ureters. J Endourol. 2011;25(10):1661–7.
37. Deliveliotis C, Chrisofos M, Gougousis E, Papatsoris A, Dellis A, Varkarakis IM. Is there a role for alpha1-blockers in treating double-J stent-related symptoms? Urology. 2006;67(1):35–9.
38. Beddingfield R, Pedro RN, Hinck B, Kreidberg C, Feia K, Monga M. Alfuzosin to relieve ureteral stent discomfort: a prospective, randomized, placebo controlled study. J Urol. 2009;181(1):170–6.
39. Park SC, Jung SW, Lee JW, Rim JS. The effects of tolterodine extended release and alfuzosin for the treatment of double-j stent-related symptoms. J Endourol. 2009;23(11):1913–7.
40. Wang CJ, Huang SW, Chang CH. Effects of specific alpha-1A/1D blocker on lower urinary tract symptoms due to double-J stent: a prospectively randomized study. Urol Res. 2009;37(3):147–52.
41. Dellis AE, Papatsoris AG, Keeley FX Jr, Bamias A, Deliveliotis C, Skolarikos AA. Tamsulosin, solifenacin, and their combination for the treatment of stent-related symptoms: A randomized controlled study. J Endourol. 2017;31(1):100–9.
42. Lee YJ, Huang KH, Yang HJ, Chang HC, Chen J, Yang TK. Solifenacin improves double-J stent-related symptoms in both genders following uncomplicated ureteroscopic lithotripsy. Urolithiasis. 2013;41(3):247–52.
43. Wang J, Zhang X, Zhang T, Mu J, Bai B, Lei Y. The role of solifenacin, as monotherapy or combination with tamsulosin in ureteral stent-related symptoms: a systematic review and meta-analysis. World J Urol. 2017;35(11):1669–80.
44. Norris RD, Sur RL, Springhart WP, Marguet CG, Mathias BJ, Pietrow PK, et al. A prospective, randomized, double-blinded placebo-controlled comparison of extended release oxybutynin versus phenazopyridine for the management of postoperative ureteral stent discomfort. Urology. 2008;71(5):792–5.
45. Maldonado-Avila M, Garduno-Arteaga L, Jungfermann-Guzman R, Manzanilla-Garcia HA, Rosas-Nava E, Procuna-Hernandez N, et al. Efficacy of tamsulosin, oxybutynin, and their combination in the control of double-j stent-related lower urinary tract symptoms. Int Braz J Urol. 2016;42(3):487–93.
46. Ragab M, Soliman MG, Tawfik A, Abdel Raheem A, El-Tatawy H, Abo Farha M, et al. The role of pregabalin in relieving ureteral stent-related symptoms: a randomized controlled clinical trial. Int Urol Nephrol. 2017;49(6):961–6.

47. Beiko DT, Watterson JD, Knudsen BE, Nott L, Pautler SE, Brock GB, et al. Double-blind randomized controlled trial assessing the safety and efficacy of intravesical agents for ureteral stent symptoms after extracorporeal shockwave lithotripsy. J Endourol. 2004;18(8):723–30.
48. Gupta M, Patel T, Xavier K, Maruffo F, Lehman D, Walsh R, et al. Prospective randomized evaluation of periureteral botulinum toxin type A injection for ureteral stent pain reduction. J Urol. 2010;183(2):598–602.
49. Tae BS, Cho S, Jeon BJ, Choi H, Park JY, Cho SY, et al. Does mirabegron relieve ureteric stent-related discomfort? A prospective, randomized, multicentre study. BJU Int. 2018;122(5):866–72.
50. Kehinde EO, Rotimi VO, Al-Hunayan A, Abdul-Halim H, Boland F, Al-Awadi KA. Bacteriology of urinary tract infection associated with indwelling J ureteral stents. J Endourol. 2004;18(9):891–6.
51. Lange D, Bidnur S, Hoag N, Chew BH. Ureteral stent-associated complications--where we are and where we are going. Nat Rev Urol. 2015;12(1):17–25.
52. El-Faqih SR, Shamsuddin AB, Chakrabarti A, Atassi R, Kardar AH, Osman MK, et al. Polyurethane internal ureteral stents in treatment of stone patients: morbidity related to indwelling times. J Urol. 1991;146(6):1487–91.
53. Hildebrandt P, Sayyad M, Rzany A, Schaldach M, Seiter H. Prevention of surface encrustation of urological implants by coating with inhibitors. Biomaterials. 2001;22(5):503–7.
54. Cauda F, Cauda V, Fiori C, Onida B, Garrone E. Heparin coating on ureteral double J stents prevents encrustations: an in vivo case study. J Endourol. 2008;22(3):465–72.
55. Laube N, Kleinen L, Bradenahl J, Meissner A. Diamond-like carbon coatings on ureteral stents—a new strategy for decreasing the formation of crystalline bacterial biofilms? J Urol. 2007;177(5):1923–7.
56. Stickler DJ, Evans A, Morris N, Hughes G. Strategies for the control of catheter encrustation. Int J Antimicrob Agents. 2002;19(6):499–506.
57. Yang L, Whiteside S, Cadieux PA, Denstedt JD. Ureteral stent technology: drug-eluting stents and stent coatings. Asian J Urol. 2015;2(4):194–201.
58. Chung HH, Lee SH, Cho SB, Park HS, Kim YS, Kang BC, et al. Comparison of a new polytetrafluoroethylene-covered metallic stent to a noncovered stent in canine ureters. Cardiovasc Intervent Radiol. 2008;31(3):619–28.
59. Lo J, Lange D, Chew BH. Ureteral stents and foley catheters-associated urinary tract infections: the role of coatings and materials in infection prevention. Antibiotics (Basel). 2014;3(1):87–97.
60. Raad I, Hanna H, Jiang Y, Dvorak T, Reitzel R, Chaiban G, et al. Comparative activities of daptomycin, linezolid, and tigecycline against catheter-related methicillin-resistant Staphylococcus bacteremic isolates embedded in biofilm. Antimicrob Agents Chemother. 2007;51(5):1656–60.
61. Rose WE, Poppens PT. Impact of biofilm on the in vitro activity of vancomycin alone and in combination with tigecycline and rifampicin against Staphylococcus aureus. J Antimicrob Chemother. 2009;63(3):485–8.
62. Bradshaw J, Khan A, Adiotomre E, Burbidge S, Biyani CS. Antegrade removal of a knotted ureteric stent: case report and review of literature. Urol Ann. 2020;12(1):96–100.
63. Eisner B, Kim H, Sacco D. Repeat knot formation in a patient with an indwelling ureteral stent. Int Braz J Urol. 2006;32(3):308–9.
64. Kim MS, Lee HN, Hwang H. Knotted stents: case report and outcome analysis. Korean J Urol. 2015;56(5):405–8.
65. Picozzi S, Carmignani L. A knotted ureteral stent: A case report and review of the literature. Urol Ann. 2010;2(2):80–2.

8 Understanding the Instruments Imaging System: Radiation Safety and Ultrasound Technique

Takaaki Inoue

Abstract

With the development of endourological technology and equipment, the procedures for stone management have become much less invasive. However, radiological occupational staff members including surgeons, nurses, medical engineers, and anesthesiologists have increased opportunities for radiation exposure during endourological operations performed under fluoroscopy. Therefore, we should learn about protective practice to increase safety with respect to radiation exposure. Although endourologists commonly use ultrasound sonography for diagnosis and intervention of urinary stones, they have not yet become accustomed to working with the machines used to perform the examinations. Many ultrasound systems with new functions have become available, so we introduce the benefits of ultrasound and explain how to use it.

Keywords

Radiation protection · Preventive methods · Radiation exposure · Ultrasound · Doppler ultrasound mode

T. Inoue (✉)
Department of Urology and Stone Center, Hara Genitourinary Hospital, Kobe, Japan

Department of Urology, Kobe University, Kobe, Japan
e-mail: inouetak@harahospital.jp

Abbreviations

ALARA	As low as reasonably achievable
FT	Fluoroscopic time
fURS	Flexible ureteroscopy
ICRP	International Commission on Radiological Protection
IR	Interventional radiology
LNT	Linear, non-threshold
NCRP	National Council on Radiation Protection and Measurements
PCNL	Percutaneous nephrolithotomy

8.1 Introduction

Generally, most endourologists have used fluoroscopic and ultrasound sonographic machines for the diagnosis and treatment of upper urinary tract stones. Especially, percutaneous puncture into the collecting system of the kidney is mostly undertaken with fluoroscopic or ultrasound guidance. Each of these guidance methods has both advantages and disadvantages.

The main advantage of fluoroscopic guidance is its status as the most frequently used technique by urologists. However, the disadvantages of fluoroscopic guidance are that it offers no real-time visualization of adjacent organs and that it exposes the operator and surgical staff to radiation. Although fluoroscopic-guided

A. C.F. Ng et al. (eds.), *Practical Management of Urinary Stone*,
https://doi.org/10.1007/978-981-16-4193-0_8

renal access is still common worldwide, ultrasound-guided renal access has also seen increased use recently, as it is associated with less bleeding, fewer complications including especially organ injuries, and perioperative advantages like shorter puncture time and higher success rate of the first puncture [1]. However, the main disadvantages of ultrasound access are its difficulty facilitating the puncture of collecting systems without distention, poor visualization of the guidewire, and (sometimes) lower visualization of the puncture needle, especially in obesity cases. In some cases, such as in patients with obesity, the ultrasonic waves may not be able to pass through the full distance between the skin and the renal capsule. This chapter explains the current understanding of fluoroscopic safety and ultrasound techniques in imaging systems.

8.2 Radiation Safety in Fluoroscopy for the Management of Urinary Calculi

The Chernobyl nuclear power plant in Ukraine had the experience of severe accident in 1986, and the Fukushima in Japan plant was similarly affected in 2011. These accidents resulted in frightful amount of radioactive fallout, which had long-term effects: the extended low-dose radiation exposure greatly influenced human health in later years. These occurrences increased the incidence of malignancies, including thyroid cancer, breast cancer, and leukemia [2].

The field of interventional radiology has been developed in the last few decades. It has been applied especially frequently in minimally invasive radiology, cardiology, gastroenterology, orthopedic surgery, and urological surgery procedures. It is a minimally invasive approach to treat various diseases, including some benign and malignant lesions, and it has some advantages, such as lower degrees of pain, complications, and cosmetic scarring.

In the urological field, endoscopic surgeries using real-time radiation imaging have been established, especially in treatment of urolithiasis. The procedures and treatment outcomes have been improved by the new surgical instruments and materials. Furthermore, polished radiological equipment has helped in spreading the use of fluoroscopy-guided interventional radiological therapy. However, concomitant to this expansion, radiation exposure to medical personnel and patients has increased. Therefore, urologists must be aware of the potential risk of harmful effects caused by radiation exposure. Knowledge about the correct and safe use of fluoroscopy in interventional radiology may be a less important interest to urologists than to radiologists and cardiologists. All urologists who use fluoroscopy should know the risks of radiation and the risk prevention techniques available.

The ICRP (International Commission on Radiological Protection) is an international academic organization that has developed, maintained, and elaborated the International Commission on Radiological Protection, which is used worldwide as the common basis for radiological protection standards, legislation, guidelines, programs, and practices [3].

According to the ICRP recommendations, three fundamental principles such as justification, protection, and dose limits are the bases of radiological protection system:

1. *Justification*: Any decision that alters the level of radiation exposure situation should do much better than harm.
2. *Protection*: The likelihood of incurring exposure, the number of people exposed, and the magnitude of their individual doses should all be kept as low as reasonably achievable, taking economic and societal factors into account.
3. *Dose limits*: The total dose to any individual from regulated sources in planned exposure situations other than medical exposure to patients should not exceed the appropriate limits specified by the ICRP.

8.3 Principle of Prevention of Radiation Exposure in Endourological Stone Management

A major source of radiation exposure to patients is caused by direct radiation which generated in the fluoroscopic field between an X-ray tube and an image intensifier. A major source of radiation exposure to surgeons and medical staffs is caused by scattered radiation that is produced from the interaction of the primary radiation beam with the patient's body and the operating table. Further, medical personnel may rarely be exposed to direct radiation when their hands enter the fluoroscopy field between the X-ray tube and the image intensifier (Fig. 8.1).

Diagnosis, evaluation and endourological procedures for upper urinary tract stones are mostly performed under fluoroscopy. Percutaneous nephrolithotomy (PCNL) using radiologic guidance was initially described by Fernstrom et al. on three patients in 1976 [4]. In the endourological field, patients with upper urinary tract stones and the surgeons and medical staff members involved in their management have opportunities for radiation exposure. Although the dose limit of medical radiation exposure for patients has not been restricted, the dose limit of occupational radiation exposure has been defined as 50 mSv per year by the National Council on Radiation Protection and Measurements [5].

Ionizing radiation exposure is a harmful risk factor for malignant cancer. The degree of harm caused by low-dose radiation exposure is unknown, but that information could be used to extrapolate the level of radiation-related cancer risk. Thus, the linear, non-threshold hypothesis is applied as the basic philosophy to consider the biological effects of radiation exposure. However, some researchers have reported that low levels of chronic occupational exposure to ionizing radiation cause an increased frequency of chromosomal micronuclei, which is a biomarker of chromosomal damage, genomic instability, and cancer risk [6]. Furthermore, occupational radiation exposure's influence on the lens of eye has currently been taken noticed with gradual increase. The ICRP recommends not exceeding a mean dose of 20 μSv/year to the eye lens. Therefore, the ICRP has recommended limiting radiation exposure to levels "as low as reasonably achievable" (ALARA) [7, 8].

The principles of medical radiation protection must be applied for both the patients and medical staffs who are involved in imaging study, the lat-

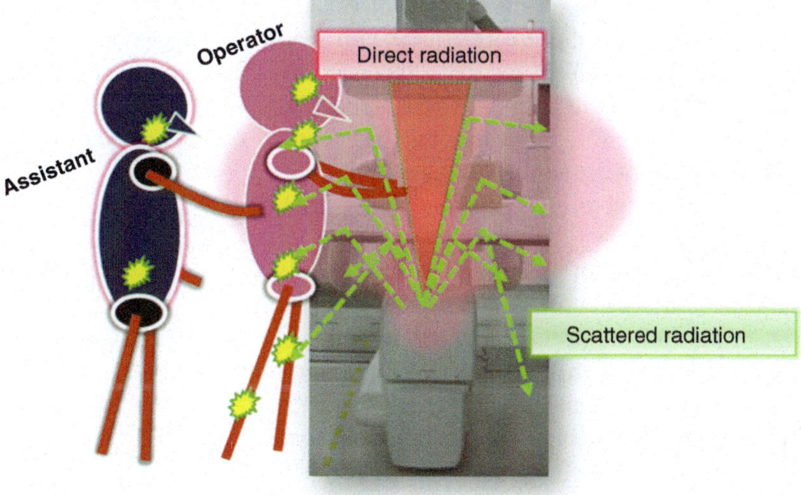

Fig. 8.1 Illustration of radiation exposure including direct and scattered radiation from C-arm

ter of which include surgeons, anesthesiologists, nurses, and medical engineers. The following are most necessary methods to optimize the protection from radiation exposure:

1. Time: The time of radiation exposure must be minimized in terms of both fluoroscopy time and the quantity of X-ray photographs acquired during procedures.
2. Distance: Medical staffs must position themselves as far as possible from the X-ray source during procedures.
3. Shielding: Medical staffs must use optimal shielding materials from radiation exposure, such as lead aprons, lead glasses, thyroid shield with lead, and lead radiation-shielding glass.

8.4 Radiation Protection During Endourological Procedures

A major source of radiation exposure to surgeons and medical staffs must be scattered radiation exposure which was produced by the interaction of the primary radiation beam with the patient's body and the operating table. Mostly, this exposure is from radiation scattering intraoperatively. Shielding instruments for such personnel is usually performed by personally wearing protective clothing. The standard protocol of lead protection requires the use of a 0.35-mm lead apron and thyroid shield for the surgeon in the operation theater and 0.25-mm lead aprons for other personnel [9]. However, the protection from scattered radiation with protective clothing might be incomplete, especially that to the arms, eyes, and brain.

The mean dose of radiation exposure for the surgeon in percutaneous nephrolithotomy (PCNL) is 12.7 mSv per procedure. This value is much higher than the 11.6 μSV per radiation exposure dose in flexible ureteroscopy (fURS) because of the longer fluoroscopic time and close distance between the surgeon and the radiation source [7, 10]. According to some literatures, the mean fluoroscopic time during PCNL has been reported as 4.5–6.04 min (range 1–12.16 min) [11]. Furthermore, the mean doses of radiation exposures to the surgeon's finger and ocular region during endourological procedures were 0.28 mSv and 0.125 mSv, respectively, because of the non-uniform radiation exposure caused by scattered radiation [12, 13]. Therefore, the surgeon's hands and eyes must also be protected from scattered radiation exposure by using gloves and glasses with lead-threading. Most endourologists generally undergo the needle puncture for access to renal collecting system under fluoroscopy when placing percutaneous nephrostomy and doing PCNL. Therefore, ultrasound-guided access is a useful approach during PCNL, as it provides better protection to surgeons from radiation exposure compared with just fluoroscopic approach.

Radiation dose of surgeon is significantly lower in URS than in PCNL in most cases because URS is characterized by shorter fluoroscopic time and longer distance between the radiation source and surgeon. Pulsed fluoroscope which was introduced to reduce the radiation dose by limiting the X-ray exposure time and number of exposures per second is quite beneficial methods during endourological procedures. The spent time of radiation exposure during URS has been decreased from the original 4.7 to 0.62 min [14], and mean fluoroscopy time during URS has been reported as 44.1 s (range 36.5–51.6 s) [15]. In addition, Kokorowski et al. and colleagues described the efficacy of a preoperative checklist related to radiation protection which was useful to decrease radiation exposure during procedures [16] (Table 8.1).

Table 8.1 One of Fluoroscopy Checklists to reduce radiation exposure

1	Are the patient's arms to the side?
2	Is the table height OK?
3	Has intensifier been brought to within one fist of patient?
4	What is the patient thickness? Has the dose rate setting been adjusted for patient size? (A) Toddler: A–P diameter < 12 cm (B) Child: A–P diameter 12–20 cm (C) Adult: A–P diameter >20 cm
5	Is the exposure mode set to digital?
6	Is everyone wearing lead?

Furthermore, Inoue et al. reported that the protectively surgical lead curtains on both sides of the operative patient table, the operating table end, and the image intensifier were quite useful tools to decrease the surgeon's radiation exposure during URS. They simulated the spatially scattered radiation dose in the operating room during procedures for management of upper urinary tract stone by using an anthropomorphic phantom and an ionization chamber and measured the dose of scattered radiation under the patient's table and image intensifier when using protective lead curtains or not. They found that the lead curtains have an effect of 75%–80% reduction of the scattered radiation dose compared with not using lead curtains [17] (Fig. 8.2a). In addition, novel shielding curtains containing **bismuth** and **antimony**, which are also suitable for radiation protection because of their high density and have potential weight savings compared with lead, have also been designed (Fig. 8.2b). Furthermore, bismuth and antimony are less toxic elements for the environment, with much lower toxicity than lead as well. In modern practice of radiation protection, active personal dosimeters are essential to satisfy the ALARA principle [18]. Most urologists have an insufficient perception of their own personal radiation protection. Some previous studies investigated that only 53.9% wore a thyroid shield and only 27.9% wore eye glasses with lead linings despite of 84.4% of urologists who were chronically exposed to ionizing radiation wearing lead aprons. Moreover, only 23.6% of urologists wore a personal dosimeter [19].

Realization of occupational radiation exposure among physicians in the urological field is still low level. Although the harmful risks of occupational radiation exposure in clinical practice may be relatively low, they should not be ignored.

Other methods to reduce or minimize the dose of occupational radiation exposure include minimizing the fluoroscopic time and number of acquired images, collimation of images, avoiding high-scatter areas, using the pulsed fluoroscopic mode, minimizing the distance between the

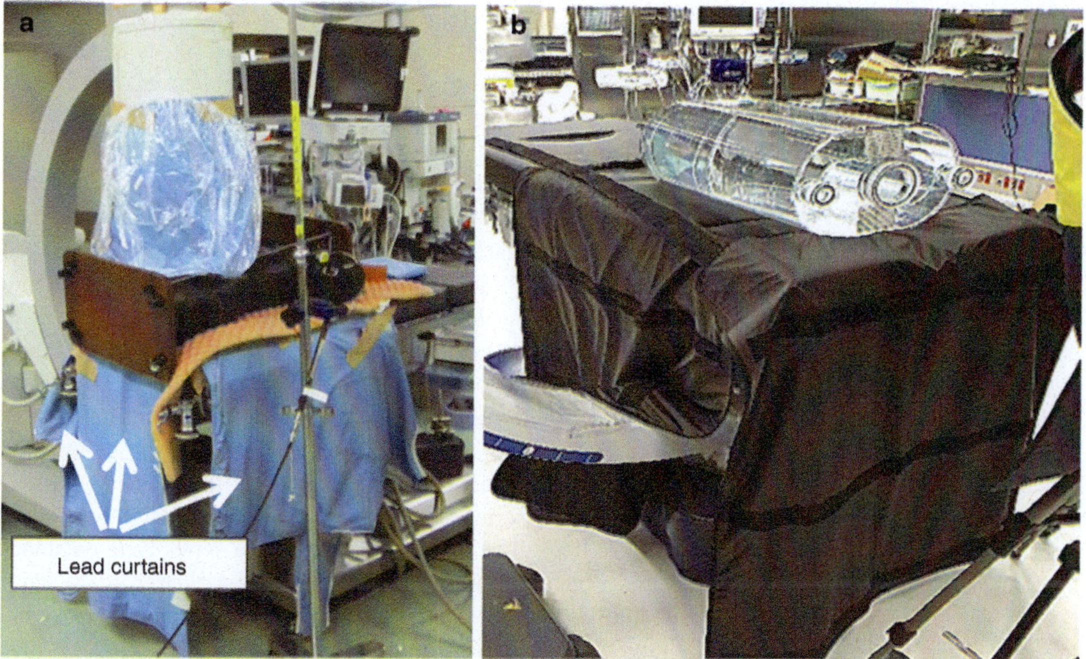

Fig. 8.2 Image picture of hand-made shielding curtain included a 0.5-mm lead (**a**) and new curtains with bismuth-antimony (**b**) to protect from radiation exposure in ureteroscopy

Table 8.2 Reduction technique from radiation exposure for patients and operators during surgery

	Methods			
Subjects	1	2	3	4
C-arm, image intensifier	Maximizing the distance between the X-ray tube and the patient	Minimizing the distance between patients and the image Intensifier	Collimating	Pulsed fluoroscopic mode
Operator	Minimizing fluoroscopy time	Protective shielding for operator	Protective shielding for patient table	
Instrument	Using ultrasound instead of fluoroscopy	Direct endoscopic vision combined with ultrasound	Last image hold	Laser guided C-arm
Others	Dedicated educational training (including preoperative checklist)			

patient and the image intensifier, maximizing the distance between the X-ray tube and the patient, using ultrasound sonography instead of fluoroscopy, using protective shielding, and wearing personal dosimeters (Table 8.2) (Fig. 8.3). To acquire the effective use of these methods, all endourologists and medical staffs are required both appropriate education, training in radiation exposure, and the availability of appropriate tools and equipment.

8.5 Ultrasound Sonography Systems

The role of ultrasound in endourological procedures is expanding as technology advances and clinicians become better educated about its clinical applications. The main use of endourological ultrasound to physicians is to examine the screening of intra-abdominal organs and to diagnose pathologic changes like tumors, stones, and hydronephrosis. Ultrasound can also be used to assist clinicians in performing interventional procedures in the endourological field. However, to successfully integrate this technology into clinical practice, physicians must be familiar with both the normal and abnormal appearances of the anatomy and the use of ultrasound machines [20]. A significant advantage of ultrasound imaging is that it is noninvasive. Its advantages over other imaging techniques include its dynamic real-time imaging capability, versatility, portability, safety, and economic feasibility.

Ultrasound imaging encompasses a wide range of imaging modes and techniques that use the interactions of sound waves with living tissues to produce images of the tissues by determining the velocity of moving tissues. Ultrasound refers to sound waves with frequencies greater than 20,000 cycles/s that are not detectable by the human ear. Diagnostic ultrasound commonly uses frequencies between 2 and 20 million cycles/sec (106 pulses/s), which urologists usually use. Generally, higher frequencies of ultrasound waves are associated with higher quality of distance resolution but larger attenuation of the reached distance. Although higher-frequency ultrasound waves can create clearer images, they reach a shorter depth. Therefore, a limitation in clinical practice is that ultrasound waves cannot easily reach deeply located target tissues in patients with obesity. Consequently, the images become rough and lack smoothness. However, currently available ultrasound machines such as the Philips EPIQ and AFFINITI series, the Hitachi ARIETTA series, the Toshiba APLIO series, the BK Medical FLEX FOCUS series, and the GE Healthcare Versana series have outstanding functions like better and clearer image quality, elastography, harmonic imaging, and high-resolution Doppler imaging.

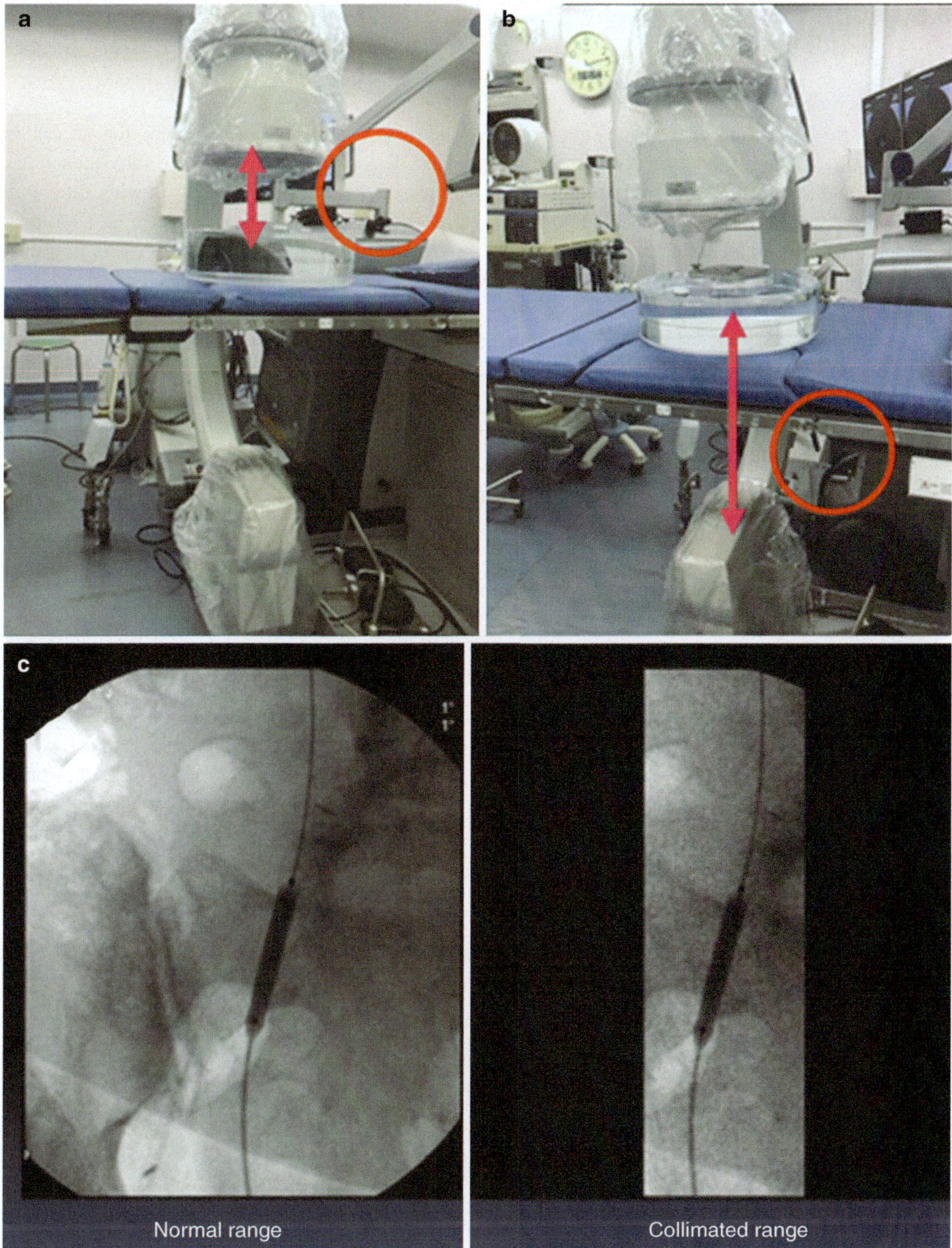

Fig. 8.3 Image picture of protective methods from radiation exposure. (**a**) Minimizing distance between patient and image intensifier. (**b**) Maximizing distance between patient and X-ray tube. (**c**) Collimation of fluoroscopic image

8.6 Ultrasound Sonography Equipment

1. Various probes

   The probe originates from the ultrasound wave and transmits and receives the ultrasound beam bounced back from obstacles like tissues or organs. Thus, it has a major role. The capabilities and frequency band of the probe influence image quality and capacity of the whole system:

   - Convex type: Standard convex and micro-convex (Fig. 8.4a, b). The convex type is commonly used in abdominal screening and percutaneous intervention. Micro-convex probes are often used alongside percutaneous puncture.

2. Regulation of ultrasound systems (Fig. 8.4c, d)

   There are various available ultrasound systems, which have many useful functions. The following are common adjustable parameters of ultrasound systems:

   - Depth of field: Adjustment of the depth of the observational field
   - Gain: Modulation of brightness in the whole-image view
   - Focus: Modulation of overall sensitivity to prevent stretching of the ultrasound beam
   - Mode: Modes include B-mode, M-mode, Doppler mode, and pulse Doppler mode

8.7 Practical Application of Ultrasound for Renal Stones

The first use of ultrasonography for access in PCNL was described in 1970, and since then, it has increased in popularity, with growing literature data demonstrating its advantages in terms of efficacy, safety, and feasibility for upper urinary tract stones [21]. Desai et al. published the first report of ultrasound-guided PCNL for pediatric stones 20 years ago [22]. The advantages of ultrasound renal access in PCNL include real-time puncture using a biplane to avoid accidental injuries to adjacent vital organs, reduced radiation exposure (especially for pregnant patients), cheaper cost of use, and reduced risk of complications like bleeding (Table 8.3). Another benefit of ultrasound guidance is that Doppler mode encompasses color Doppler, power Doppler, and wideband Doppler, all of which come enabled in standard ultrasound machines. These modes can depict the running renal vascular structure in real time and thus facilitate needle puncture without injury to significant major vessels like the interlobar vessel. However, fluoroscopy can be necessary as an adjunct for verifying correct needle placement in case ultrasound fails to facilitate renal access. It can also be used in conjunction with ultrasound for tract creation after the initial puncture [23].

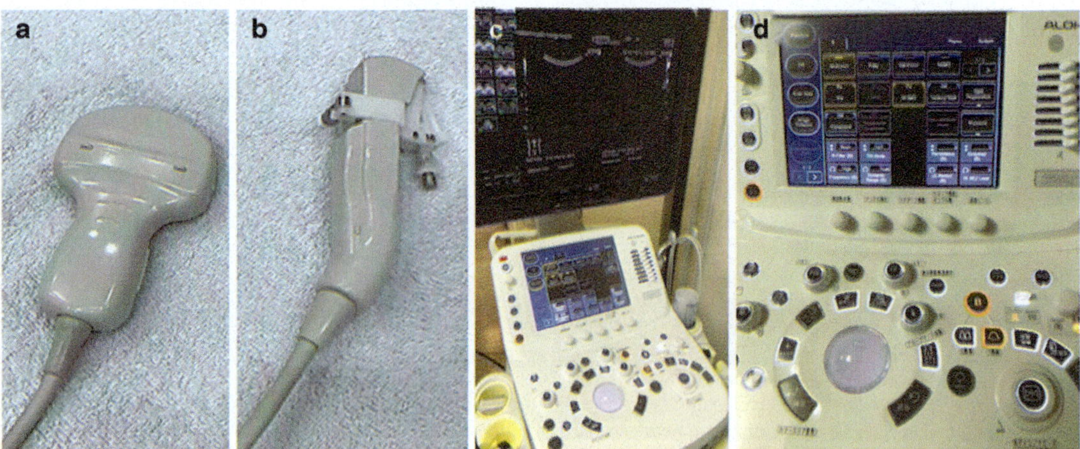

Fig. 8.4 Image picture of various ultrasound probes and (**a**) convex type (**b**) micro-convex type. (**c**) Ultrasound system. (**d**) Operation panel

Table 8.3 The advantage and disadvantage between fluoroscopic and ultrasound guidance

	Fluoroscopy	Ultrasound
Advantage	Traditional methods (bull's eye, Triangular technique)	Puncture in real-time using biplane, while avoiding accidental injuries to vital adjacent organs
		Less radiation exposure
Disadvantage	More radiation exposure to operator, medical staffs, and patients	Not easy to reach sound wave in obesity patients
	Not visualized adjacent organs during puncture	Different function between ultrasound systems
	Wide view	Limited field of view
	Need to training	Need to training

Nevertheless, ultrasound-guided renal access is a useful technique in the management of larger renal stones. Usually, urologists need training on how to use and master ultrasound systems and how to use ultrasound image monitors to recognize some organs and tissues.

8.8 The Use of Various Ultrasound Modes During Needle Puncture

1. B-mode image: This is the usual mode, in which the visualization color is monochrome. This mode's limitation is that it cannot depict running vessels or penetrate the full distance between the skin and renal capsule in some cases (Fig. 8.5a).
2. Color-power Doppler mode image: Color Doppler visualizes the direction of the running vessels, and power Doppler displays the magnitude of the running vascular flow. A blooming appearance indicates higher blood vessel thickness than the real size in both modes (Fig. 8.5b, c).
3. Wideband Doppler mode image: Wideband Doppler mode promotes temporal and spatial resolution and decreases the blooming appearance in comparison with power and color Doppler modes. Therefore, in most cases, it can visualize the clear peripheral blood vessels in renal parenchyma (Fig. 8.5d).

These Doppler modes, which are already available in current ultrasound systems, can show the vascular flow in real time through image. The use of these Doppler modes for puncture of the target calyx might result in easy detection and avoidance of renal blood vessels such as the interlobar arteries and veins and arcuate arteries and veins compared with the usual B-mode imaging. Tzeng et al., who undertook PCNL using a 30F tract sheath with B-mode or power Doppler ultrasound guidance, investigated that the hemoglobin decreases associated with each method were 2.33 ± 0.46 g/dL and 1.47 ± 0.61 g/dL, respectively [24]. Furthermore, Inoue et al. reported that the use of wideband Doppler mode during endoscopic combined intrarenal surgery for large (>30 mm) renal stones decreased hemoglobin less (0.54 ± 0.65 g/dL) [25]. The wideband Doppler mode is useful for avoiding the mis-puncture of major renal vessels (Fig. 8.6). However, these modes have some limitations, such as functional differences among various ultrasound systems and poor visualization in some patients with obesity, who have a longer distance between the skin and renal capsule.

In summary, this chapter has introduced concepts related to protection from radiation exposure and the use of ultrasound systems. Radiation safety is becoming a more important concern in the endourological field. Low-dose, long-term radiation exposure during procedures seems to be harmful to humans' long-term health, especially that of medical staff members, operators, and patients. Therefore, occupational radiological staff members should not neglect the ALARA principle. Further, current ultrasound machines are progressing in clinical usefulness and have many utilities. We should learn about the advantages of these ultrasound systems and become accustomed to them before applying them in clinical practice.

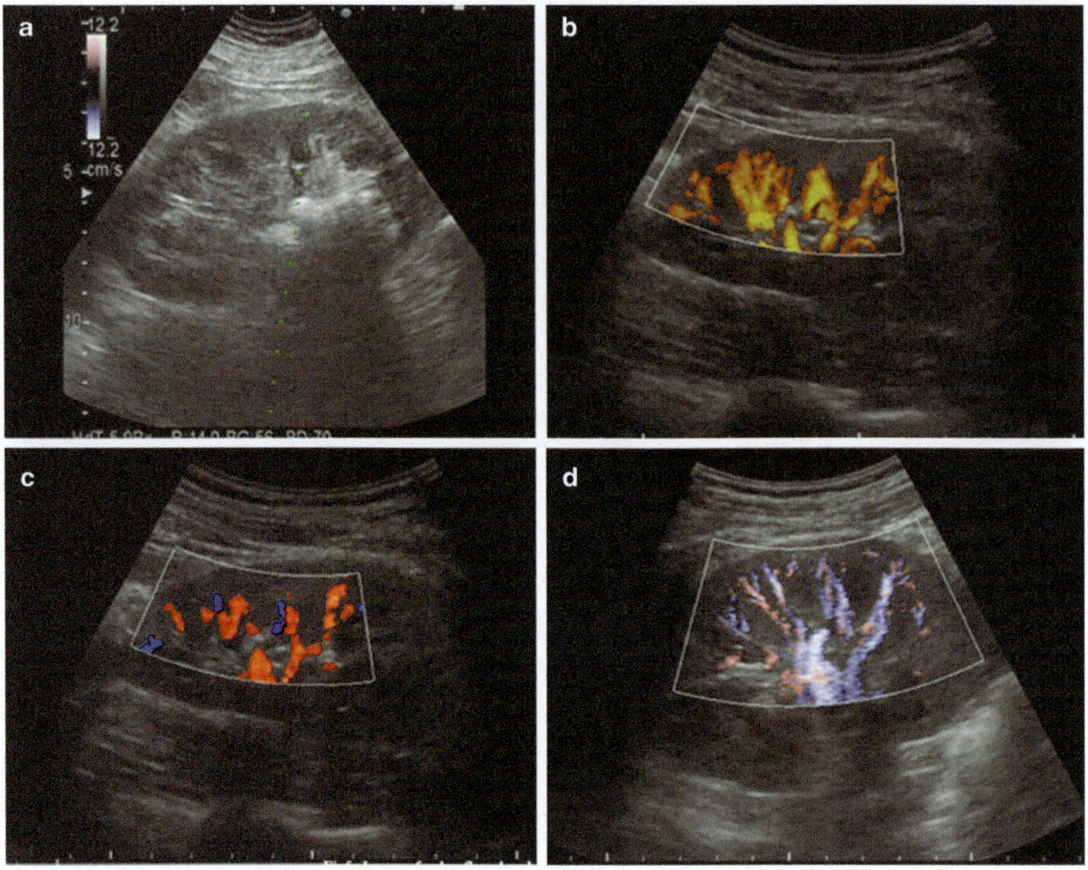

Fig. 8.5 Image picture of various modes in ultrasound sonography. (**a**) B-mode. (**b**) Power Doppler mode. (**c**) Color Doppler mode. (**d**) Wideband Doppler mode

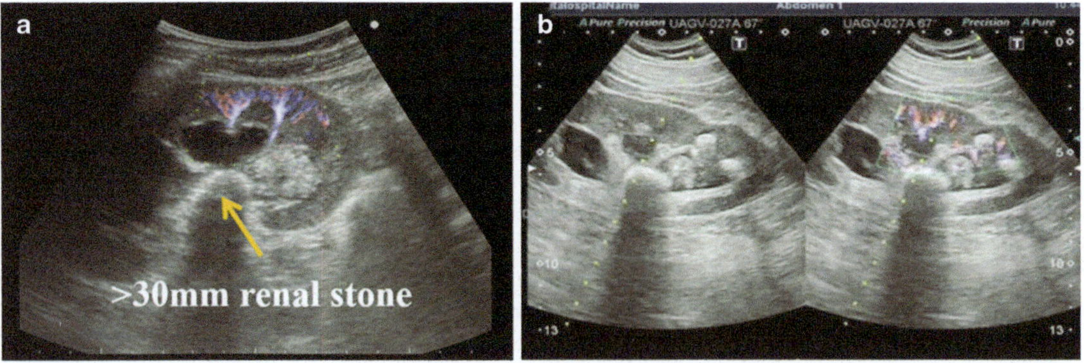

Fig. 8.6 Image view of wideband Doppler mode during renal puncture. (**a**) Appearance of clear running vessels in renal parenchyma. (**b**) Twin view image of synchronized B-mode and wideband Doppler image

References

1. Liu Q, Liang Z, Cai X, Jin T, Wang K. Fluoroscopy versus ultrasound for image guidance during percutaneous nephrolithotomy: a systematic review and Meta-analysis. Utolithiasis. 2017;45:481–7.
2. Pukkala E, Kesminiene A, Poliakov S, Ryzhov A, Drozdovitch V, Kovgan L, Kttronen P, Malakhova IV, Gulak L, Cardis E. Breast caner in Belarus and Ukraine after the Chernobyl accident. Int J Cancer. 2006;119(3):651–8.
3. ICRP. The 2007 recommendations of the International Commission on Radiological Protection. ICRP Publication 103. Ann ICRP. 2007;37(2–4):1–332.
4. Fernstrom I, Johansson B. Percutaneous pyelolithotomy. A new extraction technique. Scand. J Urol Nephrol. 1976;10:257–9.
5. Occupational dose limits for adults. In: Part 20-Standards for protection against radiation, nuclear regulatory commission regulations title 10, Code of Federal Regulation. Washington, DC: United States Nuclear Regulatory Commission; 1991.
6. Eken A, Aydin A, Erdem O, et al. Cytogenetic analysis of peripheral blood lymphocytes of hospital staff occupationally exposed to low doses of ionizing radiation. Toxicol Ind Health. 2010;26:273–80.
7. Hellawell GO, Mutch SJ, Thevendran G, et al. Radiation exposure and the urologist: what are the risks? J Urol. 2005;174:948–52.
8. Duran A, Hian SK, Miller DL, et al. Recommendations for occupational radiation protection in interventional cardiology. Cathet Cardiovasc Interv. 2013;82:29–42.
9. Medical and dental guidance notes: a good practice guide on all aspects of ionising radiation protection in the clinical environment. York: Institute of Physics and Engineering in Medicine, 2002.
10. Safak M, Olgar T, Bor D, et al. Radiation doses of patients and urologists during percutaneous nephrolithotomy. J Radiol Prot. 2009;29:409–15.
11. Kumari G, Kumar P, Wadhwa P, et al. Radiation exposure to the patient and operating room personnel during percutaneous nephrolithotomy. Int Urol Nephrol. 2006;38:207–10.
12. Majidpour HS. Risk of radiation exposure during PCNL. Urol J. 2010;7:87–9.
13. Taylor ER, Kramer B, Frye TP, et al. Ocular radiation exposure in modern urological practice. J Urol. 2013;190:139–43.
14. Bagley DH, Cubler-Goodman A. Radiation exposure during ureteroscopy. J Urol. 1990;144:1356–8.
15. Elkoushy MA, Shahrour W, Andonian S. Pulsed fluoroscopy in ureteroscopy and perctaneous nephrolithotomy. Urology. 2012;79:1230–5.
16. Kokorowski PJ, Chow JS, Strauss KJ, Pennison M, Tan W, Cilento B, Nelson CP. Prospective systematic intervention to reduce patient exposure to radiation during pediatric ureteroscopy. J Urol. 2013;190(40):1474–8.
17. Inoue T, Komemushi A, Matsuda T, et al. Effect of protective lead curtains on scattered radiation exposure to the operator during ureteroscopy for stone disease: a controlled trial. Urology. 2017;109:60–6.
18. Bolognese-Milsztajn T, Ginjaume M, Luszik-Bhadra M, et al. Active personal dosimeters for individual monitoring and other new development. Radiat Prot Dosim. 2004;112:141–68.
19. Borges CF, Reggio E, Vicentini FC, et al. How are we protecting ourselves from radiation exposure? A nationwide survey. Int Urol Nephrol. 2015;47:271–4.
20. Nassour I, Chance Spalding M, Hynan LS, Gardner AK, Williams BH. The surgeon-performed ultrasound: a curriculum to improve residents' basic ultrasound knowledge. J Surg Res. 2017;213:51–9.
21. Ng FC, Yam WL, Lim TYB, Teo JK, Hg KK, Lim SK. Ultrasound-guided percutaneous nephrolithotomy: advantages and limitation. Investig Clin Urol. 2017;58:346–52.
22. Desai M, Ridhorkar V, Patel S, Bapat S, Desai M. Pediatric percutaneous nephrolithotomy: accessing impact of technical innovations on safety and efficacy. J Endourol. 1999;13:359–64.
23. Andomian S, Scoffone CM, Louie MK, et al. Does imaging modality used for percutaneous renal access make a difference? A matched case analysis. J Endourol. 2013;27:24–8.
24. Tzeng BC, Wang CJ, Huang SW, et al. Doppler ultrasound-guided percutaneous nephrolithotomy: a prospective randomized study. Urology. 2011;78:535–9.
25. Inoue T, Kinoshita H, Okada S, Hamamoto S, Taguchi M, Murota T, Matsuda T, SMART Study Group. Wideband Doppler ultrasound-guided mini-endoscopic combined intrarenal surgery as an effective and safe procedure for management of large renal stones: a preliminary report. Urology. 2016;95:60–6.

Part III

Ureteroscopy

9 How to Perform Semi-rigid Ureteroscopy: Step by Step

Yung-Ting Cheng and Chen-Hsun Ho

Abstract

Semi-rigid ureteroscopy is a fundamental procedure with high success rate that all urologists should be familiar with. Even if the ureteroscopy is commonly performed, there are many details between each step. We summarized the tips and tricks for both diagnostic and therapeutic uses. Follow these surgical steps to help surgeons avoid unwanted complications.

Keywords

Ureteroscopy · Endourology · Urolithiasis
Ureteral stricture · Ureteral obstruction

Y.-T. Cheng
Department of Urology, National Taiwan University Hospital Hsin-Chu Branch, Taipei, Taiwan

Graduate Institute of Anatomy and Cell Biology, College of Medicine, National Taiwan University, Taipei, Taiwan

C.-H. Ho (✉)
Division of Urology, Department of Surgery, Shin Kong Wu Ho-Su Memorial Hospital, Taipei, Taiwan

School of Medicine, College of Medicine, Fu Jen Catholic University, New Taipei City, Taiwan

9.1 Introduction

Semi-rigid ureteroscopy (URS) was firstly introduced in 1989 and had become a standard treatment for ureteral stones, urothelial carcinoma, and ureteral strictures [1]. This chapter aims to introduce the basic techniques of semi-rigid URS as well as some tips and tricks of overcoming some challenging conditions during the procedure.

9.2 Preoperative Preparations

Before operation, it is imperative to evaluate patients individually. Personal medical history should include prior ureteral calculus history, cancer history (lymphoma, colon cancer, cervical cancer, transitional cell carcinoma, etc.), autoimmune disease (IgG4 disease), infectious disease (tuberculosis), endometriosis, or abdominal aortic aneurysm. Radiation or surgery to the pelvic region should also be taken into consideration in order to judge the risk of associated ureteral stricture [2]. Laboratory investigation includes renal function and coagulation assays. Renal ultrasound or kidney, ureter, and bladder X-ray study (KUB) arranged in the morning of surgery ensuring the persistence of opaque stone can be useful, especially for the ureterovesical junction (UVJ) stone. Intravenous pyelography or computed tomography scan helps delineate the anatomy of collecting system. Reviewing the radiographic

A. C.F. Ng et al. (eds.), *Practical Management of Urinary Stone*,
https://doi.org/10.1007/978-981-16-4193-0_9

studies preoperatively is mandatory to plan the procedure in detail, including the size, location, and density of the stones. Preoperative ureteric stenting is not always necessary, while it has more pronounced benefit in treating renal stones than the ureteral stones on the stone-free rate and complications [3, 4].

While there were no strong evidences to support the benefit of antibiotic prophylaxis in reducing clinical urinary tract infection (UTI), the incidence of pyuria and bacteriuria after URS can still be reduced [5]. Peri-operative antibiotic prophylaxis to all the endourological treatment is now recommended by the American Urological Association (AUA) and European Association of Urology (EAU) guideline to prevent sepsis or kidney infection [6]. Single dose is sufficient for preoperative administration [7]. Prophylactic fluoroquinolone is supported by Knopf et al. to reduce post-procedure UTI [8]. The increased risk of infections can be caused by trauma to the mucosa, prolonged surgical duration, elevated intra-renal pressure due to irrigation, or infected stones. For patients with suspected infection or high-risk of infection, it is recommended to check urine culture and complete antimicrobial treatment course preoperatively. Risks of instrumentation should always be mentioned with informed consent, for example, failed access to the ureter, ureteral trauma, postoperative infection, and ureteral stricture.

The patient is placed in lithotomy position. General anesthesia is more recommended for prolonged procedure than the spinal anesthesia, since its breathing movement is lesser disruptive and can be stopped temporarily if needed during the procedure. In selected patients, intravenous sedation or local anesthesia is also suitable with high satisfaction and short postoperative recovery time [9]. Unwanted patient movement throughout the procedure can result in ureteral trauma.

9.3 Ureteral Orifice Cannulation

At the beginning of the procedure, focusing the scope and white balance is essential. Bladder is thoroughly inspected by cystoscopy to confirm no bladder stone or tumor has been missed. Unnecessary trauma to the bladder neck should be avoided. Bleeding site should be well cauterized to keep better visual field during the operation, especially patients with enlarged and vascular prostate. Bilateral ureteral orifices (UO) could be identified symmetrically 1–2 cm from the midline along the inter-ureteric ridge. Difficulties could be met in patients with protruding prostate median lobe, severe bladder trabeculation, re-implanted ureter, duplicated urinary system, ureterocele, diverticulum, or the presence of UVJ tumor. Once the UO is hardly to be identified, release the distended bladder to avoid bilateral UO being compressed by bladder pressure on the intramural ureter. Then, withdraw the cystoscopy back to the bladder neck to better localize the inter-ureteric ridge. Urine jet from UO and periodical peristalsis of the ureter can help in exploring the entrance of UO. Otherwise, trace along the intra-ureteric ridge slowly by protruding the guidewire tip from the cystoscopy. Intravenous indigo carmine or methylene blue injection from the nephrostomy tube if the tube has already been placed can also be attempted. Obliteration of the UO by tumors may require transurethral tumor resection over the orifice by bipolar loop to lessen over-cauterization of the orifice.

After the position of UO being noted, keep the beak close to the UO, and turn it parallel to the orifice, aiding safety guidewire insertion (Fig. 9.1a). Estimate the distance of wire being inserted and no more insertion when the resistance is sensed. Additional force may cause unnecessary push-back of the stone or trauma to the urothelium. Occasionally, the guidewire can be blocked at the segment of UVJ. A hydrophilic tip wire with the assistance of an open-ended 5 Fr ureteral catheter can help the wire pass through the tortuous curve (Fig. 9.2a). The hydrophilic wire tends to find its way with lower risk of false lumen, and the ureteral catheter can be advanced over the wire for additional guidance. If the difficulty still persists, fluoroscopy can be used to define the anatomy of the lower ureter. For instance, fishhook ureter may appear in patients with prostate enlargement (Fig. 9.2b) [1]. Try to avoid poking the UO repeatedly, which will cause further ureteral edema and bleeding. Place the guidewire

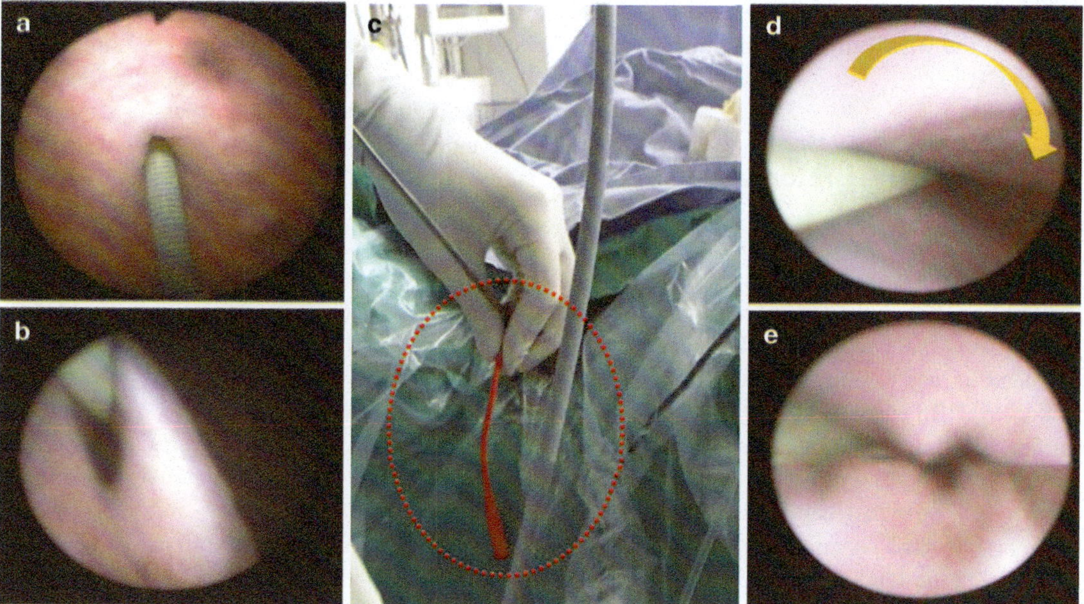

Fig. 9.1 Insert the guidewire into the ureter by approaching cystoscopic beak to the ureteral orifice along the axis of intramural ureter (**a**). Advance the URS by "riding above" or "creeping forward" along the guidewire (**b**). Make the left hand as a pivot to assist the stability of URS during scope insertion. Maintain Nelaton tube with constant drainage when entering the ureter to keep low intrarenal pelvic pressure (**c**). Rotating clockwise may help the URS pass through the intramural part of the right ureter (**d**). Mucosa fold during peristaltic movements can sometimes stop the URS from going forward. Stop and wait the peristalsis was over (**e**)

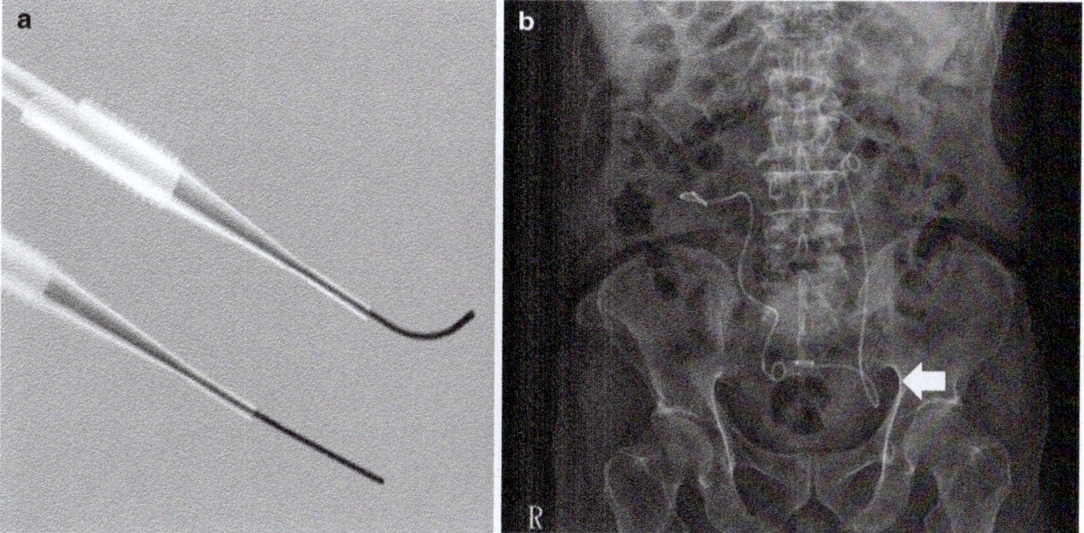

Fig. 9.2 Nitinol core hydrophilic guidewire: BiWire® by Cook Company is designed to provide two options for ureteral access, having the value of being straight at one end and angled at the other. Permission for use granted by Cook Medical, Bloomington, Indiana (**a**), Fishhook ureters, also called "J-shaped ureters," indicate the configuration of distal ureter in patients associated with prostate enlargement (**b**)

into the rigid URS in advance, and then insert the tip of the wire to the UO under direct vision by the URS [10].

9.4 Enter the Ureter with URS

Before entrance of the URS into the urethra, fully lubrication of the shaft is necessary to lessen the resistance. Although the necessity of safety guidewire is controversial, EAU guidelines recommend its use to allow repeated access to the ureter [6]. URS carried out by the dominant hand approaches the UO and then moves forward by riding onto the guidewire or creeping below the guidewire (Fig. 9.1b). Stability can be maintained with the left-hand support as a pivot at the anterior part of the URS (Fig. 9.1c). Slight rotating the URS clockwise for the right ureter and counter-clockwise for the left ureter to aid its passage through the horizontal segment of the UVJ (Fig. 9.1d). Alternatively, a second guidewire passed through the URS will be needed to open up the ureter, enabling URS to pass between the two guidewires, also called "railroading" (Fig. 9.3b). If it is still difficult to pass the intramural ureter, consider pulsed irrigation via a 20-ml syringe simultaneously or dilation with serial dilators/a balloon catheter to expand the ureter (Fig. 9.4a). In some cases, UVJ stone could block the negotiation of the orifice. Picking the protruding stone out with graspers or stone fragmentation by laser could be considered. In addition, incision of the stenotic ureteral orifice or flicking the stone out with a Collins loop can also be used. Once the URS is placed into the ureter smoothly, Nelaton catheter provides urine flow during the procedure, in order to keep the bladder being emptied without compressing the intramural part of the ureter and lower intraureteral pressure.

Occasionally, failure of ureteral access due to ureteral stricture could be encountered during the procedure for 8–10% [11]. Smaller-diameter URS can be attempted first. Care should be taken that in those with ureteral stricture, stricture site will severely encase the URS or the guidewire. PTFE coating guidewire fragmentation could happen if inappropriate pulling force is given to the guidewire. If sudden loss of tension was sensed during the procedure, apply stable pulling force gently to the guidewire. Then, check the integrity of the guidewire tip after fully withdrawn. Hydrophilic guidewire is usually made of Nitinol, being more flexible and resistant to kinking. With either straight tip or angled tip, the

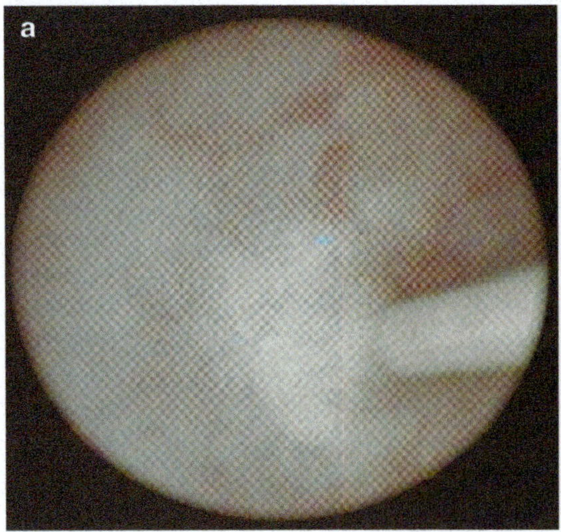

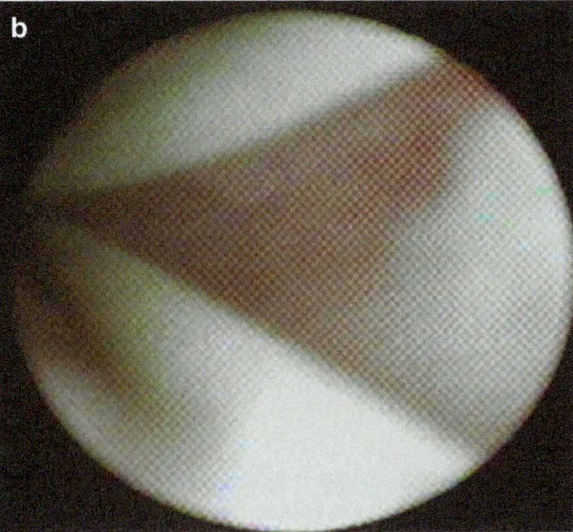

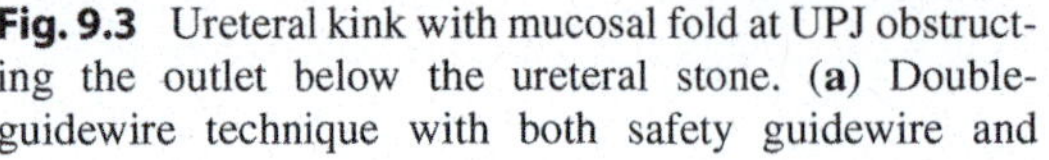

Fig. 9.3 Ureteral kink with mucosal fold at UPJ obstructing the outlet below the ureteral stone. (**a**) Double-guidewire technique with both safety guidewire and working guidewire was used to expand and then straighten the ureter. Then, URS crawls forward between the guidewires (**b**)

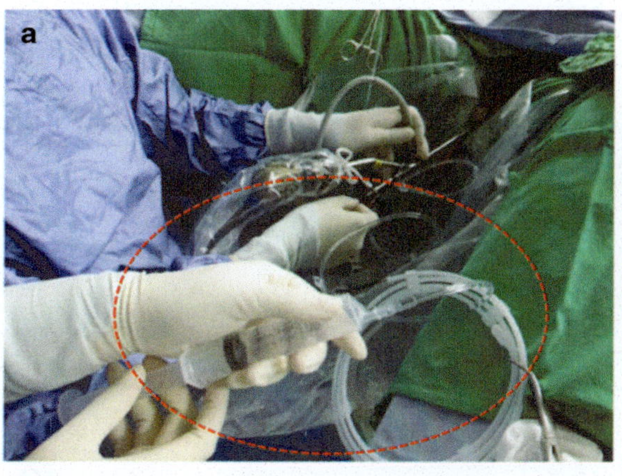

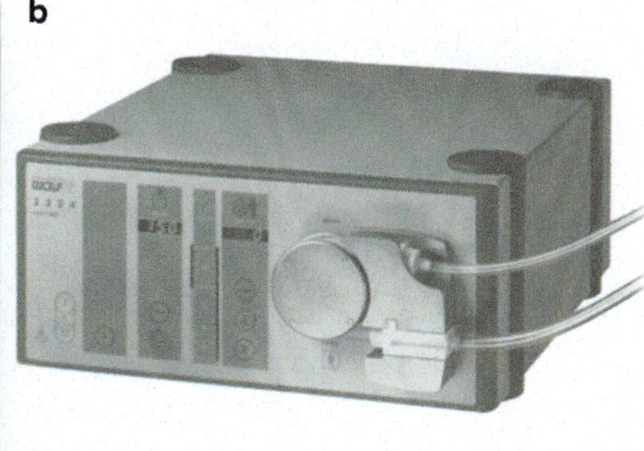

Fig. 9.4 Hand pump with a 20-ml/50-ml syringe by an assistant. (**a**) Uro-Pump by Richard Wolf Company achieves pressure-controlled fluid irrigation, allowing an excellent view by selectable continuous pressure and flow. Pressure measurement optimizes the pressure control intra-operatively (**b**)

Nitinol core wire allows the physician to navigate difficult anatomy. Thus, it usually acts as a savior when being blocked by the ureteral stricture or tortuous ureter. The hydrophilic coatings made these wires particularly slippery and easy to slide out of the patient. Whenever the initial access is established by the hydrophilic wire, exchange to the standard guidewire is a safer way to maintain the access. Some wires can adjust the length of the flexible tip by withdrawing the movable core. It is important for the surgeon to be familiar with the advantages and disadvantages between varied wire designs, which may help in overcoming difficult circumstances.

When needed, some physicians would decide to perform passive ureteric dilatation by ureteral stent and reschedule the operation 7–14 days later, which take more procedures and time for definitive surgery [1, 12]. Others would like to perform dilation actively by dilating catheters or balloon dilators. Compared to coaxial dilators, the balloon dilators appear to be safer and have fewer perforations [13, 14]. These dilators are placed through a wire under the cystoscopy. Image guidance is important to assure that the stenotic segment is being covered by the radiopaque markers of the balloon (Fig. 9.5). Thus, contrast medium is used to inflate the balloon. Confirm the balloon being fully dilated without waist to achieve adequate dilation. The maximum inflation pressure could be tolerated up to 20 atmospheres depending on the balloon designs.

Moving URS forward with a constant and gentle force is suggested. During the advance of the URS, keep the lumen in the central part of the view with little protrusion of the guidewire to straighten the ureter. Pause for a moment during the ureteral peristalsis (Fig. 9.1e). It is important not to push hard when resistance is met or add unnecessary force to bend the shaft. Any mucosa tear or perforation will cause possible traumatic ureteral stricture. Appropriate irrigation by hand pump or machine pump helps dilate the ureter properly and maintain clear visual field (Fig. 9.4).

9.5 Bypass the Obstruction with Guidewire and URS

Safety guidewire is usually suggested during URS for immediate stent insertion in case any trouble is met. Either standard PTFE wire or hydrophilic tip wire is accepted and passed beyond an impacted stone. The safety guidewire should be secured as close to the urethral meatus to avoid accidental displacement. Once the obstruction with impacted stone is impassable by the guidewire, "Billiard Cue" technique can be applied to dislodge the stone proximally to a wider space, especially for UVJ stones (Fig. 9.6). If such maneuver failed, careful fragmentation of

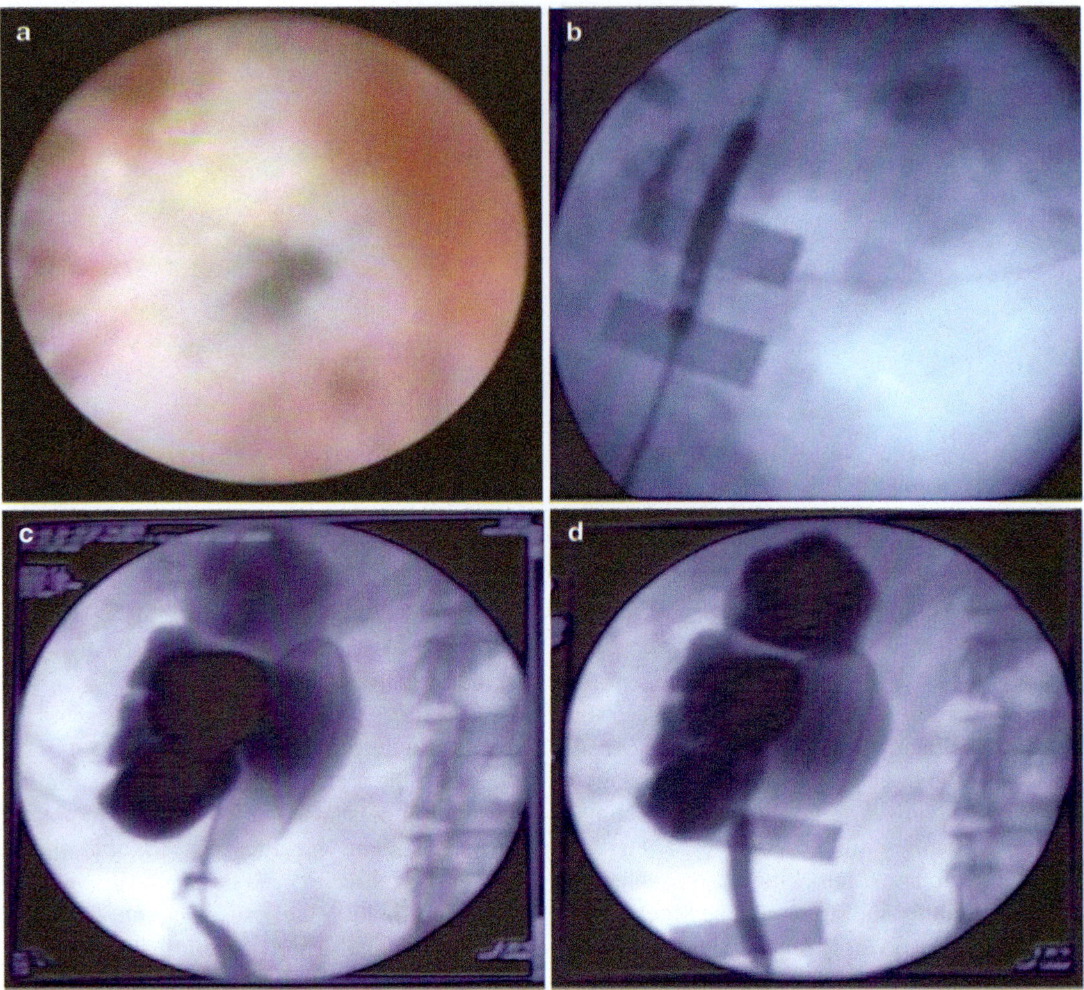

Fig. 9.5 Primary access up to the ureter is failed due to ureteral stricture. (**a**) The segment of ureteral stricture is marked by a tape and dilated by a balloon dilator under the guidance of fluoroscopy. (**b**) Severely dilated renal pelvis with tortuous upper ureter. (**c**) Confirm the stricture length being well covered by the balloon dilator (**d**)

the stone can be considered in experienced hands. After that, insert the guidewire as soon as possible when the channel is unplugged. Any suspicious infection with cloudy pus noticed above the stone decompresses the hydronephrosis immediately and is sent for urine culture (Fig. 9.7). A stent needs to be placed as soon as possible, and the procedure should be postponed until the infection is well-treated. Monitor vital signs closely in the recovery room to detect early signs of sepsis.

Obstructed ureter can result in "Z-shape" proximal ureteric dilation and kidney enlargement, which increase the difficulties in the advancement of the URS (Fig. 9.8a). When the tortuous ureter is encountered, firstly, insert the guidewire to identify the correct direction. Then, keep the URS to the side of the ureter at the corner, followed by horizontal movement to straighten the ureter (Fig. 9.8b). Aspirating the urine with syringe may sometimes help release the hydroureter. Otherwise, shifting the patient to Trendelenburg position may straighten the ureter with gravity to the enlarged kidney. Mertz maneuver by pushing the kidney upward and medially with a fist on the flank below the costal margin is also a useful technique to straighten the ureter.

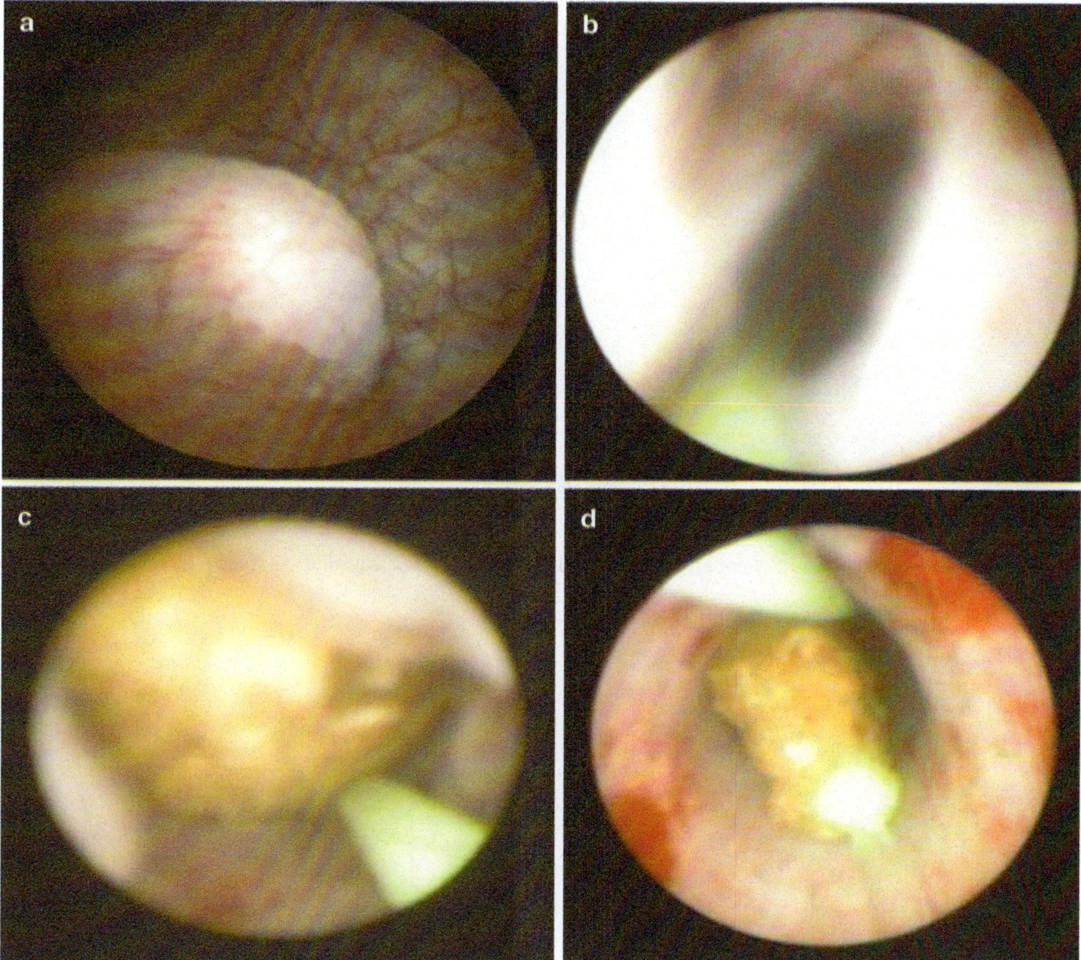

Fig. 9.6 Enlarged intramural ureter because of the impacted UVJ stone. Stenotic ureteral orifice was noted due to suspected secondary inflammatory response. (**a**) Stenotic orifice was dilated subsequently after URS passage. (**b**) Attempt to insert the guidewire beyond the impacted stone as a safety guidewire. (**c**) Lithotripsy by laser fiber (**d**)

9.6 Stone Fragmentation and Extraction

Before the operation, fragmentation and extraction devices should be ensured according to the stone size and its position to lessen the retropulsed fragments. Holmium YAG laser is the most commonly used and effective technique (Fig. 9.9). Appropriate laser fiber size should be chosen if flexible URS or basket is planned to be used. Based on different circumstances, laser settings, such as fragmentation, popcorn, or dusting mode, can be adjusted according to different pulse duration, energy, and frequency [15]. As the energy rises, thermal injury might happen with different irrigation rates. Thus, keep the laser power as low as possible in efficient range with continuous irrigation flow [16]. Pneumatic/ballistic and ultrasound devices, on the other side, have a greater risk of retropulsion up to 5–40% [17].

For a good visibility, it is essential to keep adequate irrigation flow by opening up and turn-

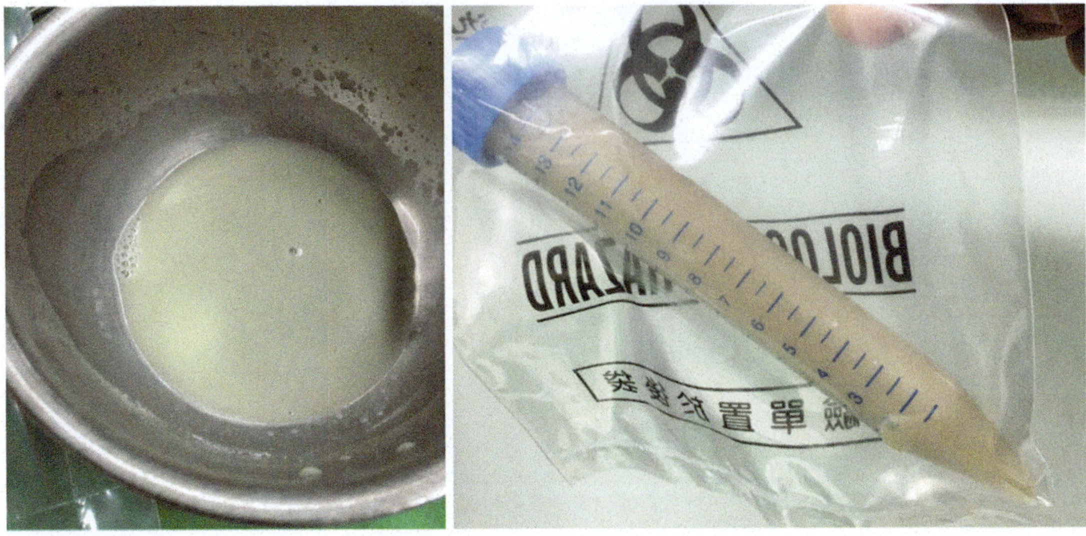

Fig. 9.7 Pus appeared as the URS went across the obstruction site. Immediate aspiration of the pus from the ureter was done and sent for urine culture

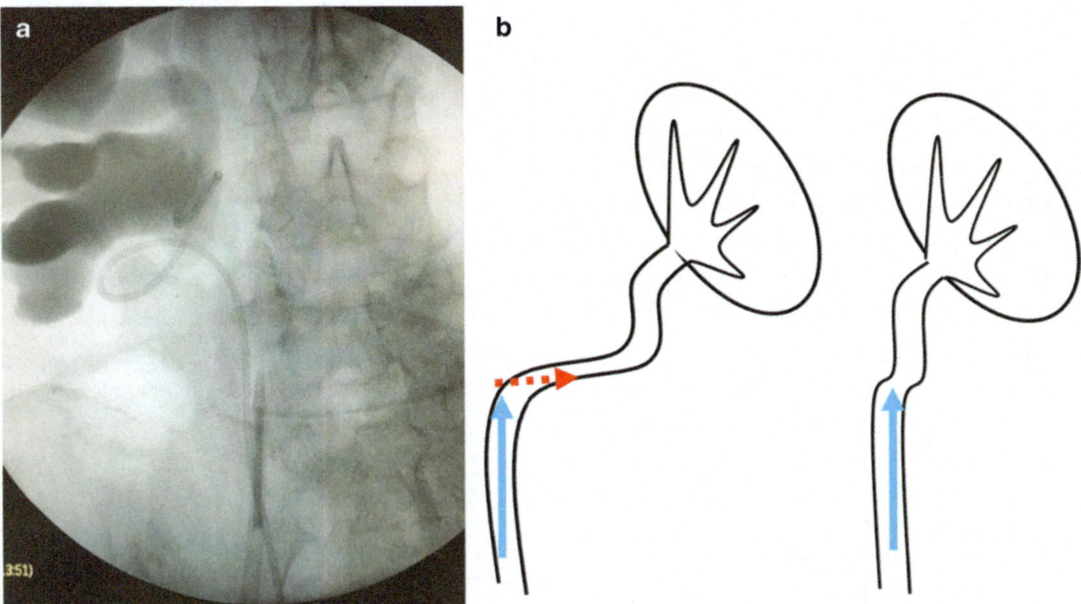

Fig. 9.8 Tortuous upper ureter with Z loop because of elongated hydroureter. (**a**) Stay steady at the corner since breathing usually causes strong heave to the ureter. Move horizontally toward the direction of the guidewire, and then advance forward when the route to proximal ureter is seen (**b**)

ing off the flow control stopcock skillfully (Fig. 9.10). Most of the time, saline irrigation with gravity is adequate for simple procedure under a pressure less than 40 cm water (30 mmHg) [15]. Increase the irrigation pressure to improve the views in situations such as stones with dusts, ureteral polyps or any bleeding affecting the visual field. Such maneuver, however, will increase intra-ureteral and intra-renal pressure, causing calculus being pushed-back to the renal pelvis. Further acute pressure related renal damage or complications have also been observed in the previous studies. Therefore, maintaining low pressure in the renal system during the procedure

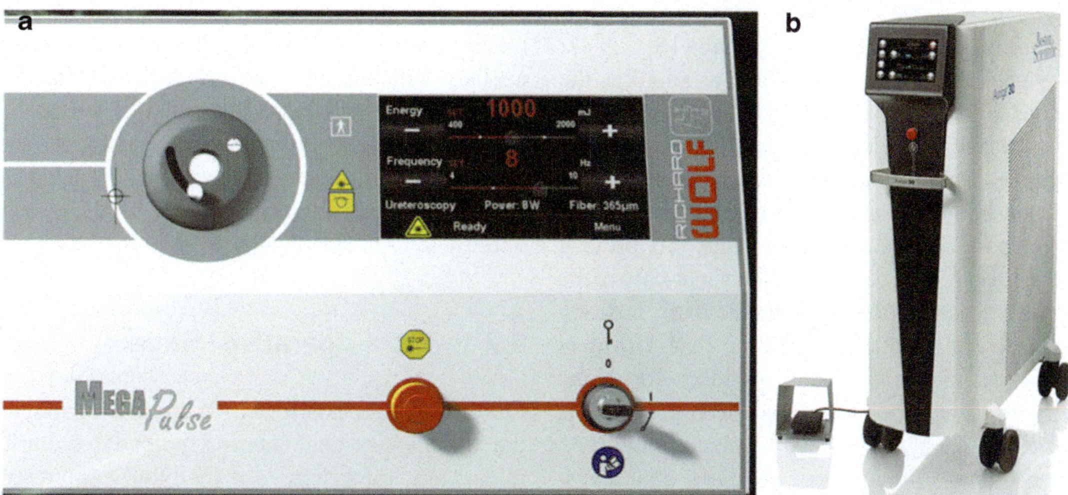

Fig. 9.9 Holmium YAG laser by Richard Wolf Company has outstanding benefits in stone lithotripsy, elimination of strictures, and vaporization of tumors with 230 V, 50/60 Hz energy settings. (**a**) Auriga™ 30 Holmium laser by Boston Scientific Company is suited for stone procedures and ablation with powerful energy and three pulse width modes for different indications (**b**)

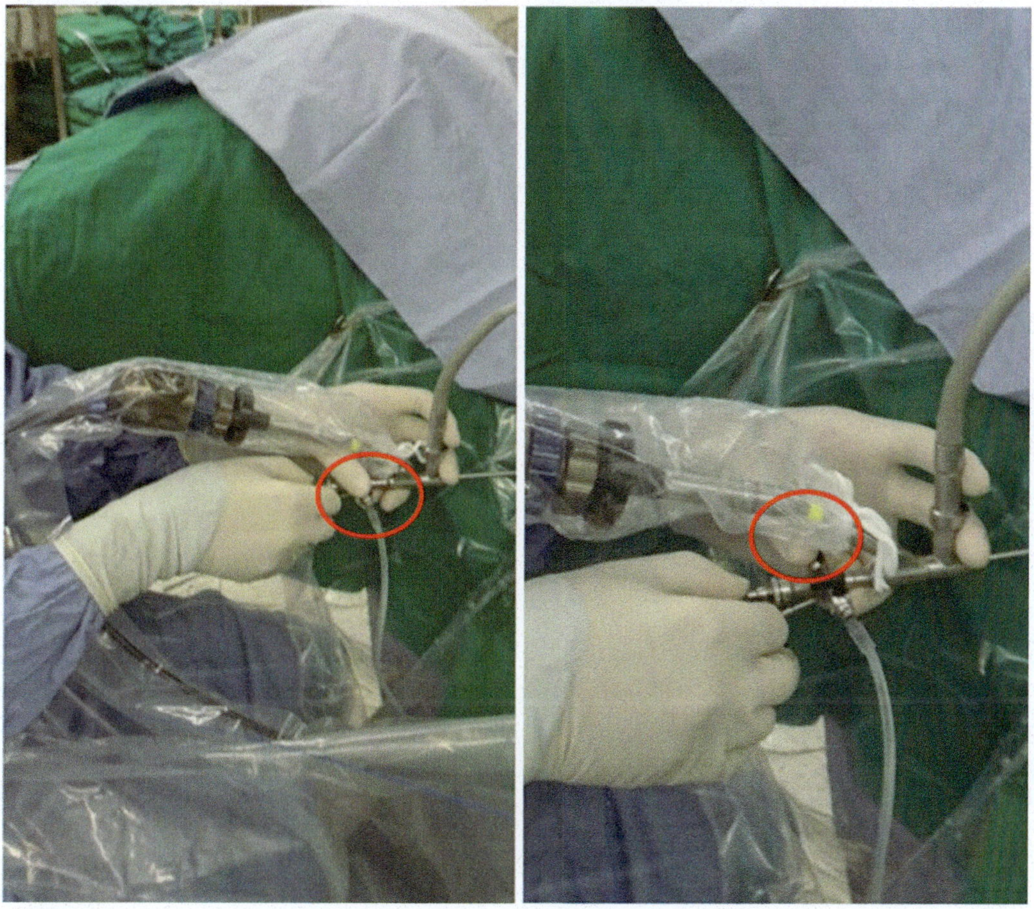

Fig. 9.10 Keep adequate irrigation flow by controlling the flow control stopcock

is important to prevent postoperative pain, pyelovenous backflow, and fornix rupture [18].

Stones need to be fragmented as small as the diameter size of laser fiber below 5 mm. For those stones with larger size or higher risk of retrograde propulsion, basket extraction can be attempted if no ureteric stricture appears at the distal part of the obstruction site. To prevent migration of the stones into the renal calyx, the patient can be shifted to Trendelenburg position with the effected side rotating upward. Graspers are considered the safest products for stone retrieval. Diversified shapes are seen in the stone baskets. Helical baskets can be made of double-, three-, four-, or five-wire designs, making it much easier to rotate and then capture the stone fragments. Recent innovation in tipless baskets not only aids calyceal stone capture without the interference from the tip but also reduces further mucosa trauma.

During stone extraction, keep the basket tip closed beyond the stone, then open the basket in the upper ureter and then drag back slowly to allow the stone being captured and repositioned (Fig. 9.11). The basket and stone should be clearly seen close to the URS tip when withdrawing, which allows the ureteral mucosa to be observed at all times. "Blind basketing" should be avoided. Keeping the stone in a favorable orientation or small enough to be removed will facilitate removal. Fragment the stones simultaneously with laser if they are still too large to pass through the lumen. But make sure that the basket remains intact without being damaged by the laser [8]. If the basket is stuck and unable to dislodge after stone fragmentation, cut the basket wire by laser to free it [1].

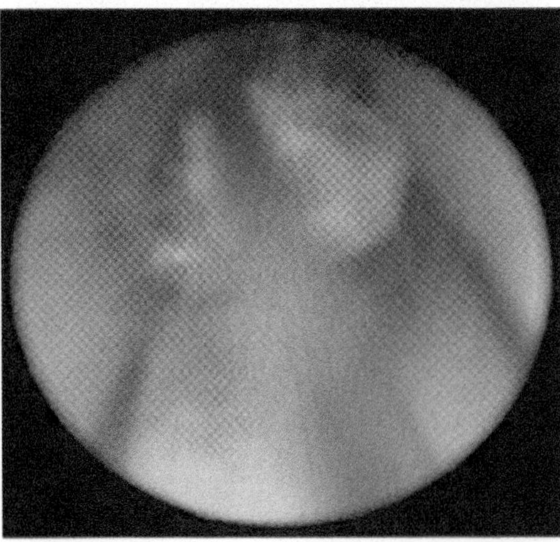

Fig. 9.11 Extract the stone by basket in proper orientation. Keep the basket under vision directly to avoid mucosal avulsion along the ureter

9.7 Intra-operative Image

Fluoroscopy is best used when being uncertain to the orientation, encountering potential ureteric injury, ureteral stricture, or the blind-end ureter. Diluted contrast medium can be injected from retrograde URS or antegrade nephrostomy tube to be used as a road map to depict the anatomy and stone position (Fig. 9.12) [10]. If any extravasation of the contrast is noticed, it is best not to proceed any further and terminate the procedure with immediate stent placement. Otherwise, a smaller URS can be introduced further by using the irrigation pressure to cannulate the false lumen with safety guidewire in the channel.

The length of stricture can be measured under fluoroscopy to decide further treatment plan (Fig. 9.12a). For those with short segment of stricture, balloon dilators can be attempted to enable URS advancement. Meanwhile, guidewire can be inserted under the guidance of fluoroscopy to ensure its position to the renal pelvis, instead of the extraureter space. If the URS is still being unable to advance, place a ureteric stent and delay the intervention [1].

9.8 Management of the Ureteral Strictures

As the progress of URS techniques, endourologic therapy acts as an option for treating ureteric strictures, including retrograde balloon dilation and endoureterotomy. Basically, short stricture segment less than 2 cm and ipsilateral renal moiety accounted for more than 25% of the renal function are more suitable for such techniques. Balloon dilation demonstrated good outcomes

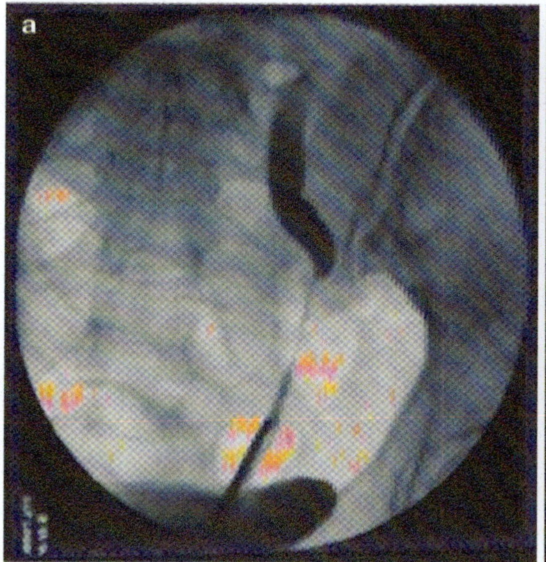

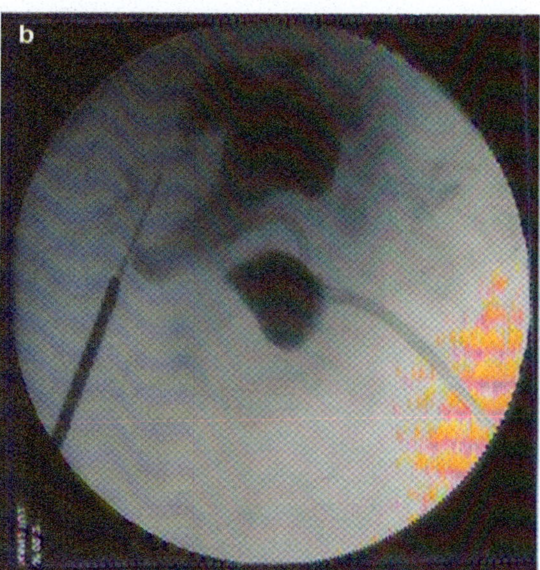

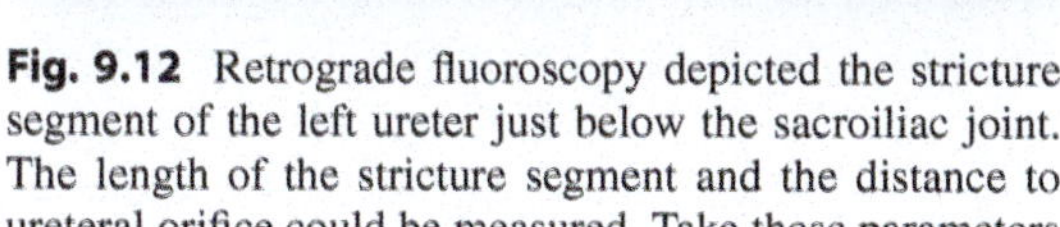

Fig. 9.12 Retrograde fluoroscopy depicted the stricture segment of the left ureter just below the sacroiliac joint. The length of the stricture segment and the distance to ureteral orifice could be measured. Take these parameters into consideration for the treatment plan in the future. (**a**) URS combined antegrade fluoroscopy showed complete left ureteropelvic junction obstruction. Guidewire punctured to the false way was noticed (**b**)

with success rate up to 48–82% [19]. Laser endoureterotomy is mostly performed by Holmium YAG laser with low morbidities and short recovery time [20]. Incision is made anteriorly at the distal to middle ureter and laterally at the proximal ureter under direct vision. Adequate depth is required until the extraureteric fat is seen. Postoperative ureteral stenting is recommended to promote ureteral healing and reduce recurrent stricture. Patients with active infection, longer stricture segment more than 2 cm, or poor renal function are contraindicated for ureteroscopic treatment [19].

9.9 Diagnostic and Therapeutic URS for Urothelial Pathology

URS allows complete visualization of the ureter, renal pelvis, and collecting system. Minimize scope and guidewire-related trauma during the process that could be mistaken as a pathological finding. Urine cytology can be collected selectively with high sensitivity in high-grade tumors and carcinoma in situ. Tumors in collecting system can be biopsied by using a stone basket or biopsy forceps [1]. Cancer staging based on ureteroscopic biopsies is usually inaccurate. Endoscopic ablation with Holmium YAG laser can be considered in patients with low-risk cancer. A ureteral catheter can be placed for postsurgical intrapelvic chemotherapy or Bacillus Calmette-Guerin (BCG). Vigilant endoscopic surveillance program should be informed for the risk of recurrences [21].

9.10 Withdraw the URS

Once the procedure is completed, withdraw the URS gently and slowly especially if the tight lower ureter has been passed over previously. Since the stricture site can encase the shaft of the URS, rotate the URS back and forth when drawing backward to avoid ureteric avulsion or injury (Fig. 9.13). Inspect possible mucosa injury or intramural stones carefully that might have been missed during the way upward. Also, immobile visual field along the way down may highly suggest the risk of ureteric trauma. Safety guidewire should be in position immediately to confirm stent insertion in safe.

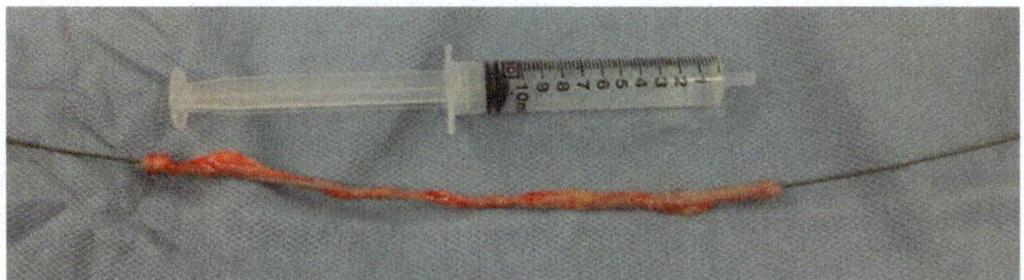

Fig. 9.13 Ureteral avulsion may occur during scope withdrawal, mostly along with the stone basket or lower ureteral stricture

9.11 Ureteric Stent Placement

Ureteric stent is not necessary after uncomplicated URS as no difference has been seen in stone-free rate and stricture formation. On the contrary, more stent-related urinary symptoms, postoperative pain, infection, and higher costs were detected in stented patients [22, 23]. Alternatively, ureteral catheter for shorter indwelling time or tethered stent can be considered that are more easily to be removed postoperatively to reduce stent-related morbidities [24]. For those who are at increased risk of complications, such as ureteral trauma, bleeding, residual fragments, UTIs, possible secondary URS, renal functional impairment, or pregnancy, stents should be inserted to avoid potential emergencies.

Choosing a correct stent should consider many aspects, including its length, size, material, estimated indwelling time, type of procedures, and physician preferences. Patients may suffer from postoperative lower urinary tract symptoms due to redundant stent coil or migration risk because of short stent. Patient's height and CT measurements of the ureteral length are reliable methods to predict the best stent length [25, 26]. Special stent length needs to be considered in children or transplanted kidney. Patient's age in years +10 has been reported as a formula in children [27]. 6 French is the standard size for ureteral stents. Larger diameter stents are usually recommended for infection or severe stricture. Whether different sizes associate with urinary symptoms and pain is controversial. Several studies demonstrated that 5Fr stents may cause fewer symptoms but tend to dislodge more often [28].

Different materials, coatings, and designs can affect the ease of placement, patient's comfort, and variable levels of encrustation. With hydrophilic coatings designed in most ureteric stents, it is suggested to soak the stents with saline to lessen the resistance during placement. Adequate tension should be applied to the guidewire by assistant and fixed on a table to make the axis as straight as possible. Once the stent failed to slide over the guidewire, make sure that the guidewire is right on the axis of the working channel. Then, try to keep the beak of the cystoscopy close to the UO to avoid stent looping in the bladder (Fig. 9.14). If such maneuver still failed, examine the ureter again to affirm no residual stones stop the stent from inserting. A smaller caliber stent can be attempted in ureteral stricture.

The ideal duration of stenting is not known and often decided by the urologists according to the findings during URS. One to two weeks is mostly favored. The position of the stent should be checked by KUB to ensure that a good curl is obtained in the kidney and bladder. If the patient had a nephrostomy tube previously, it is also prudent to check the presence of entwinement between the nephrostomy tube and ureteric stent. Subsequent nephrostomy removal needs to be performed by a guidewire to straighten the curl tip of nephrostomy tube under the fluoroscopy. Alpha-blockers and anti-muscarinic therapy can help in reducing the stent discomfort and morbidities [29].

9.12 Conclusions

URS has become a standard diagnostic and therapeutic intervention for the ureter with high success rates. Endourologists should be familiar with its equipment and technical skills. Adherence to the basic principles of endourology with cau-

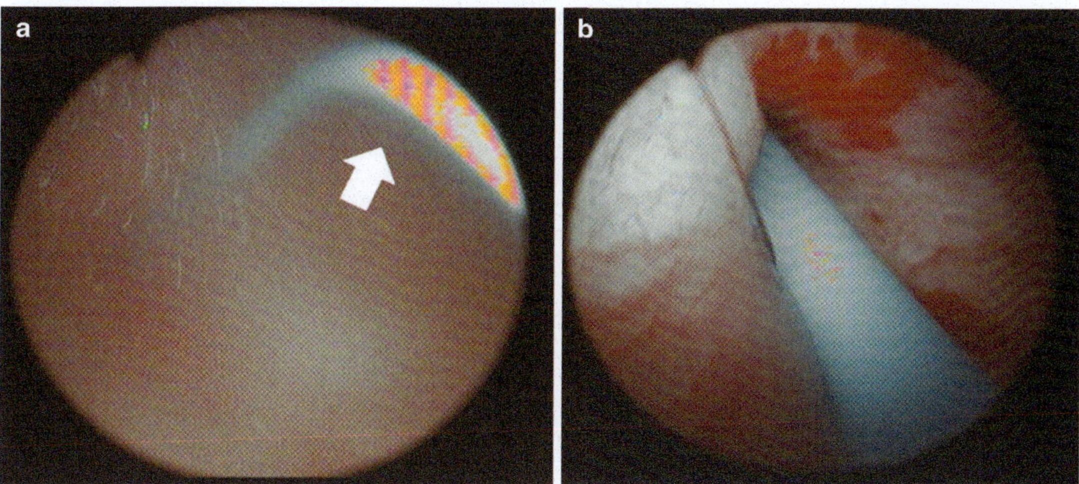

Fig. 9.14 Far distance from the UO or inadequate tension to the guidewire makes the stent insertion distract from the axis with stent loop in the bladder. (**a**) Keep the scope close to the UO to better applicate the force to the stent (**b**)

tion and patience can prevent potential complications. Meanwhile, innovations in adjunct devices allow surgeons to expand the indications of URS and overcome challenging cases.

Acknowledgments Author's contributions: All the authors contributed to the chapter. Yung-Ting Cheng collected the references and completed manuscript editing. Chen-Hsun Ho critically reviewed the manuscript and offered the materials.

References

1. Whitehurst LA, Somani BK. Semi-rigid ureteroscopy: indications, tips, and tricks. Urolithiasis. 2018;46(1):39–45. https://doi.org/10.1007/s00240-017-1025-7.
2. Tran H, Arsovska O, Paterson RF, Chew BH. Evaluation of risk factors and treatment options in patients with ureteral stricture disease at a single institution. Can Urol Assoc J. 2015;9(11–12):E921–4. https://doi.org/10.5489/cuaj.3057.
3. Jessen JP, Breda A, Brehmer M, Liatsikos EN, Millan Rodriguez F, Osther PJ, et al. International collaboration in endourology: multicenter evaluation of prestenting for ureterorenoscopy. J Endourol. 2016;30(3):268–73. https://doi.org/10.1089/end.2015.0109.
4. Assimos D, Crisci A, Culkin D, Xue W, Roelofs A, Duvdevani M, et al. Preoperative JJ stent placement in ureteric and renal stone treatment: results from the Clinical Research Office of Endourological Society (CROES) Ureteroscopy (URS) Global Study. BJU Int. 2016;117(4):648–54. https://doi.org/10.1111/bju.13250.
5. Lo CW, Yang SS, Hsieh CH, Chang SJ. Effectiveness of prophylactic antibiotics against post-ureteroscopic lithotripsy infections: systematic review and meta-analysis. Surg Infect. 2015;16(4):415–20. https://doi.org/10.1089/sur.2014.013.
6. El-Faqih SR, Shamsuddin AB, Chakrabarti A, Atassi R, Kardar AH, Osman MK, et al. Polyurethane internal ureteral stents in treatment of stone patients: morbidity related to indwelling times. J Urol. 1991;146(6):1487–91. https://doi.org/10.1016/s0022-5347(17)38146-6.
7. Chew BH, Flannigan R, Kurtz M, Gershman B, Arsovska O, Paterson RF, et al. A single dose of intraoperative antibiotics is sufficient to prevent urinary tract infection during ureteroscopy. J Endourol. 2016;30(1):63–8. https://doi.org/10.1089/end.2015.0511.
8. Knopf HJ, Graff HJ, Schulze H. Perioperative antibiotic prophylaxis in ureteroscopic stone removal. Eur Urol. 2003;44(1):115–8. https://doi.org/10.1016/s0302-2838(03)00189-1.
9. Cybulski PA, Joo H, Honey RJ. Ureteroscopy: anesthetic considerations. Urol Clin North Am. 2004;31(1):43–7., viii. https://doi.org/10.1016/s0094-0143(03)00087-9.
10. Rukin NJ, Somani BK, Patterson J, Grey BR, Finch W, McClinton S, et al. Tips and tricks of ureteroscopy: consensus statement part I. basic ureteroscopy. Cent European J Urol. 2015;68(4):439–46. https://doi.org/10.5173/ceju.2015.605a.
11. Cetti RJ, Biers S, Keoghane SR. The difficult ureter: what is the incidence of pre-stenting? Ann R Coll Surg Engl. 2011;93(1):31–3. https://doi.org/10.1308/003588411x12851639106990.

12. Ambani SN, Faerber GJ, Roberts WW, Hollingsworth JM, Wolf JS Jr. Ureteral stents for impassable ureteroscopy. J Endourol. 2013;27(5):549–53. https://doi.org/10.1089/end.2012.0414.
13. Bourdoumis A, Tanabalan C, Goyal A, Kachrilas S, Buchholz N, Masood J. The difficult ureter: stent and come back or balloon dilate and proceed with ureteroscopy? What does the evidence say? Urology. 2014;83(1):1–3. https://doi.org/10.1016/j.urology.2013.08.073.
14. Kuntz NJ, Neisius A, Tsivian M, Ghaffar M, Patel N, Ferrandino MN, et al. Balloon dilation of the ureter: a contemporary review of outcomes and complications. J Urol. 2015;194(2):413–7. https://doi.org/10.1016/j.juro.2015.02.2917.
15. Somani BK, Ploumidis A, Pappas A, Doizi S, Babawale O, Dragos L, et al. Pictorial review of tips and tricks for ureteroscopy and stone treatment: an essential guide for urologists from PETRA research consortium. Transl Androl Urol. 2019;8(Suppl 4):S371–80. https://doi.org/10.21037/tau.2019.06.04.
16. Wollin DA, Carlos EC, Tom WR, Simmons WN, Preminger GM, Lipkin ME. Effect of laser settings and irrigation rates on ureteral temperature during holmium laser lithotripsy, an in vitro model. J Endourol. 2018;32(1):59–63. https://doi.org/10.1089/end.2017.0658.
17. Ahmed M, Pedro RN, Kieley S, Akornor JW, Durfee WK, Monga M. Systematic evaluation of ureteral occlusion devices: insertion, deployment, stone migration, and extraction. Urology. 2009;73(5):976–80. https://doi.org/10.1016/j.urology.2008.12.048.
18. Jung H, Osther PJ. Intraluminal pressure profiles during flexible ureterorenoscopy. Springerplus. 2015;4:373. https://doi.org/10.1186/s40064-015-1114-4.
19. Tyritzis SI, Wiklund NP. Ureteral strictures revisited…Trying to see the light at the end of the tunnel: a comprehensive review. J Endourol. 2015;29(2):124–36. https://doi.org/10.1089/end.2014.0522.
20. Emiliani E, Breda A. Laser endoureterotomy and endopyelotomy: an update. World J Urol. 2015;33(4):583–7. https://doi.org/10.1007/s00345-014-1405-3.
21. Petros FG, Li R, Matin SF. Endoscopic approaches to upper tract urothelial carcinoma. Urol Clin North Am. 2018;45(2):267–86. https://doi.org/10.1016/j.ucl.2017.12.009.
22. Song T, Liao B, Zheng S, Wei Q. Meta-analysis of postoperatively stenting or not in patients underwent ureteroscopic lithotripsy. Urol Res. 2012;40(1):67–77. https://doi.org/10.1007/s00240-011-0385-7.
23. Haleblian G, Kijvikai K, de la Rosette J, Preminger G. Ureteral stenting and urinary stone management: a systematic review. J Urol. 2008;179(2):424–30. https://doi.org/10.1016/j.juro.2007.09.026.
24. Moon TD. Ureteral stenting—an obsolete procedure? J Urol. 2002;167(5):1984.
25. Pilcher JM, Patel U. Choosing the correct length of ureteric stent: a formula based on the patient's height compared with direct ureteric measurement. Clin Radiol. 2002;57(1):59–62. https://doi.org/10.1053/crad.2001.0737.
26. Barrett K, Foell K, Lantz A, Ordon M, Lee JY, Pace KT, et al. Best stent length predicted by simple CT measurement rather than patient height. J Endourol. 2016;30(9):1029–32. https://doi.org/10.1089/end.2016.0105.
27. Palmer JS, Palmer LS. Determining the proper stent length to use in children: age plus 10. J Urol. 2007;178(4 Pt 2):1566–9. https://doi.org/10.1016/j.juro.2007.03.191.
28. Kim BS, Choi JY, Jung W. Does a ureteral stent with a smaller diameter reduce stent-related bladder irritation? A single-blind, randomized, controlled, multicenter study. J Endourol. 2020;34(3):368–72. https://doi.org/10.1089/end.2019.0482.
29. Lamb AD, Vowler SL, Johnston R, Dunn N, Wiseman OJ. Meta-analysis showing the beneficial effect of alpha-blockers on ureteric stent discomfort. BJU Int. 2011;108(11):1894–902. https://doi.org/10.1111/j.1464-410X.2011.10170.x.

10 How to Perform Flexible Ureteroscopy: Step by Step

Shimpei Yamashita and Takaaki Inoue

Abstract

In recent decades, flexible ureteroscopy (fURS) has become a standard and popular surgical treatment for kidney and ureteral stones. As novel surgical devices have been developed, including flexible endoscopes, laser devices and fibers, stone baskets, and access sheathes, surgical techniques of fURS have also evolved and improved. Meanwhile, manipulation of these scopes and devices can be difficult for trainees. To master the fURS procedure, it is necessary to acquire a broad base of knowledge and skill. Simulation-based training is also useful for trainees to improve their surgical skills. In this section, we describe the current standard surgical fURS techniques.

Keywords

Flexible ureteroscopy · Technique · Renal stones · Ureteral stones · Urolithiasis

S. Yamashita
Department of Urology, Wakayama Medical University, Wakayama, Japan

T. Inoue (✉)
Department of Urology and Stone Center, Hara Genitourinary Hospital, Kobe, Japan

Department of Urology, Kobe University, Kobe, Japan
e-mail: inouetak@harahospital.jp

Abbreviations

fURS	Flexible ureteroscopy
Ho:YAG	Holmium:yttrium-aluminum-garnet
IPA	Infundibular pelvic angle
QOL	Quality of life
UAS	Ureteral access sheath

10.1 Introduction

Surgical management of kidney or ureteral stones has benefited from many technological advances in recent decades, a prime example being the development of flexible ureteroscopy (fURS) and holmium:yttrium-aluminum-garnet (Ho:YAG) laser. This facilitates access to the upper urinary tract including renal pelvis and calyces, resulting in a widening of its indication for surgical management of urolithiasis. Currently, fURS is a popular standard treatment option for kidney or proximal ureteral stones, but to safely and efficiently perform it, extensive knowledge and a high level of skills are required. The steps of fURS procedure are shown in Fig. 10.1. This section describes surgical techniques using fURS, with tips and tricks.

A. C.F. Ng et al. (eds.), *Practical Management of Urinary Stone*,
https://doi.org/10.1007/978-981-16-4193-0_10

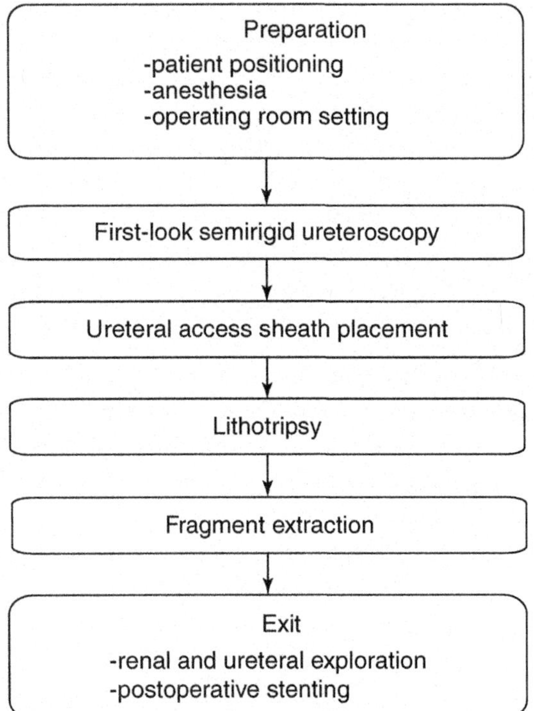

Fig. 10.1 Flowchart of fURS procedure

10.2 Patient Positioning, Anesthesia, and Operating Room Settings

The patient is placed in lithotomy position, so to prevent postoperative complications linked to this position, such as deep vein thrombosis, neural damage, and compartment syndrome, it is important to hold the patient's posture appropriately.

Spinal anesthesia is a feasible option [1], but general anesthesia is recommended for fURS for several reasons. Renal movement caused by respiration can affect navigation and lithotripsy. Under general anesthesia using apnea, these issues can be temporarily avoided. Moreover, in patients with large stones, the time frame for spinal anesthesia can be exceeded, requiring addition of general anesthesia to complete the procedure.

Surgeons should plan the operating room setting to comfortably perform each task. We usually set the endoscopic tower on the right side of the patient and C-arm fluoroscopy on the left side. A long table should be present close to the surgeons so they can easily pick up scopes and disposable equipment. Irrigation system and laser-generating device are also prepared to facilitate the procedures. These operating room settings need to be arranged according to the facilities in each institution.

As the position of surgeons, both standing position and sitting position during fURS are acceptable depending on the surgeon's preference. Although standing position is a common use in fURS, prolonged standing, over 2 h, would be tiring for surgeon. On the other hand, sitting position is more comfortable for surgeon ergonomics. However, surgeon's manipulation during procedure might be limited.

10.3 Access to the Upper Urinary Tract (Including Ureteral Access Sheath Placement)

We recommend an initial examination of the ureter by semirigid ureteroscopy before placement of ureteral access sheath (UAS). Surgeons need to advance endoscope until checking the whole upper ureter. This step enables us to check the diameter, the compliance, the relax of ureters, the patient's genitourinary anatomy, and the presence of migrated stones and to assess the appropriate UAS size for the patient. Moreover, by the insertion of semirigid ureteroscope, the whole ureter can be passively dilated under direct vision. In our experience, although the global standard size in UAS is 12–14Fr, the Asian standard size may be less than 11–13Fr because of influence of body size between Caucasian and non-Caucasian.

The procedure therefore usually starts with semirigid ureteroscopy to place a guidewire into the kidney. In cases with ureteral stent placement, a guidewire is placed after the stent removal, and semirigid ureteroscopy is performed. If there is difficulty to advance the semirigid ureteroscope further because of ureteral stricture or ureteric tightness, it is safer to place a ureteral stent for passive ureteral dilation and plan for a second procedure session at later date (at least 7–14 days later).

Next, UAS is placed under fluoroscopic control. This step is delicate because careless insertion of UAS could lead to ureteral injury. Ureteral wall injury caused by UAS was reported to be found in 46.5% of cases of retrograde intrarenal surgery [2]. It is important not to apply excessive force, although there is a proper feeling of resistance during UAS placement. The choice of UAS, its size, and diameter depend on the result of the initial semirigid ureteroscopy, the type of endoscope used, and the surgeon's preferences. In previous study, 12/14 Fr UAS was considered to be a universal UAS that fits all currently available flexible ureteroscopes in the endourology field [3]. Smaller-diameter endoscopes have been developed; however, we expect UAS with smaller diameters will become the new standard. To avoid ureteral damage, if flexible ureteroscopy with small diameter is available, the 10/12 Fr UAS is suggested as the new first-line choice [4]. The best position of UAS depends on the location of stones. In ureteral stone cases, the position of UAS needs to be adjusted to facilitate access to the stones. In renal stone cases, the tip of UAS should be placed in the proximal ureter or just below the ureteropelvic junction. To judge whether the position of UAS is appropriate or not, it is also important to confirm the flow-out of urine or irrigation fluid from the sheath. After placement of UAS, flexible ureteroscope can be navigated to the upper urinary tract.

10.4 Irrigation

The fURS is usually performed with continuous saline irrigation through the working channel. Irrigation is very important to maintain endoscopic visibility. In addition to gravity irrigation, additional devices including syringes and manual pressure pumps are useful to improve the visibility, especially when stone dust disturbs the endoscopic view or if venous bleeding occurs. Moreover, these devices can be helpful to flush and move stone fragments to facilitate lithotripsy or basketing. Attention must be paid, however, to the rise of intrarenal pressure generated by these devices. The rise of intrarenal pressure could lead to urosepsis due to the backflow of irrigation saline into blood vessels and lymph vessels. This backflow is considered to be caused by the rise of intrarenal pressure to 30–40 cmH_2O [5]. Therefore, to prevent urosepsis, it is necessary to maintain low intrarenal pressure. The level of intrarenal pressure differs depending on the irrigation system used, the application of power by operators or assistants, the diameter of UAS, the type of ureteroscope, and the instruments inserted into the working channel [6]. Automated irrigation systems for urological endoscopic procedures have also recently become available. These systems may be useful to maintain irrigation pressure within a safe range and to provide clear visualization during surgery [7]. In addition, for prevention of urosepsis, it is also a good clinical practice to decompress the upper urinary tract regularly, as well as limited the operation time [8].

10.5 Lithotripsy

Laser lithotripsy by using Ho:YAG laser has become the gold standard method for stone lithotripsy during fURS procedure [9].

To prevent any eye damage caused by lasers, proper eye protection should be considered. Ho:YAG laser could cause damage to the cornea when set to high energy from close distance in the absence of eye protection, although eyeglasses have been shown to be as effective as laser safety glasses in preventing eye damage caused by lasers [10]. Eye lenses are highly radiosensitive, and prolonged radiation exposure may lead to the development of cataracts, so wearing lead-lined glasses is recommended to avoid any eye damage during lithotripsy procedure.

Regarding laser fiber used in fURS procedures, we recommend small-diameter fibers (200–275 μm) for several reasons; they provide better irrigation, better scope deflection, and less retropulsion than large-diameter fibers. It has been shown that fiber diameter does not affect fragmentation efficiency. On the other hand, small-diameter fibers are more fragile and prone to fiber-tip degradation because of the burn-back effect. During laser fragmentation, a regular laser stripping and cleaving should therefore be considered.

When laser fiber is inserted into the working channel, the scope should be straightened to prevent scope damage caused by the fiber. After the insertion of laser fiber, to avoid laser damage, it is recommended to keep the laser fiber tip at one-quarter of the endoscopic screen, which is named by "safety distance" [11]. When laser firing, operators should avoid mucosal damage due to laser shots, and extra care is necessary for ureteral stone cases because of limited space in the ureter. In ureteral stone cases, pushing up stones may be pushed into a wide space, the renal pelvis, or renal calyces. Also, in impacted ureteral stone, the stone should be peeled away to the upper ureter of the renal pelvis. In kidney stone cases, if access to the stones is difficult, repositioning of stones by using stone baskets can also be useful.

When using the majority of laser lithotripters, operators need to set two laser parameters, the pulse energy and pulse frequency. The total power output (W) is calculated as pulse energy (J) × pulse frequency (Hz). These laser settings depend on lithotripsy strategies. The conventional lithotripsy strategy is stone fragmenting; stones are fragmented to a suitable size, and the stone fragments are then extracted using stone baskets. In recent years, a new strategy, stone dusting, has been advocated and has become popular, especially in Europe and the United States [12]. The stones are reduced to a dust-like state, which are intended to be passed spontaneously. To properly use these different lithotripsy strategies, it is necessary to understand the characteristics of laser setting and laser-generating devices. For stone fragmenting, the laser output is usually set to high energy (0.5–1.0 J) and low frequency (5–15 Hz) and is then gradually adjusted during surgery. The stones need to be reduced to small fragments, which can be extracted using UAS. For stone dusting, meanwhile, the laser output is set to low energy (0.2–0.5 J) and high frequency (30–50 Hz) and requires arrangement according to the stone hardness. The stones should be reduced to fine dust which is intended to be passed spontaneously without the need for stone baskets. The laser tip should be moved along the stone surface avoiding prolonged contact at the same place [13]. It is important to note that some low-power laser devices do not offer high-frequency settings. In addition to these two laser lithotripsy options, a unique lithotripsy technique called "popcorn technique" is also useful for reducing stone burden. Using this technique, the laser tip does not directly contact the stones and is instead positioned near a collection of stones in a dependent calyx. Firing the laser at relatively high frequency induces a whirlpool-like phenomenon, which displaces stone fragments within the calyx [13]. For popcorn technique, the laser output is set to high energy (0.5–1.0 J) and relatively high frequency (10–20 Hz). Moreover, some lithotripsy techniques have been introduced in the previous article [13]. Dancing technique is best applied to soft stones. In this technique, the tip of laser fiber is brushed back and forth across the stone surface, ablating it layer by layer. The laser output is set to 0.8–1.0 J and 8–10 Hz. Chipping technique is the most commonly used. The laser is aimed at the stone periphery and fired continuously until a small fragment chipped off. This technique is until the stone is whittled down to a small core fragment. For this technique, the laser output is also set to 0.8–10 J and 8–10 Hz. A recent prospective study compared stone fragmenting and stone dusting and reported that the stone-free rate in fragmenting plus active basketing group was higher than that in the dusting group on univariate analysis, but not on multivariate analysis [14]. There was no difference between the two groups in postoperative complication rates. The method of lithotripsy should be determined depending on stone size, stone location, stone hardness, patient anatomy, the laser lithotripter used, and the operator's skill. If possible, the operators should dynamically use these different techniques during surgery according to the situation without favoring a particular technique.

A new generation of laser lithotripters provides a third parameter following pulse energy, pulse frequency, and pulse duration. Operators can choose between short-pulse and long-pulse modes. The difference in these two modes is the period of time of one laser shot; and the period is 180–330 μs in short-pulse mode and 650–1215 μs in long-pulse mode [15]. While the fragmentation rates for long- and short-pulse durations are at a comparable level, it has been reported that long-pulse duration reduces stone retropulsion, which is one of the factors that affects lithotripsy efficiency [16]. If pulse duration can be selected, long-pulse duration is therefore recommended in most cases, while short-pulse duration might be useful depending on stone hardness.

The technology associated with lithotripsy is undergoing remarkable advances. For example, high-power Ho:YAG laser (100–120 W) has been available and becoming the standard device for ureteroscopic lithotripsy. It enables dusting and pop-dusting techniques using high-frequency and long-pulse length laser setting. The first stage starts with dusting using a low-pulse energy (0.2–0.5 J), high frequency (40–50 Hz), and long-pulse length in a contact mode. If the stone is hard, the next stage allows pop-dusting using a low energy (0.5–0.6 J), high frequency (20–40 Hz), and long-pulse length in a non-contact mode. Pietropaolo et al. reported that, in the treatment of large stones (≥15 mm) using high-power laser machine (100 W), the initial and final stone-free rates were 93% and 98%, respectively [17]. In addition, a novel laser technology, Moses technology, was recently developed, which enables two-step firing of laser. The first shot draws the stones nearby negative pressure, and the second shot then breaks the stones. This technology was shown to result in more efficient laser lithotripsy and smaller-stone retropulsion compared with the conventional mode of lithotripsy. Elhilali et al. reported a significant reduction in retropulsion when using the Moses mode [18]. The stone movement was reduced by 50 times at 0.8 J and 10 Hz. The pronounced reduction in retropulsion in the Moses mode was clearly observed also at dusting setting (0.5 J and 50 Hz). In addition, stone fragmentation tests revealed that the Moses modes resulted in a significantly higher ablation volume compared with the regular mode (160% higher). Other novel laser technologies, such as vapor tunnel, virtual basketing, and bubble blast technologies, have been also recently developed. It has been already shown that these technologies can lead to retropulsion reduction, lithitripsy optimization, and theoretically a shorter stone ablation time [19]. Large-scale clinical trials are needed to confirm their efficacy and advantages. Moreover, next-generation laser technology in the place of Ho:YAG laser, thulium fiber laser, has recently been explored. Traxer et al. have shown that this innovative laser technology offers several advantages: fourfold higher absorption coefficient in water, smaller operating laser fibers (50–150 μm core diameter), lower energy per pulse (as low as 0.025 J), higher maximal pulse repetition rate (up to 2000 Hz), 1.5–4 times faster stone ablation, and 2–4 times less stone retropulsion without heat increase [20]. Therefore, this next-generation laser is expected to become an important milestone for urinary stone treatment. The introduction of these new technologies may greatly influence future lithotripsy strategy.

10.6 Fragment Extraction

When stone fragmenting techniques are performed, stone fragments need to be extracted, mainly using stone baskets. Stone basketing requires advanced skills, which is thought to be one of the main reasons for dusting technique preference. Regarding fragment extraction, the following two points are important: identification of the fragment size and choice of stone baskets. The size of fragments can be estimated from the comparison with the size of laser fiber or stone baskets and by fluoroscopic images. When there are many stone fragments, small fragments should be extracted as priority. If the fragments become stuck, without pulling them forcefully, the surgeons should reposition them and add additional lithotripsy. Tip-less nitinol baskets have become the standard instruments, and multiple types are commercially available. The type of baskets should be chosen according to the size and location of fragments and the surgeon's preference.

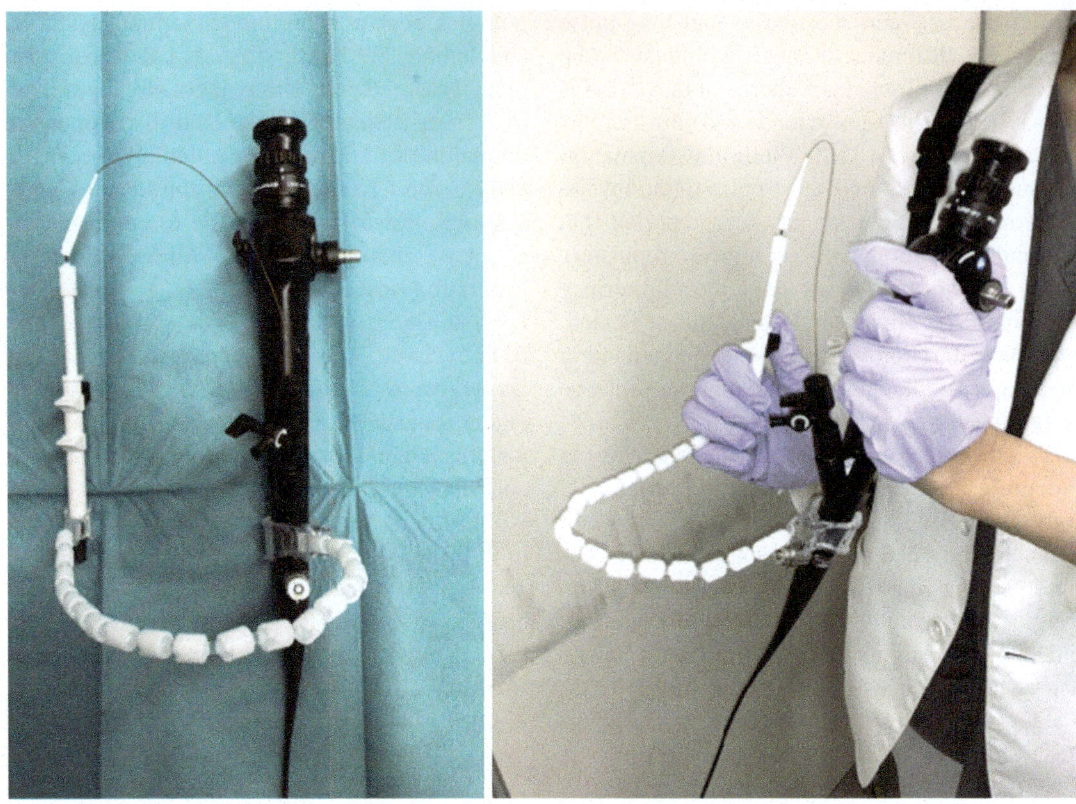

Fig. 10.2 One-person basketing technique using M-arm

In most institutions, stone retrieval with baskets is performed by two people; the operator manipulates the ureteroscopy, and the assistant opens and closes stone baskets. This method requires harmonious cooperation between two people, however, and mainly depends on the actions of stone baskets. In our experience, retrieval of stone fragments by this two-person method leads to the increase in the number of basket opening/closing actions. In addition, the stone basket usually is opened widely regardless of fragment size, because it is difficult for the assistant to open the stone basket to meet with fragment size. In our clinical practice, we therefore usually perform stone retrieval by one-person method; the operator performs both the manipulation of ureteroscope and the opening/closing operations of stone baskets. This method requires an advanced ureteroscope handling technique, but stone fragments can be retrieved with fewer basket operations. In Japan, M-arm (MC medical, Tokyo, Japan), which can fix the stone basket to flexible ureteroscope, is commercially available and is very useful for one-person performance of basketing technique (Fig. 10.2). The worldwide distribution of this device is expected to make one-person basketing techniques more popular.

10.7 Exit Strategy Including Postoperative Stenting

At the end of operation, careful renal and ureteral exploration should be performed before the complete retrieval of the scope and UAS. During the UAS retrieval, the tip of the scope should be kept a few centimeters out of UAS to detect remaining fragments, ureteral stricture, and eventual ureteral lesions due to UAS placement. It is also necessary to check for any damage to the ureteral orifice. This procedure is important to determine whether or not to place the postoperative ureteral stent and the duration of stenting. According to the guidelines, routine postoperative stenting after uncomplicated ureteroscopy is not necessary [21]. Postoperative stenting rates actually differ between countries (93% in the United States, 70% in European countries) [22]. There is no specific indication or criteria for stent omission after uncomplicated ureteroscopy, but the use of UAS has been reported to be a risk factor for emergency room visits [23]. Postoperative stenting is therefore currently recommended when a UAS has been used. If the procedure is uneventful, the duration of stenting can be short. In our opinion, because the UAS with small diameter (10–12Fr or less) tends to be used, routine postoperative stenting may not be necessary, even when UAS has been used. Future studies are required to examine the necessity of postoperative stenting after fURS with small-diameter UAS.

10.8 Preoperative Ureteral Stenting

Routine preoperative stenting before fURS is not desired because of the deterioration in patient's quality of life (QOL) caused by stent-related symptoms including bladder irritability, pain and hematuria, and the extra costs.

Preoperative stenting may still be considered for several purposes, however, such as treatment for infected hydronephrosis, control for persistent colic pain, treatment for renal insufficiency, and passive dilation of the ureter. Notably, preoperative stenting facilitates the dilation of the ureter, which is an advantage of performing fURS. Preoperative stenting was shown in a previous study to improve stone-free rates and to decrease intra-operative complications in patients with renal stones receiving ureteroscopy [24]. In addition, placement of a postoperative ureteral stent after uncomplicated fURS with preoperative stenting may not be necessary. The patient's preoperative QOL may deteriorate by preoperative stent-related symptoms, but the improvement of surgical outcomes and the avoidance of postoperative stenting can result in improvement of patient's overall QOL. It should be noted, however, that there are several disadvantages of preoperative stenting in addition to the deterioration of preoperative QOL and the extra costs. First, there is a risk for placing the stent into submucosal ureter. Second, long ureteral stent dwelling time has been reported to be associated with increasing rates of postoperative urosepsis (>30 days vs ≤30 days) [25]. When there is a period more than 30 days from stent placement to surgery, ureteral stent replacement may be recommended before surgery.

10.9 Strategy for Complicated Cases

(a) Lower-Pole Stones

The fURS procedure for lower-pole stone cases is often difficult because of the patient's pelvicalyceal anatomy. Infundibular pelvic angle (IPA) was shown in previous studies to be the most important predictor of treatment outcomes, and treatment success rates in patients' sweep IPA are low (<30°) because the approach to inferior calyces is difficult in such cases [26, 27]. Digital flexible scopes have been reported to be less effective in approaching the sharp-angled inferior calyx and had lesser end-tip deflection compared with the fiber-optic scopes [28]. In difficult lower-pole stone cases, it may therefore be better to use fiber-optic scopes. In addition, taking into account the risk of ureteroscope damage, the use of single-use disposable scopes can also be considered [29]. The location of UAS is also important, and the tip of UAS should not be located near the renal pelvis considering the bending of flexible scopes.

If possible, the stones should be relocated with stone baskets to a more easily approachable location, for example, the upper pole or renal pelvis [30]. This technique can reduce the risk of scope damage and can make stone targeting during lithotripsy and basketing easier and more effective. In patients with large stones >10 mm, however, it is impossible to relocate them, so laser lithotripsy is required before relocating. In such cases, it is necessary to pay full attention to ureteroscope damage caused not only by scope deflection but also by insertion of laser fiber. To avoid scope damage, laser fiber must be inserted into the working channel with minimal deflection of the ureteroscope. The use of small-diameter laser fiber is also recommended to get better scope deflection.

(b) Impacted Stones

The fURS procedure for impacted ureteral stones can also present troubles for surgeons. In impacted ureteral stone cases, clear endoscopic visualization may not be possible because of mucosal edema, ureteral polyp, and worse irrigation due to stone impaction. Surgeons should therefore be careful not to injure the ureteral mucosa by laser shots, and if possible, placement of safety guidewires is recommended to ensure the correct urinary tract pathway. When performing laser lithotripsy, we recommend the "peeling off and push-back" technique (Fig. 10.3). First, we break the center of stones, not the edge near the mucosa, until the stones become movable. Stones are then peeled off and removed from the stone bed by using the tip of the endoscope. After repeated lithotripsy and peeling off, fragmented stones can be finally pushed back to the wide space, for example, the upper ureter or renal pelvis. We believe that this technique is safe and can minimize the risk of ureteral injury. Ureteral injury by laser can lead to severe postoperative ureteral stricture, so when the procedure is too difficult, the operators should finish the surgery with ureteral stent placement and prepare for a second session.

10.10 Simulation-Based Ureteroscopic Training

The fURS procedure has a steep learning curve and cannot be easily mastered. Simulation-based ureteroscopic training to learn the basic skills is therefore receiving an increased attention, and various models, including a bench model and a virtual reality model, are currently available for simulation-based ureteroscopic training [31], although these models cannot entirely recreate actual clinical situations. Although advanced models, such as animal models and human tissue (cadaver) models, may be especially useful to learn endoscopic techniques, repeated training using these models is difficult to facilitate. There are also several complications, such as cost, legal issues, ethics, and the need for animal licenses [32].

With this background, a novel model for simulation-based fURS training is expected. Our colleagues recently introduced a new advanced bench model for fURS training called the smart simulator (Olympus, Tokyo, Japan) (Fig. 10.4) [33]. This simulator features portability, similar structure to actual human anatomy, and the ability to simulate breathing-induced kidney movements. This model can therefore facilitate a

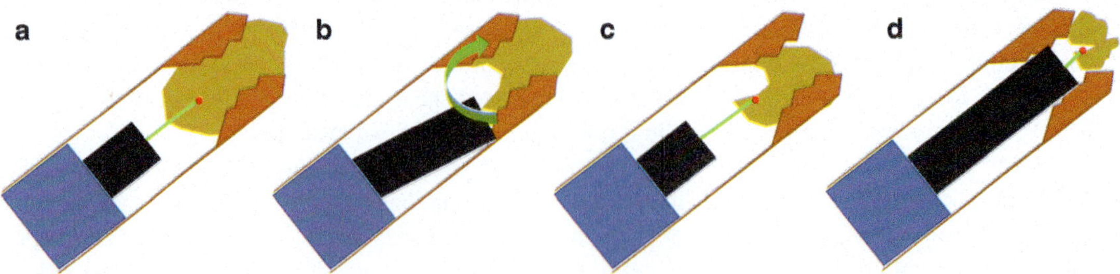

Fig. 10.3 "Peeling off and push-back" technique in cases with impacted stones. (**a**) Break the center of stones, (**b**) peel off and remove the stone from the stone bed by using the tip of the ureteroscope, (**c**) break the stones again, and (**d**) push back

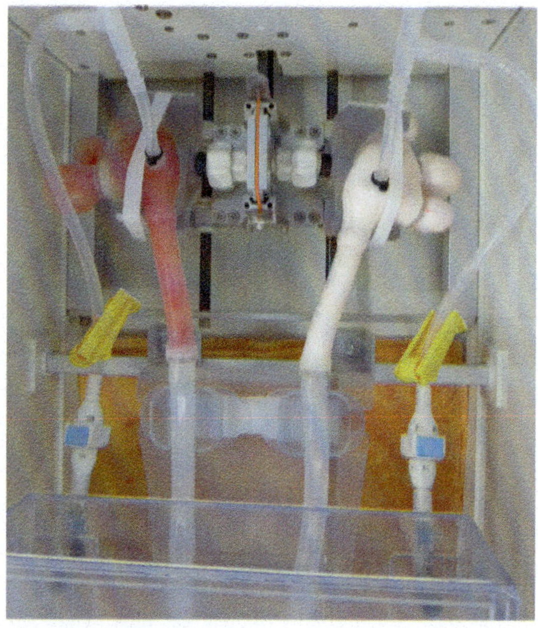

Fig 10.4 Smart simulator

situation closer to actual clinical settings than other bench models, and trainees' technical skills may be improved. Development of more advanced simulation-based training for fURS is expected.

10.11 Conclusions

The fURS procedure has become popular worldwide, but to become skilled at this procedure, the ability to overcome various difficulties is required. In this section, we reviewed the current standard method of fURS, but development of novel ureteroscopes, laser devices, and optional instruments is expected. Endourologists must adapt to changes in endourological technologies.

References

1. Zeng G, Zhao Z, Yang F, Zhong W, Wu W, Chen W. Retrograde intrarenal surgery with combined spinal-epidural vs general anesthesia: a prospective randomized controlled trial. J Endourol. 2015;29(4):401–5. https://doi.org/10.1089/end.2014.0249.
2. Traxer O, Thomas A. Prospective evaluation and classification of ureteral wall injuries resulting from insertion of a ureteral access sheath during retrograde intrarenal surgery. J Urol. 2013;189(2):580–4. https://doi.org/10.1016/j.juro.2012.08.197.
3. Al-Qahtani SM, Letendre J, Thomas A, Natalin R, Saussez T, Traxer O. Which ureteral access sheath is compatible with your flexible ureteroscope? J Endourol. 2014;28(3):286–90. https://doi.org/10.1089/end.2013.0375.
4. Sener TE, Cloutier J, Villa L, Marson F, Butticè S, Doizi S, Traxer O. Can we provide low intrarenal pressures with good irrigation flow by decreasing the size of ureteral access sheaths? J Endourol. 2016;30(1):49–55. https://doi.org/10.1089/end.2015.0387.
5. Rehman J, Monga M, Landman J, Lee DI, Felfela T, Conradie MC, Srinivas R, Sundaram CP, Clayman RV. Characterization of intrapelvic pressure during ureteropyeloscopy with ureteral access sheaths. Urology. 2003;61(4):713–8. https://doi.org/10.1016/s0090-4295(02)02440-8.
6. Proietti S, Dragos L, Somani BK, Butticè S, Talso M, Emiliani E, Baghdadi M, Giusti G, Traxer O. In vitro comparison of maximum pressure developed by irrigation systems in a kidney model. J Endourol. 2017; https://doi.org/10.1089/end.2017.0005.
7. Fedrigon D III, Alshara L, Monga M. Comparison of automated irrigation systems using an in vitro ureteroscopy model. Int Braz J Urol. 2020;46(3):390–7. https://doi.org/10.1590/s1677-5538.ibju.2019.0230.
8. Scotland KB, Lange D. Prevention and management of urosepsis triggered by ureteroscopy. Res Rep Urol. 2018;10:43–9. https://doi.org/10.2147/rru.s128071.
9. Gupta PK. Is the holmium:YAG laser the best intracorporeal lithotripter for the ureter? A 3-year retrospective study. J Endourol. 2007;21(3):305–9. https://doi.org/10.1089/end.2006.0247.
10. Villa L, Cloutier J, Compérat E, Kronemberg P, Charlotte F, Berthe L, Rouchausse Y, Salonia A, Montorsi F, Traxer O. Do we really need to wear proper eye protection when using holmium:YAG laser during endourologic procedures? Results from an ex vivo animal model on pig eyes. J Endourol. 2016;30(3):332–7. https://doi.org/10.1089/end.2015.0232.
11. Talso M, Emiliani E, Haddad M, Berthe L, Baghdadi M, Montanari E, Traxer O. Laser fiber and flexible ureterorenoscopy: the safety distance concept. J Endourol. 2016;30(12):1269–74. https://doi.org/10.1089/end.2016.0209.
12. Dauw CA, Simeon L, Alruwaily AF, Sanguedolce F, Hollingsworth JM, Roberts WW, Faerber GJ, Wolf JS Jr, Ghani KR. Contemporary practice patterns of flexible ureteroscopy for treating renal stones: results of a worldwide survey. J Endourol. 2015;29(11):1221–30. https://doi.org/10.1089/end.2015.0260.
13. Hecht SL, Wolf JS Jr. Techniques for holmium laser lithotripsy of intrarenal calculi. Urology. 2013;81(2):442–5. https://doi.org/10.1016/j.urology.2012.11.021.
14. Humphreys MR, Shah OD, Monga M, Chang YH, Krambeck AE, Sur RL, Miller NL, Knudsen BE,

Eisner BH, Matlaga BR, Chew BH. Dusting versus basketing during ureteroscopy—which technique is more efficacious? A prospective Multicenter trial from the EDGE Research Consortium. J Urol. 2018;199(5):1272–6. https://doi.org/10.1016/j.juro.2017.11.126.
15. Kronenberg P, Traxer O. Update on lasers in urology 2014: current assessment on holmium:yttrium-aluminum-garnet (Ho:YAG) laser lithotripter settings and laser fibers. World J Urol. 2015;33(4):463–9. https://doi.org/10.1007/s00345-014-1395-1.
16. Bader MJ, Pongratz T, Khoder W, Stief CG, Herrmann T, Nagele U, Sroka R. Impact of pulse duration on Ho:YAG laser lithotripsy: fragmentation and dusting performance. World J Urol. 2015;33(4):471–7. https://doi.org/10.1007/s00345-014-1429-8.
17. Pietropaolo A, Jones P, Whitehurst L, Somani BK. Role of 'dusting and pop-dusting' using a high-powered (100 W) laser machine in the treatment of large stones (≥15 mm): prospective outcomes over 16 months. Urolithiasis. 2019;47(4):391–4. https://doi.org/10.1007/s00240-018-1076-4.
18. Elhilali MM, Badaan S, Ibrahim A, Andonian S. Use of the Moses Technology to improve holmium laser lithotripsy outcomes: a preclinical study. J Endourol. 2017;31(6):598–604. https://doi.org/10.1089/end.2017.0050.
19. Pulse Modulation for Holmium Laser: Vapor Tunnel–Virtual Basket–Bubble Blast. Videourology. 2020;34(3). https://doi.org/10.1089/vid.2020.0018
20. Traxer O, Keller EX. Thulium fiber laser: the new player for kidney stone treatment? A comparison with holmium:YAG laser. World J Urol. 2020;38(8):1883–94. https://doi.org/10.1007/s00345-019-02654-5.
21. Türk C, Petřík A, Sarica K, Seitz C, Skolarikos A, Straub M, Knoll T. EAU guidelines on interventional treatment for urolithiasis. Eur Urol. 2016;69(3):475–82. https://doi.org/10.1016/j.eururo.2015.07.041.
22. Muslumanoglu AY, Fuglsig S, Frattini A, Labate G, Nadler RB, Martov A, Wong C, de la Rosette J. Risks and benefits of postoperative double-J stent placement after ureteroscopy: results from the Clinical Research Office of Endourological Society Ureteroscopy Global Study. J Endourol. 2017;31(5):446–51. https://doi.org/10.1089/end.2016.0827.
23. Rapoport D, Perks AE, Teichman JM. Ureteral access sheath use and stenting in ureteroscopy: effect on unplanned emergency room visits and cost. J Endourol. 2007;21(9):993–7. https://doi.org/10.1089/end.2006.0236.
24. Assimos D, Crisci A, Culkin D, Xue W, Roelofs A, Duvdevani M, Desai M, de la Rosette J. Preoperative JJ stent placement in ureteric and renal stone treatment: results from the Clinical Research Office of Endourological Society (CROES) Ureteroscopy (URS) Global Study. BJU Int. 2016;117(4):648–54. https://doi.org/10.1111/bju.13250.
25. Nevo A, Mano R, Baniel J, Lifshitz DA. Ureteric stent dwelling time: a risk factor for post-ureteroscopy sepsis. BJU Int. 2017;120(1):117–22. https://doi.org/10.1111/bju.13796.
26. Karim SS, Hanna L, Geraghty R, Somani BK. Role of pelvicalyceal anatomy in the outcomes of retrograde intrarenal surgery (RIRS) for lower pole stones: outcomes with a systematic review of literature. Urolithiasis. 2020;48(3):263–70. https://doi.org/10.1007/s00240-019-01150-0.
27. Inoue T, Murota T, Okada S, Hamamoto S, Muguruma K, Kinoshita H, Matsuda T. Influence of pelvicaliceal anatomy on stone clearance after flexible ureteroscopy and holmium laser lithotripsy for large renal stones. J Endourol. 2015;29(9):998–1005. https://doi.org/10.1089/end.2015.0071.
28. Dragos LB, Somani BK, Sener ET, Buttice S, Proietti S, Ploumidis A, Iacoboaie CT, Doizi S, Traxer O. Which flexible ureteroscopes (digital vs. fiber-optic) can easily reach the difficult lower pole calices and have better end-tip deflection: in vitro study on K-box. A PETRA Evaluation. J Endourol. 2017;31(7):630–7. https://doi.org/10.1089/end.2017.0109.
29. Hennessey DB, Fojecki GL, Papa NP, Lawrentschuk N, Bolton D. Single-use disposable digital flexible ureteroscopes: an ex vivo assessment and cost analysis. BJU Int. 2018;121(Suppl 3):55–61. https://doi.org/10.1111/bju.14235.
30. Auge BK, Dahm P, Wu NZ, Preminger GM. Ureteroscopic management of lower-pole renal calculi: technique of calculus displacement. J Endourol. 2001;15(8):835–8. https://doi.org/10.1089/089277901753205852.
31. Brunckhorst O, Aydin A, Abboudi H, Sahai A, Khan MS, Dasgupta P, Ahmed K. Simulation-based ureteroscopy training: a systematic review. J Surg Educ. 2015;72(1):135–43. https://doi.org/10.1016/j.jsurg.2014.07.003.
32. Ogan K, Jacomides L, Shulman MJ, Roehrborn CG, Cadeddu JA, Pearle MS. Virtual ureteroscopy predicts ureteroscopic proficiency of medical students on a cadaver. J Urol. 2004;172(2):667–71. https://doi.org/10.1097/01.ju.0000131631.60022.d9.
33. Inoue T, Okada S, Hamamoto S, Matsuda T. New advanced bench model for flexible ureteroscopic training: the smart simulator. J Endourol. 2017; https://doi.org/10.1089/end.2017.0430.

11 Management of Complications Related to Ureteroscopy

Hyung Joon Kim

11.1 Introduction

The incidence of complications after the ureteroscopic surgery is reported at 7–25%. A recent study of 11,885 patients in 32 countries and 114 institutions reported that the most common complications during URS were bleeding, ureteral perforation, and failure of ureteroscope insertion, with 1.41%, 1.05%, and 1.67%, respectively [1]. Most postoperative complications are minor, and very few require additional treatment [1–3]. However, some complications could be of significance. The most relevant perioperative complications are urinary tract infection (UTI), sepsis, ureteral injury, and ureteral stricture. This chapter will provide advice on how to prevent and manage the complications related to ureteroscopy.

11.2 Intraoperative Complications

The incidence of complications during the ureteroscopic surgery is around 0.5% to 20% [4]. Significant complications occur in 1.5–5%. Among them, most of the complications are related to the ureteral injury. Utilization of safety guidewire is recommended to reduce ureteral damage and perforation during ureteroscopy.

11.2.1 Ureteral Bleeding

Bleeding occurs in 1.9% of ureteroscopic surgeries, which is the second most common complication [4]. It is usually related to the ureteral orifice trauma during the insertion of the ureteroscope. Mucosal injury is expected during the insertion of the guidewire. Advancing guidewire too far upward can pierce the collecting system entering the parenchyma. Overdistention of the renal pelvis or calyx by increased intrarenal pressure can induce hematuria as well. Bleeding can also be caused during ureteral dilation and lithotripsy or from the target lesion itself. Such minor bleeding is mostly self-limited. Bleeding risk can be reduced by utilizing a smaller-diameter ureteroscope. A hydrophilic guidewire may ease the engagement into the orifice and lessen the chance of ureteral damage. Forceful or blind insertion should be avoided. Extensive bleeding is rare, but it might occur after endopyelotomy or endoscopic tumor resection of the ureteral tumor. If bleeding is too severe to be controlled by active irrigation for a certain period, the procedure should be terminated, and place a ureteral stent. Angioembolization is required in rare situations.

H. J. Kim (✉)
Department of Urology, Konyang University, Daejeon, Republic of Korea
e-mail: hjkim@kyuh.ac.kr

A. C.F. Ng et al. (eds.), *Practical Management of Urinary Stone*,
https://doi.org/10.1007/978-981-16-4193-0_11

11.2.2 Ureteral Injury

Ureteral injury is the most frequent complication which can mostly be managed with the insertion of a ureteral stent. However, in some severe cases, it may require immediate or delayed surgical repair. Delayed sequelae of urine extravasation include prolonged ileus, urinary obstruction, urinoma, azotemia, fever, persistent flank pain, fistula formation, and sepsis. Thermal injury can be caused by direct contact with an electrohydraulic probe or laser fiber. Mechanical injury can be induced by a guidewire, ureteral access sheath (UAS), or the retropulsion of the stone. As for the injury caused during the insertion of a UAS, it has been reported that the rate of ureteral injury can be significantly reduced if pre-stented [5]. Several retrospective studies have reported that preoperative ureteral stent insertion can increase the stone-free rate and shorten the surgical time [6, 7]. However, most of the guidelines do not recommend pre-stenting due to lack of evidence [8, 9]. A recent study reported that the rapid insertion of UAS or the application of a force greater than 600G results in the damage to the ureter. Preoperative use of alpha-blockers lowers the insertion force, thus helping to reduce the chance of ureteral injury [10].

Utilization of safety guidewire is recommended to reduce ureteral injury and perforation during ureteroscopy. Some studies have reported that the URS was safely and successfully performed without a safety guidewire [11–13]. Still, experts consider it safer to perform the operation with a safety guidewire inserted and recommend its use [8, 9]. When exiting the ureteroscope, identification of ureteral damage is necessary. The tip of the ureteroscope should be kept a few centimeters out of the sheath to detect eventual ureteral lesions due to UAS placement and determine the most appropriate stenting duration. Stent is routinely placed whenever a UAS has been used. It is not necessary to place the ureteral stent in all cases. However, it is recommended to insert and leave the stent for 1 to 2 weeks if residual stones remain or ureteral injury, bleeding, perforation, and urinary tract infections are suspected during surgery. The meta-analysis on the postoperative ureteral stent insertion showed that it causes various urinary symptoms, such as postoperative urinary tract infection and pain [14]. Therefore, many guidelines do not recommend postoperative stenting when the complications are not expected [8, 9, 14]. On the contrary, a ureteral stent is indicated in cases with ureteral injury expected to result in ureteral stricture, decreased contralateral or overall renal function, and scheduled staged operation [8, 9]. However, it has been reported that without the insertion of the ureteral stent, the probability of unexpected visit to an outpatient clinic or emergency room after discharge increases, and for this reason, the majority of urologists still prefer to insert the stent after ureteroscopic surgery [12, 13]. There is a controversy over the insertion period of the ureteral stent, but the majority of urologists prefer to maintain it for 1 or 2 weeks postoperatively [8, 9].

Several groups have proposed grading systems on the degree of ureteral injury (Table 11.1). The management plan for each grade is recommended, but it depends on each case by case [16].

11.2.2.1 Low-Grade Ureteral Injury

Low-grade ureteral injuries consist of contusion, mucosal erosion, or false passage. It could be induced while manipulating scopes or accessories such as UAS, guidewires, or baskets. Misfire of the energy may also be the cause. The procedure can proceed even after a low-grade ureteral injury like mucosal erosion, but care must be taken not to perforate the erosion site. If there is a concern for the worsening of the injury degree, it would be reasonable to abort the operation and place a ureteral stent. Stricture rate after a low-grade injury is rare (0.3%) [4].

Table 11.1 Grading systems for ureteral injury

	Grade	Description	Management
PULS [15]	0	No lesion or insignificant mucosal abrasions: Contusions with minimal hematoma, mucosal molding via guidewire	No intervention required
	1	Superficial mucosal lesion and/or significant mucosal edema/hematoma: Superficial bleeding/tears of the mucosa and/or mucosal edema or hematoma	No intervention required, consider ureteral stent <1 week in some cases
	2	Submucosal lesion: Deep tear of the mucosal and submucosal layer (ureteral integrity, no extravasation)	Ureteral stent 1–2 weeks
	3	Perforation <50% (partial transection)	Ureteral stent 3–4 weeks
	4	Perforation 50–99% (partial transection)	Ureteral stent 6–12 weeks
	5	Complete transection	Surgical reconstruction
Traxer and Thomas [5]	0	No lesion found or only mucosal petechiae	No intervention required, consider ureteral stent 1–2 weeks
	1	Ureteral mucosal erosion without smooth muscle injury	Ureteral stent 1–2 weeks
	2	Ureteral wall injury involving the mucosa and smooth muscle (periureteral fat not seen)	Ureteral stent 3–6 weeks
	3	Ureteral wall injury involving adventitial perforation (periureteral fat seen)	Ureteral stent (and/or nephrostomy) Surgical reconstruction in some cases
	4	Total ureteral avulsion	Surgical reconstruction

PULS, post-ureteroscopic lesion scale (modified from reference [16])

11.2.2.2 High-Grade Ureteral Injury

High-grade ureteral injury includes ureteral perforation, intussusception, and avulsion. Perforation is an injury to the whole layers of the ureter involving adventitia or periureteral fat. The cause of injury is similar to that of mucosal erosion, but the degree is more severe. The rate of perforation is around 1% [4]. Insertion of UAS does not increase the risk of ureteral perforation. Once a perforation is identified, the procedure should be aborted and stented. The ureteral stent should be kept for several weeks. Ureteral stricture is rare, but extrusion of the stone fragment via perforation site can be more of a concern. Intramural stone extrusion sometimes results in submucosal stone, which may be the predisposing factor for stricture or nidus for stone growth. Fragments may imbed within perforation site as they pass down the ureter or during the insertion of UAS. Extramural stone migration, known as "lost stone," may result in more severe sequelae such as stricture, fluid extravasation, and retroperitoneal abscess. In the case of failed conservative management or high-grade injuries, surgical repair is needed. An immediate repair can be done within 5 days, and deferred treatment should be performed at least 6 weeks postoperatively with PCN in situ.

A ureteral avulsion is the most critical complication which can be encountered during the ureteroscopy. Such complications can be induced by attempting forceful insertion of the ureteroscope. It is reported in 0.1% of cases [4]. The proximal part of the ureter is at greater risk, and previous perforations are the most critical risk factors for this complication. It usually occurs when a stone too large to be removed is engaged within a basket and then an excessive force is applied to remove it. The ureter can be trapped during removal and torn from its attachment. Then it is externalized with the basket and ureteroscope as withdrawn. Another possible explanation for this complication is when the proximal part of the ureteroscope, which is wider than the distal tip, becomes wedged in the narrow distal ureter resulting in friction and mucosal dislocation.

To prevent such complications, care must be taken while removing the stone or inserting the instrument. The mucosa must always be visualized when retrieving the stone fragments. The distance between the stone fragment and the tip of the scope should always be kept close. Blind basketing should always be avoided. If the stone fragment grabbed with the stone basket is stuck during pull-back, removal must be aborted immediately. If gentle push-back to the upper wider portion of the ureter or renal pelvis is possible, release the stone free from the basket to fragment the stone into smaller pieces. If not, place the basket in situ, and insert the laser alongside it to break the stone or the wire of the stone basket. Sometimes the stone basket needs to be disintegrated to pull out the scope.

Once ureteral avulsion occurs, a nephrostomy tube should be inserted immediately. The open or laparoscopic repair is required depending on the location of the injury afterward. The type of surgery ranges from simple ureteroneocystostomy, psoas hitch, and Boari flap to ileal ureter, autotransplantation, or even nephrectomy.

11.3 Failure to Reach the Stone

During retrograde approaches for ureteral or renal stone, surgeons sometimes encounter situations where access to the ureter or stone cannot be achieved. Failure and conversion are reported as complications in many studies, with an overall rate of 1.6% and 0.1% [4]. Failure is more common when the stone is multifocal or located in the proximal part. Failure to access the upper tract occurs in 1.6–1.8% with flexible URS and 8% with semirigid ureteroscopy. Risk factors are stones >15 mm, proximal stones, intrinsic or extrinsic ureteral narrowing, stone impaction, ureteral edema, and iatrogenic or pathologic lesions. The ureter course should be visualized by retrograde ureterography. Switching to a curved tip guidewire may ease the insertion to the difficult ureter. Gentle probing with hydrophilic guidewire can be helpful. When stricture (or tight ureter) is encountered, dilation using tapered or balloon-dilator can also be considered. Even though failure and conversion are categorized into complications, it might be viewed as an appropriate treatment choice to minimize the risk of more severe complications. In that situation, inserting a ureteral stent and terminating the procedure for stage operation are highly recommended. If there is resistance inserting the scope, the stent should be indwelled for at least 1–2 weeks. The passive dilation effect of stenting eases the insertion of the ureteroscope, increases the stone-free rate, and reduces the complications rate.

11.3.1 Postoperative Complications

Most of the postoperative complications are minor. Bleeding or lower urinary tract symptoms related to stent can be conservatively managed. However, cerebrovascular complications, acute myocardial infarction, or even death can occur at a rate of less than 0.02%. Such major complications may be unpredictable, but as for prevention, the patient's medical condition should be thoroughly evaluated before the surgery. More common postoperative complications, infection (early), and stricture (late) will be dealt with in this part.

11.3.2 Urinary Tract Infection

Infection occurs in the early postoperative period. Fever is the most common immediate postoperative complication with a rate of 1.8% [4]. The incidence of urinary tract infection after ureteroscopic stone surgery is 1–3.7%. UTI risk factors are older age, obesity, female gender, nutrition or immune system impairment, diabetes mellitus, smoking, coexisting bodily infection, and increased bacterial load. Urine analysis must be conducted before surgery to prevent and minimize infection-related complications. Urine culture should be performed if urinary tract infection is suspected or if pyuria or bacteriuria is present. Proper antibiotic treatment should precede if the UTI is confirmed [8, 17, 18]. Even in patients who do not have bacteriuria or UTI before surgery, prophylactic antibiotics have been found to help prevent postoperative fever and other complications [19]. A single preoperative dose or duration of less than 24 h is sufficient to prevent infection after URS [8, 17, 20]. If the obstruction is the cause of UTI, it should be drained by placing either a ureteral stent or percutaneous nephrostomy.

Among all the infectious complications, sepsis is the most fearful since it can be life-threatening if not recognized and managed early. The incidence of a septic condition after URS is reported at 0.3% [4]. Sepsis is associated with retrograde seeding of bacteriuria or infected calculi. Therefore, in the case with a higher risk of UTI, renal urine aspirate and stone culture should be obtained intraoperatively.

Intrarenal reflux occurs when the intrarenal pressure rises above 40cmH2O (30 mmHg) [21]. If the pressure in the kidneys rises above this threshold, the risk of postoperative fever and systemic inflammatory response syndrome (SIRS) increases [22, 23]. Therefore, to prevent the occurrence of infection-related complications, it is important to lower the pressure in the kidneys during ureteroscopic stone surgeries. It is necessary to lower the inflow rate of irrigation fluid or outflow resistance. The most effective way of reducing intrarenal pressure during ureteroscopic stone surgery is to place UAS. The risk of sepsis can be reduced to 50% when UAS is used [21, 24].

11.3.3 Ureteral Stricture

Ureteral stricture is secondary to inflammatory processes following devascularization or ischemic injury to the urothelium. Direct mechanical trauma, iatrogenic mucosal lesions, perforation, submucosal dissection, ischemia, radiation, impacted stone, and periureteral fibrosis are the risk factors for ureteral stricture.

Ureteral perforation at the stone impaction site is the most significant primary risk factor for stricture. Thus, an alternative approach, such as antegrade or laparoscopic surgery, should be considered when dealing with impacted stones. Stenting for 2–3 weeks after surgery may decrease the risk of stenosis. It is shown that the

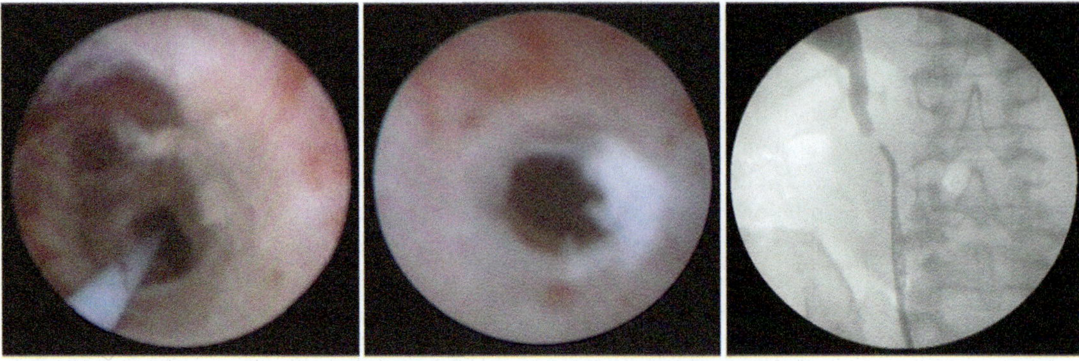

Fig. 11.1 Ureteral stricture after URS for impacted ureteral stone

use of UAS does not seem to increase the risk of stricture formation significantly. Routine postoperative ultrasound is recommended for cases suggested of ureteral stricture.

Once ureteral stricture is identified, the type of repair will depend on the location and extent of the injury, comorbid medical conditions, and the surgeon's experience (Fig. 11.1). Endoscopic management can be applied in nonischemic, nonradiation-induced, short (less than 1.5 cm in length) benign stricture. If endoscopic repair is not applicable, open or laparoscopic surgical repair must be considered.

11.4 Conclusion

Ureteroscopy is a relatively safe procedure for the treatment of ureteral stones with a low incidence of complications. Proper patient selection, case preparation, and sound endoscopic technique are critical to minimize the potential for complications. Always visualize the actions of your instruments and energy sources, and never force the scope or device. When ureteral stricture is suspected, procedure should be aborted, and a ureteral stent should be placed for staged operation.

References

1. Somani BK, Giusti G, Sun Y, Osther PJ, Frank M, De Sio M, et al. Complications associated with ureterorenoscopy (URS) related to treatment of urolithiasis: the Clinical Research Office of Endourological Society URS Global study. World J Urol. 2017;35:675–81.
2. Geavlete P, Georgescu D, Nita G, Mirciulescu V, Cauni V. Complications of 2735 retrograde semirigid ureteroscopy procedures: a single-center experience. J Endourol. 2006;20:179–85.
3. Perez Castro E, Osther PJ, Jinga V, Razvi H, Stravodimos KG, Parikh K, et al. Differences in ureteroscopic stone treatment and outcomes for distal, mid-, proximal, or multiple ureteral locations: the Clinical Research Office of the Endourological Society ureteroscopy global study. Eur Urol. 2014;66:102–9.
4. De La Rosette J, Denstedt J, Geavlete P, Keeley F, Matsuda T, Pearle M, CROES URS Study Group. The clinical research office of the endourological society ureteroscopy global study: indications, complications, and outcomes in 11,885 patients. J Endourol. 2014;28:131–9.
5. Traxer O, Thomas A. Prospective evaluation and classification of ureteral wall injuries resulting from insertion of a ureteral access sheath during retrograde intrarenal surgery. J Urol. 2013;189:580–4.
6. Rubenstein RA, Zhao LC, Loeb S, Shore DM, Nadler RB. Prestenting improves ureteroscopic stone-free rates. J Endourol. 2007;21:1277–80.
7. Netsch C, Knipper S, Bach T, Herrmann TR, Gross AJ. Impact of preoperative ureteral stenting on stone-free rates of ureteroscopy for nephroureterolithiasis: a matched-paired analysis of 286 patients. Urology. 2012;80:1214–9.
8. Turk C, Petrik A, Sarica K, Seitz C, Skolarikos A, Straub M, et al. EAU guidelines on interventional treatment for urolithiasis. Eur Urol. 2016;69:475–82.
9. Assimos D, Krambeck A, Miller NL, Monga M, Murad MH, Nelson CP, et al. Surgical management of stones: American Urological Association/ Endourological Society guideline, PART II. J Urol. 2016;196:1161–9.
10. Koo KC, Yoon JH, Park NC, Lee HS, Ahn HK, Lee KS, et al. The impact of preoperative alpha-adrenergic antagonists on ureteral access sheath insertion force and the upper limit of force required to avoid ureteral

mucosal injury: a randomized controlled study. J Urol. 2018;199:1622–30.

11. Dickstein RJ, Kreshover JE, Babayan RK, Wang DS. Is a safety wire necessary during routine flexible ureteroscopy? J Endourol. 2010;24:1589–92.
12. Eandi JA, Hu B, Low RK. Evaluation of the impact and need for use of a safety guidewire during ureteroscopy. J Endourol. 2008;22:1653–8.
13. Ulvik O, Rennesund K, Gjengsto P, Wentzel-Larsen T, Ulvik NM. Ureteroscopy with and without safety guide wire: should the safety wire still be mandatory? J Endourol. 2013;27:1197–202.
14. Wang H, Man L, Li G, Huang G, Liu N, Wang J. Meta-analysis of stenting versus non-stenting for the treatment of ureteral stones. PLoS One. 2017;12:e0167670.
15. Schoenthaler M, Buchholz N, Farin E, Ather H, Bach C, Bach T, et al. The post-Ureteroscopic lesion scale (PULS): a multicenter video-based evaluation of inter-rater reliability. World J Urol. 2014;32(4):1033–40.
16. Smith AD, Preminger GM, Kavoussi LR, Badlani GH, Rastinehad AR. Smith's textbook of endourology. 4th ed. Wiley; 2018. https://doi.org/10.1002/9781119245193.
17. Assimos D, Krambeck A, Miller NL, Monga M, Murad MH, Nelson CP, et al. Surgical Management of Stones: American Urological Association/Endourological Society guideline, PART I. J Urol. 2016;196:1153–60.
18. Mariappan P, Smith G, Bariol SV, Moussa SA, Tolley DA. Stone and pelvic urine culture and sensitivity are better than bladder urine as predictors of urosepsis following percutaneous nephrolithotomy: a prospective clinical study. J Urol. 2005;173:1610–4.
19. Lo CW, Yang SS, Hsieh CH, Chang SJ. Effectiveness of prophylactic antibiotics against post-ureteroscopic lithotripsy infections: systematic review and meta-analysis. Surg Infect. 2015;16:415–20.
20. Chew BH, Flannigan R, Kurtz M, Gershman B, Arsovska O, Paterson RF, et al. A single dose of intraoperative antibiotics is sufficient to prevent urinary tract infection during ureteroscopy. J Endourol. 2016;30:63–8.
21. Rehman J, Monga M, Landman J, Lee DI, Felfela T, Conradie MC, et al. Characterization of intrapelvic pressure during ureteropyeloscopy with ureteral access sheaths. Urology. 2003;61:713–8.
22. Uchida Y, Takazawa R, Kitayama S, Tsujii T. Predictive risk factors for systemic inflammatory response syndrome following ureteroscopic laser lithotripsy. Urolithiasis. 2018;46:375–81.
23. Zhong W, Leto G, Wang L, Zeng G. Systemic inflammatory response syndrome after flexible ureteroscopic lithotripsy: a study of risk factors. J Endourol. 2015;29:25–8.
24. Auge BK, Pietrow PK, Lallas CD, Raj GV, Santa-Cruz RW, Preminger GM. Ureteral access sheath provides protection against elevated renal pressures during routine flexible ureteroscopic stone manipulation. J Endourol. 2004;18:33–6.

Part IV

Percutaneous Nephrolithotomy

Percutaneous Nephrolithotomy: Preparation and Procedure Overview

12

Bannakij Lojanapiwat

Abstract

Patient's preparation is the important step of PCNL procedure. Hemostasis and urine bacteriologic and radiologic assessment are the key procedure of patient's preparation. Patient's selection, experience of the surgeon, and surgical steps including anesthesia, positioning, renal access, tract dilatation, stone disintegration, and nephrostomy tube placement are the important factors of the surgical outcome.

Keywords

Percutaneous nephrolithotomy · Preparation Procedure

Patient's preparation is one of the important steps of PCNL procedure to achieve the best surgical outcome of high success rate and low complication.

12.1 Patient's Preparation

Complete history and physical examination are the important initial evaluation in all patients who are being considered for PCNL. This information can identify patients who have absolute contraindication for this procedure such as active urinary tract infection, uncorrected coagulopathy, the current usage of medication that affect coagulogram (aspirin, coumadin, and other anti-platelet medications), and general conditions that are suitable for anesthesia of procedure.

All patients need appropriate hemostasis evaluation, urine bacteriologic assessment, and radiologic assessment. General preoperative laboratory evaluation is essential for all patients including a complete blood count (CBC), serum electrolyte, renal function tests, and urinalysis.

12.2 Hemostasis Assessment

Hemostasis evaluation with any bleeding problem such as prothrombin time (PT), partial thromboplastin time (PTT), and platelet count should be done especially in patients who are predisposing to coagulopathy, history of prolonged bleeding, and liver disease. Aspirin should be discontinued 1 week prior to the procedure. A platelet count should be corrected above 80,000 cells per ml prior procedure. Coumadin must be discontinued and monitored with PT and PTT level. Subcutaneous heparin should be administered in patients with the high risk of venous thrombosis.

B. Lojanapiwat (✉)
Chiang Mai University, Chiang Mai, Thailand

A. C.F. Ng et al. (eds.), *Practical Management of Urinary Stone*,
https://doi.org/10.1007/978-981-16-4193-0_12

12.3 Urine Bacteriologic Assessment

PCNL is categorized as clean-contaminated or contaminated procedure. Postoperative bacteriuria can occur even in patient with preoperative sterile urine especially in those without prophylactic antibiotic. The incidence of post-PCNL fever is 20–35%, and post-PCNL bacteremia is 0–59%, so the postoperative fever is not an indicator of postoperative urinary tract infection. Several studies demonstrated the important role of intraoperative urine and stone culture. This information is very helpful for choosing appropriate postoperative antibiotic regimen [1–3].

Two multicenter global studies under the Clinical Research Office of the Endourological Society (CROES) reported the complication following PCNL. Among all complications, fever is the most common complication. However, most of them were minor and can be managed with medication. The criteria of postoperative fever were the body temperature higher than 38.5 °C, which was noted in 10% of the cases even if the patients received preoperative antibiotic prophylaxis. The percentage of post-PCNL fever in patients with positive and negative urine culture was 18.2% and 8.8%, respectively. Most patients with post-PCNL fever were significantly increased with several factors such as long duration of hospitalization and post-PCNL nephrostomy placement [2, 3]. Risk factors affecting infection complication following PCNL divided into preoperative factors (positive preoperative urine culture, positive intraoperative urine culture, stone size), intraoperative factors (renal pelvic pressure, operative time), and postoperative factors (nephrostomy tube placement, antibiotic administration) [1, 3].

Prophylaxis antibiotics are recommended in all patients with PCNL procedure and even negative preoperative urine cultures. The European Association of Urology (EAU) guideline supports the administration of prophylactic antibiotic in all PCNL patients (level 1 b, grade A), and long-term postoperative antibiotic at least 4 days should be given in patients with infected stones, recent history of UTI, and positive urine culture [4].

The common organisms are enterobacteria, enterococci, and staphylococci. The recommended antibiotic prophylaxis is trimethoprim/sulfamethoxazole, cephalosporin, aminopenicillin/beta-lactamase inhibitor, or fluoroquinolone. The best choice of prophylactic antibiotic is a susceptible one of antibiogram of each hospital [4].

12.4 Radiologic Assessment

Radiologic assessment of anatomy and function of both kidneys for the detail of stone, degree of hydronephrosis, and anatomy of pelvicalyceal system is very important prior to the procedure. Recent preoperative plain kidney–urinary–bladder (KUB) radiography and retrograde pyelography are for patients with decreased renal function. These radiographic investigations demonstrate the detail of size, number, and location of the stone as well as establishing the preoperative renal function and other pathologies.

The recent practice, the routine usage of helical computed tomography (CT) (Fig. 12.1) for preoperative radiographic assessment of patients with urolithiasis, has eliminated the use of intravenous pyelography (IVP) or retrograde pyelography (RP). CT urography can demonstrate all details of anatomy and renal function. The main advantage of helical CT over the other investigation is the ability of CT for assessing the spatial relation of the kidney to the stone and also the relationship of the kidney to adjacent retroperitoneal and peritoneal structure. CT urography is a very important tool in patients who are suspecting to have a retrorenal colon (less than 1% of all patients) especially patients with history of jejunoileal bypass, spinal cord injury, and spinal deformities such as severe scoliosis. This information is very important to the prevention of colon injury during the procedure. The benefit of CT urography is also found in patients with ectopic kidneys that are both congenital and iatrogenic (renal allograft, autotransplantation) and patients with dysmorphic body habitus (spinal dysraphism).

Retrograde pyelography may be required to demonstrate renal anatomy in patients with impaired kidney function and performed at the time in the surgical field for detail of calyceal anatomy in selection of renal access. Radionuclide may be required in selected patients such as impaired renal function to evaluate differential renal function especially in patients with staghorn calculi. If there is concern about stone migration, immediate plain kidney–urinary–bladder (KUB) film should be obtained at the time of procedure.

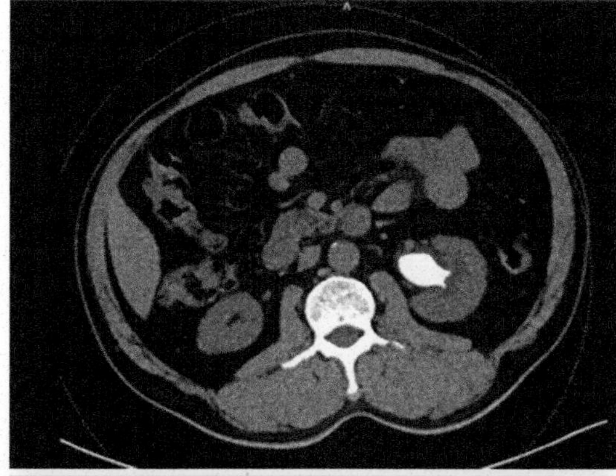

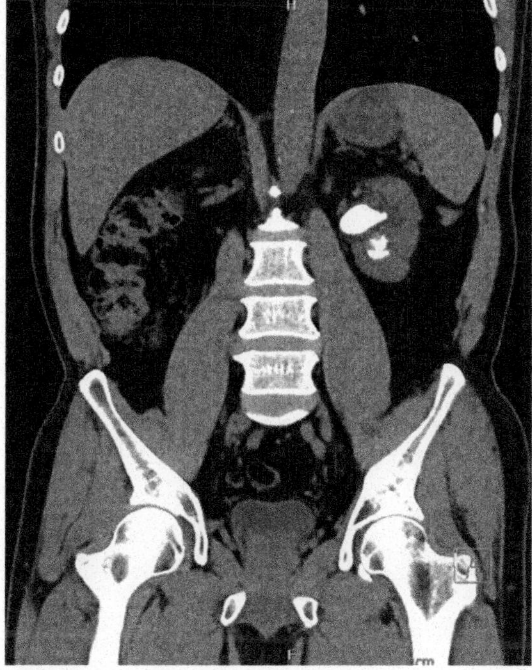

Fig. 12.1 Non-contrast CAT scan demonstrated left partial staghorn stone

12.5 Assessment of Elderly Patients

There is high prevalence of comorbidity and single kidney in elderly patients (age >65 years old). Mainly comorbidities are diabetes mellitus, hypertension, and high level of ASA classification. The study demonstrates no difference in success rate, operative time, length of hospital stays, auxiliary treatment, and general complication. Only sepsis is a more frequent common complication, so preoperative evaluation for prevention of infectious complication is very important in elderly PCNL patients [5].

12.6 Classification Patient for General Assessment by Stone Nomogram

Despite advances in surgical techniques and technology, PCNL for treatment of large renal stone may not always result in the optimal goal of stone free (success rate) and risk of complication. Nowadays, in research and clinical practice, the information of success rate and complication can be predicted by nomogram. This is very important for both surgeons and patients in surgical planning and patient's counseling. Nomograms are consisted of the Guy's Stone Scoring (GSS) system, the STONE nephrometry scoring system, and the CROES (Clinical Research Office of Endourological Society) nomogram [6, 7]. Guy's Stone Score (GSS) is quite simple and reliable nomogram in prediction success rate and possible complication in general PCNL procedure and upper pole access PCNL. GSS nomogram is classified into four grades according to the complexity of the stone and anatomy of the collecting system. More complex cases are usually being in grade 3 or grade 4. PCNL in patients with GSS grade 3 or grade 4 stone should be performed in high patient volume center and more expertise [6].

12.7 Anesthesia

PCNL can be performed under general, epidural block or local anesthesia. Teamwork of surgeons and anesthesia are very important in optimizing the outcome of PCNL.

General anesthesia is the technique of choice of PCNL anesthesia especially in long operative time due to its best way of protecting the airway in the prone position. Of the upper pole access, general anesthesia is preferred due to the permission of an anesthesiologist controlling the respiratory movement in the prevention of pulmonary complication.

Regional epidural anesthesia is an alternative technique compared to general anesthesia. The advantages of regional anesthesia are less early postoperative pain, less adverse effects from medication of general anesthesia, and more patient satisfaction. The disadvantage of this technique is the chance of high block to control renal pain. The problem with vasovagal reaction can occur when the renal pelvis is distending during regional epidural anesthesia [8].

Local anesthesia is usually performed with intravenous sedation and analgesics. It may be an option if regional or general anesthesia is contraindicated. The technique of local anesthesia could be done by using a 23-gauge spinal needle injection along the access tract from the skin to the renal capsule or using an 8.3Fr anesthetic injection catheter with multiple side holes.

A meta-analysis and review demonstrated that there were several advantages of regional anesthesia compared to general anesthesia in terms of fluoroscopy time, surgical duration, blood transfusion, postoperative pain/analgesic requirement, and length of hospital stay without the increase of complication. Due to regional anesthesia's favorable hemodynamic profile and lower cost, this technique may be an alternative anesthesia in PCNL [9].

12.8 The Role of Anesthesiologist in Upper Access PCNL

After the upper pole access PCNL, surgeons and anesthesiologists should be aware about pulmonary complication including hydrothorax or pneumothorax. Carefully monitoring the airway pressures, tidal carbon dioxide level, and oxygen saturation is necessary. Hemodynamic assessment should be frequently performed to detect acute blood loss or blood dilution.

12.8.1 Position

Prone position is the position of choice since the establishment of PCNL procedure. Recently, the alternative positions are the supine and lateral positions. There are no clear overall benefits for one position over another; each modality is equally feasible and safe. The surgeon's preference is the prime indication to one over the other. There are some PCNL cases in which supine PCNL is preferable for obese patients (Fig. 12.2) [10].

12.8.2 Renal Access

A general overview of the procedure will be given here with more detail discussion in the following chapters.

The perfect percutaneous tract into the collecting system is one of the most important steps for the PCNL procedure. This step required radiographic imaging guidance such as ultrasonographic guidance, fluoroscopic guidance, endoscope guidance, and CT/MRI guidance. Each percutaneous renal guidance technique has

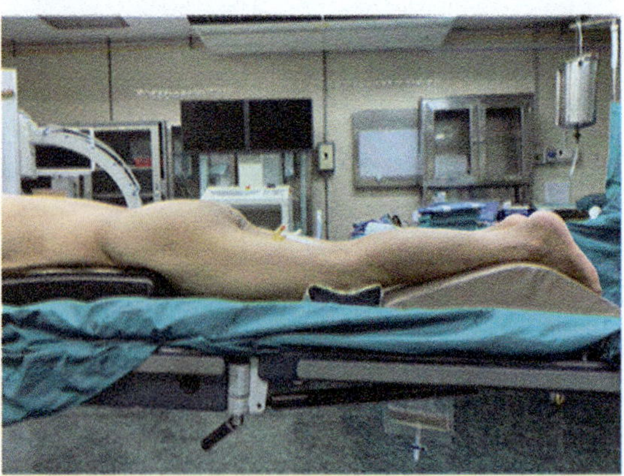

Fig. 12.2 Prone position of PCNL

its advantage and disadvantage compared with the other. No single technique is ideal for all situations [11].

12.8.3 Ultrasonographic Guidance

Primary advantages of ultrasonographic guidance are less radiation, the ability to image structure between the skin and kidney, and no need of contrast media. This technique is safe for pregnancy and pediatric patients. This guidance can avoid intrarenal vascular injury when combined with color Doppler ultrasound. However, ultrasonographic guidance needs operator skill and technical difficulty especially in none or mild dilated collecting system.

12.8.4 Fluoroscopic Guidance

Fluoroscopic guidance is quite familiar to most urologists and can demonstrate anatomical details. Radiation safety is one of the concerns during this technique (Fig. 12.3).

12.8.5 Endoscopic Guidance

As the principle of flexible ureteroscope-assisted retrograde nephrostomy, the advantage of the technique is continuous visualization of all steps of PCNL. The desired calyx can be selected under direct vision. The tip of the needle is visualized and monitored by fluoroscopy and endoscope. This technique improves safety of renal access, but the cost and operator experience are the disadvantages of this technique.

12.8.6 Computed Tomography (CT) Guidance/MRI Guidance

Computed tomography guidance is essential in specific patients with morbid obesity and organomegaly such as splenomegaly/hepatomegaly, history of previous major intra-abdominal surgery, severe skeletal anomalies of scoliosis, or kyphosis. The advantage of MRI guidance over CT guidance is no radiation exposure, but limitation of the technique is routine clinical practice.

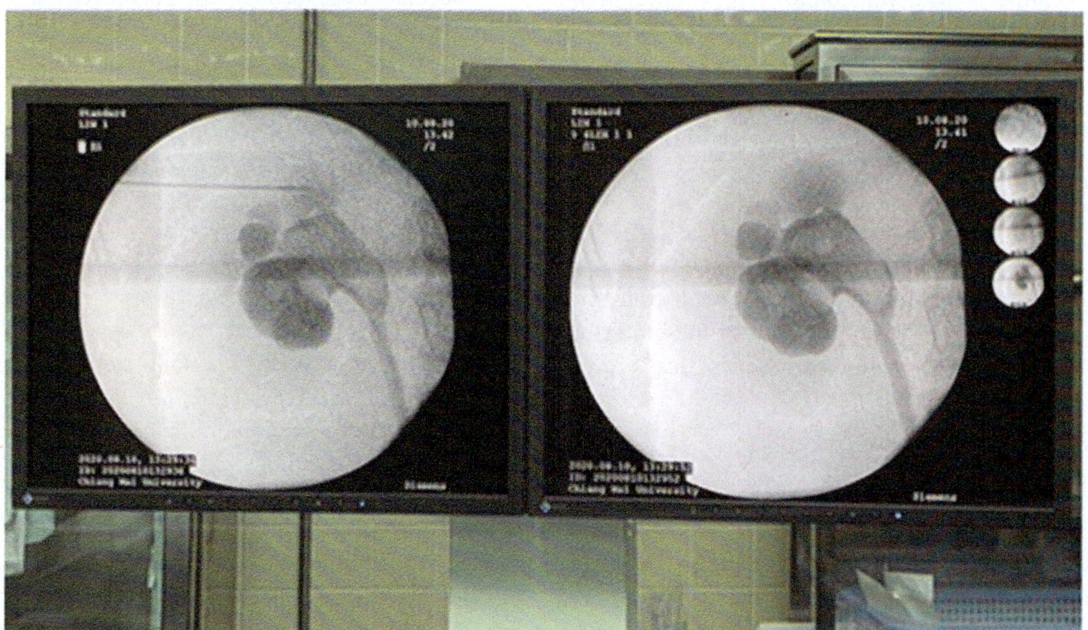

Fig. 12.3 Intraoperative fluoroscopy before upper pole access

The two most common modalities in renal access guidance are ultrasonography and fluoroscopy with each advantage and disadvantage over the other. Additional color Doppler ultrasound shows advantage in avoidance vascular injury resulting in decreasing intraoperative and postoperative hemorrhage. CT guidance is only for complex cases. Endoscope guidance is the most safe technique in renal access, but cost and experience of surgeons need to be considered [11].

12.8.7 The Ideal Puncture Site

The ideal site of puncture of PCNL depends on the position of the stone and choice of associated procedure to obtain the best surgical outcome:

- Stone in the renal pelvis: Tract is through the middle or lower calyx.
- Stone in the calyx: Tract is through the stone-bearing calix peripheral to the stone.
- Staghorn stone: Tract is through the upper calyx.
- Upper ureteric stone: Tract is through the middle or upper pole.
- Stone in the diverticulum: Tract is through the diverticulum.
- Ureteropelvic junction obstruction or upper ureteral structure: Tract is through the middle or upper calyx for endopyelotomy/ endoureterotomy.

One of the important steps for the success in PCNL procedure is renal access. The causes of access failure are non-dilated renal collecting system, obscuring the location of the collecting system, and the impacted stones that prevent guidewire manipulation.

12.8.8 Upper Pole Renal Access

Upper pole access is a shorter and easier access route due to upper pole of the kidney aligned medially and posterior to the lower pole. The upper pole access provides a straight tract along the long axis of the kidney and the ability to reach most part of the collecting system during manipulation of the rigid nephroscope. The upper pole access technique needs coordination with anesthetists for controlling breathing to prevent intercostal vessel and pulmonary injury [12].

The indication of upper pole access is:

- Staghorn calculi
- Buck of large upper pole calculi
- Obesity patients
- Anomaly kidney such as horseshoe kidney
- Multiple separate lower pole calculi
- Large upper ureteric stone
- Ureteropelvic junction or proximal ureteral pathology

The details of the upper pole access technique are as follows:

- Need of coordination with the anesthetists for controlling inspiration/expiration.
  - The point of the puncture should be done in the lower half of intercostal space to avoid intercostal vessel injury.
  - The needle is passed through the retroperitoneum during full expiration, while the needle passes through renal parenchyma to the collecting system during deep inspiration for downward displacement of the kidney.
  - An Amplatz sheath should be used in all cases to maintain low-pressure irrigation (Fig. 12.4).

12.8.9 Tract Dilatation

Tract dilatation is the important step during PCNL procedure. The most common used instruments are metal telescopic dilatation (MTD), Amplatz sheath dilation, high-pressure balloon dilation, and one-shot dilation [13–15].

Standard PCNL with standard size PCNL is challenging with bleeding complication. A systematic review and meta-analysis demonstrated that the shorter fluoroscopy time and lesser hemoglobin level decrease in one-shot dilation compared with metal telescope dilatation [14].

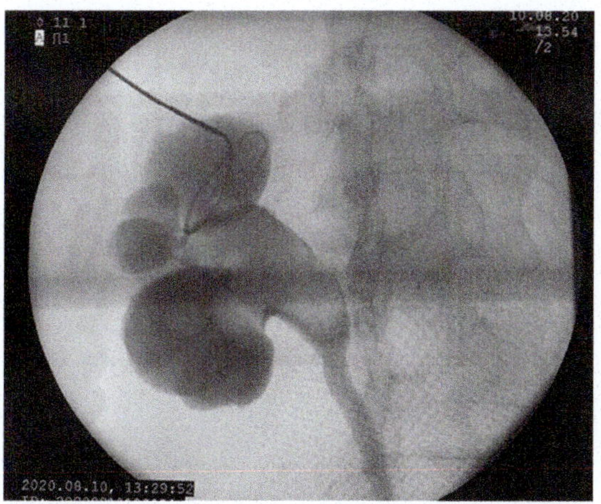

Fig. 12.4 Upper pole access during PCNL of partial staghorn calculi

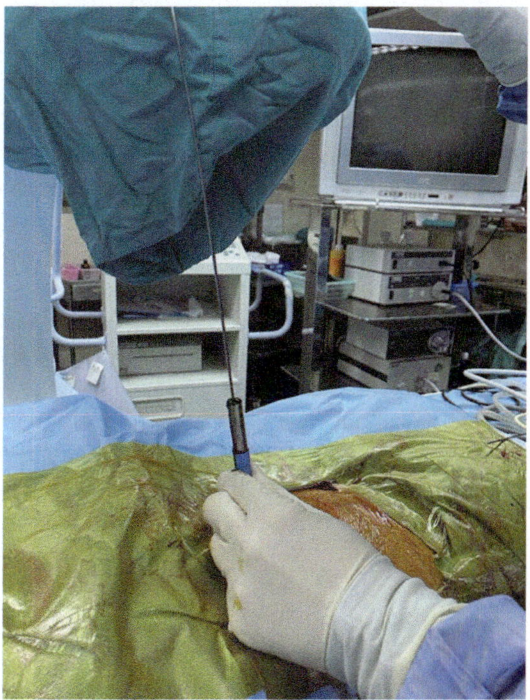

Fig. 12.5 Telescopic metal dilator in the step of renal dilatation

Previous open renal surgery is one key factor for choosing the type of dilators. Among patients without previous open surgery, balloon dilator shows a lower transfusion rate and shorter surgical time compared with Amplatz dilator. For patients with a history of open surgery, one-shot dilator and metal telescope dilator are used due to scar around the kidney. One-shot dilator is safer in the aspect of shorter tract dilation fluoroscopy time and a lesser decrease in blood loss. Recently, one-shot dilator can be applied for most patients who undergo PCNL procedure (Fig. 12.5) [16, 17].

For detailed discussion of individual devices, please refer to the previous chapter.

12.8.10 Intracorporeal Lithotripters

PCNL for removing large renal calculi usually needs intracorporeal lithotripsy to permit the safe extraction of calculus fragment. The efficacy of lithotripter is very important followed by the size and flexibility of the probe [18–20].

Nowadays, the intracorporeal lithotripter consists of:

- Ballistic lithotripsy
- Ultrasonic lithotripsy
- Combined ballistic and ultrasonic lithotripsy
- Laser lithotripsy
- Electrohydraulic lithotripsy

12.8.11 Technique of Intracorporeal Lithotripsy

All instruments should be activated only when the operative field is clear. Surgeons should see the stone and position before activation. Fixation of the stone in the kidney is not difficult for ballistic lithotripsy. For ultrasonic lithotripsy, the stone should be trapped between the probe and urothelium; then make a gentle pressure to the stone to enhance fragmentation followed by evacuation of the small stone.

The technique of laser lithotripsy is simple by just placing the fiber contact to the stone surface before activation. A short break is necessary between activations due to “the snowstorm” by stone fragments. These techniques of laser lithotripsy are fragmentation, vaporization, and popcorn technique that was used in different situations.

12.9 Nephrostomy Tube Placement

Nephrostomy tube is usually placed at the end of the PCNL procedure. The purpose of nephrostomy tube placement is the tamponade of nephrostomy tract to prevent postoperative bleeding and adequate drainage following the procedure. The tract can be used for the secondary nephroscope to remove retained stone. Recently, in selected cases, tubeless PCNL can be performed without the increase of complications. Several techniques of tubeless placement are reported such as tubeless PCNL with only postoperative external ureteral catheter [21], postoperative DJ stent [22–24], or total tubeless PCNL [25, 26].

The indication for tubeless PCNL is for selected patients who has no significant bleeding or extravasation, only single access, no obstructed renal unit and secondary nephroscope is not required. Tubeless PCNL is a good option in noncomplicated PCNL patients with more cost effectivity. This technique significantly reduced hospital stay time, postoperative analgesic requirement, lower urine leakage, and shorter time returning normal activities without compromising the efficacy. This technique also can be applied in challenging PCNL cases such as patients with staghorn stones, horseshoe kidney, ectopic kidney, elderly, and patients who required supracostal access [27]. Hemostatic agents might not be necessary in tubeless PCNL (Fig. 12.6).

Standard PCNL with postoperative normal-size nephrostomy tube causes significant postoperative pain. Postoperative pain affects postoperative quality of life with the increase of postoperative complication, delayed mobilization, and prolonged hospitalization. Several techniques have been used to overcome post-PCNL pain such as PCNL with small-size nephrostomy tube, various postoperative analgesic regimens, tubeless PCNL, mini-PCNL, 0.5% bupivacaine intercostal nerve block, and local or capsule analgesic infiltration (Fig. 12.7).

Even tubeless PCNL demonstrates the advantage of less postoperative pain, but this technique can be used only selected patients with specific indication. The study demonstrated the beneficial

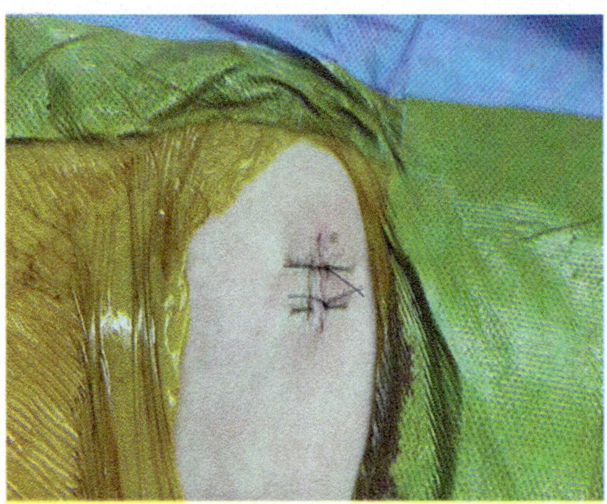

Fig 12.7 Skin closure during tubeless PCNL

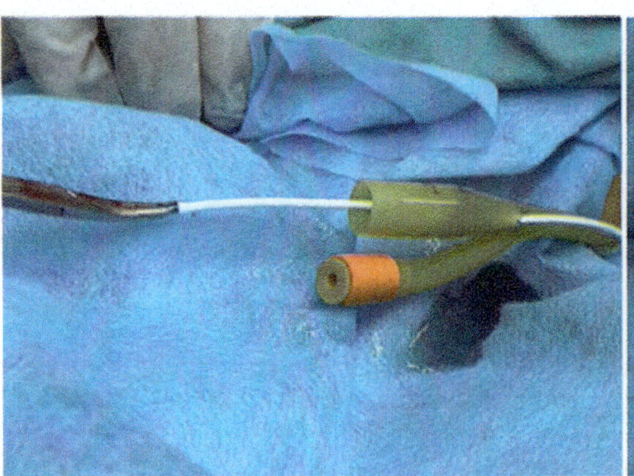

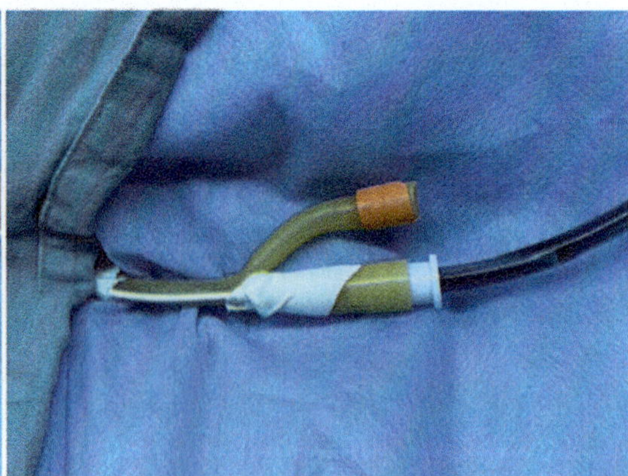

Fig. 12.6 Tubeless PCNL with an external ureteral catheter

effect of 0.25% peritubal local anesthetic infiltration with bupivacaine in alleviating immediate postoperative pain following PCNL and even supracostal access. Lower early postoperative pain, lower number of anesthetic usage, longer time of the first analgesic requirement, and increase patient's satisfaction were found in patients following standard PCNL with peritubal local infiltration. This technique is performed under fluoroscopic guidance, and the 23-gauge, 90-mm spinel needle was inserted to the renal capsule along the nephrectomy tube at 6 and 12 o'clock from the renal capsule, muscle, subcutaneous tissue, and skin [28].

References

1. Lojanapiwat B, Kitirattrakarn P. Role of preoperative and intraoperative factors in mediating infection complication following percutaneous nephrolithotomy. Urol Int. 2011;86:448–52.
2. Gonen M, Turan H, Ozturk B, et al. Factors affecting fever following percutaneous nephrolithotomy: a prospective clinical study. J Endourol. 2008;22:2135–8.
3. Lojanapiwat B. Infective complication following percutaneous nephrolithotomy. Urological Science. 2016;27:8–12.
4. Türk C (Chair), Neisius A, Petrik A, et al. EAU guideline 2020: urolithiasis
5. Nakamon T, Kitirattrakarn P, Lojanapiwat B. Outcomes of percutaneous nephrolithotomy: comparison of elderly and younger patients. Int Braz J Urol. 2013;39:692–700.
6. Lojanapiwat B, Rod-Ong P, Kitirattrakarn P, Chongruksut W. Guy's Stone Score (GSS) based on intravenous pyelogram (IVP) findings predicting upper pole access percutaneous nephrolithotomy (PCNL) outcomes. Adv Urol. 2016; https://doi.org/10.1155/2016/5157930.
7. Elkoushy MA, Metwally AH, Noureldin YA. Implications of different nephrolithometry scoring systems on clinical practice of endourologists: an international web-based survey. Arab J Urol. 2016;14:216–22.
8. Tangpaitoon T, Nisoog C, Lojanapiwat B. Efficacy and safety of percutaneous nephrolithotomy (PCNL): a prospective and randomized study comparing regional epidural anesthesia with general anesthesia. Int Braz J Urol. 2012;38:504–11.
9. Pu C, Wang J, Tang Y, et al. The efficacy and safety of percutaneous nephrolithotomy under general anesthesia versus regional anesthesia: a systemic review and meta-analysis. Urolithiasis. 2015;43:455–66.
10. Astroza G, Lipkin M, Neisius A, CROES PNL Study Group, et al. Effect of supine vs prone position on outcomes of percutaneous nephrolithotomy in staghorn calculi: results from the Clinical Research Office of the Endourology Society Study. Urology. 2013;82:1240–4.
11. Lojanapiwat B. The ideal puncture approach for PCNL: fluoroscopy, ultrasound or endoscopy? Indian J Urol. 2013;29:208–13.
12. Lojanapiwat B, Lojanapiwat B, Prasopsuk S. Upper-pole access for percutaneous nephrolithotomy: comparison of supracostal and infracostal approaches. J Endourol. 2006;20:491–4.
13. Dehong C, Liangren L, Huawei L, et al. A comparison among four tract dilation methods of percutaneous nephrolithotomy: a systematic review and meta-analysis. Urolithiasis. 2013;41:523–30.
14. Peng PX, Lai SC, Ding ZS, et al. One-shot dilation versus serial dilation technique for access in percutaneous nephrolithotomy: a systematic review and meta-analysis. BMJ Open. 2019;9:e025871.
15. Srivastava A, Singh S, Dhayal IR, et al. A prospective randomized study comparing the four tract dilation methods of percutaneous nephrolithotomy. World J Urol. 2017;35:803–7.
16. Lojanapiwat B. Does previous open nephrolithotomy affect the efficacy and safety of tubeless percutaneous nephrolithotomy? Urol Int. 2010;85:42–6.
17. Lojanapiwat B. Previous open nephrolithotomy: does it affect percutaneous nephrolithotomy techniques and outcome? J Endourol. 2006;20:17–20.
18. Scotland KB, Kroczak T, Pace KT, et al. Stone technology: intracorporeal lithotripters. World J Urol. 2017;35:1347–51.
19. Lowe G, Knudsen BE. Ultrasonic, pneumatic and combination intracorporeal lithotripsy for percutaneous nephrolithotomy. J Endourol. 2009;23:1663–8.
20. York NE, Borofsky MS, Chew BH, et al. Randomized controlled trial comparing three different modalities of lithotrites for intracorporeal lithotripsy in percutaneous nephrolithotomy. J Endourol. 2017;31:1145–51.
21. Lojanapiwat B, Soonthornphan S, Wudhikarn S. Tubeless percutaneous nephrolithotomy in selected patients. J Endourol. 2001;15:711–3.
22. Xun Y, Wang Q, Hu H, et al. Tubeless versus standard percutaneous nephrolithotomy: an update meta-analysis. BMC Urol. 2017;17(1):102.
23. Tirtayasa PMW, Yuri P, Birowo P, et al. Safety of tubeless or totally tubeless drainage and nephrostomy tube as a drainage following percutaneous nephrolithotomy: a comprehensive review. Asian J Surg. 2017;40:419–23.
24. Agrawal MS, Agarwal M. Percutaneous nephrolithotomy: large tube, small tube, tubeless, or totally tubeless? Indian J Urol. 2013;29:219–24.
25. Zhong Q, Zheng C, Mo J, et al. Total tubeless versus standard percutaneous nephrolithotomy: a meta-analysis. J Endourol. 2013;27:420–6.
26. Choi SW, Kim KS, Kim JH, et al. Totally tubeless versus standard percutaneous nephrolithotomy for

renal stones: analysis of clinical outcomes and cost. J Endourol. 2014;28:1487–94.
27. Jun-Ou J, Lojanapiwat B. Supracostal access: does it affect tubeless percutaneous nephrolithotomy efficacy and safety? Int Braz J Urol. 2010;36:171–6.
28. Lojanapiwat B, Chureemas T, Kittirattarakarn P. The efficacy of peritubal analgesic infiltration in postoperative pain following percutaneous nephrolithotomy - a prospective randomized controlled study. Int Braz J Urol. 2015;41:945–52.

How to Perform Renal Puncture: Fluoroscopic Approach

13

Palaniappan Sundaram, Henry Ho Sun Sien, and Michael Y.C. Wong

Abstract

Percutaneous access is performed in a variety of positions; however, most commonly this is done in the prone position. Access can be guided with various modalities. Fluoroscopy remains the most readily and widely available resource in the operating room. Hence the knowledge of gaining percutaneous access using fluoroscopy is essential for the endourologist. We describe the two techniques often used in the routine practice. Training under a mentor and case volume is crucial in learning this technique as the primary aim is to target a calyx at an unknown depth using only two-dimensional images obtained with fluoroscopy.

P. Sundaram
Department of Urology, Sengkang General Hospital, Sengkang, Singapore
e-mail: palaniappan.sundaram@singhealth.com.sg

H. H. S. Sien
Department of Urology, Singapore General Hospital, Singapore, Singapore
e-mail: henry.ho.s.s@singhealth.com.sg

M. Y.C. Wong (✉)
International Urology, Fertility and Gynecology Centre, Mount Elizabeth Hospital, Singapore, Singapore
e-mail: email@drmichaelwong.com

13.1 Introduction

Access to the collecting system is essential in percutaneous nephrolithotomy (PCNL). Without the perfect access, the majority of the surgery will be fraught with multiple problems. In this chapter, we endeavour to lay out the principles of percutaneous access using fluoroscopy. This is the most preferred method of access by most endourologists.

13.2 Accurate Renal Access Is Crucial to the Outcome of Surgery

PCNL has indeed come a long way since its humble beginnings in the 1980s when it was proposed as an alternative to open nephrolithotomy. The technology associated with the technique has also evolved tremendously with miniaturisation, better optics and lithotriptors. However, the most integral part of PCNL will always be the puncture and entry into the pelvicalyceal system. This enables the procedure to progress without the dreaded vascular injuries and complete the procedure with a better stone-free rate. Other access-related complications include injury to adjacent organs and failure of access which may prevent the planned procedure altogether. Many strategies were evaluated to achieve an ideal

A. C.F. Ng et al. (eds.), *Practical Management of Urinary Stone*,
https://doi.org/10.1007/978-981-16-4193-0_13

access. The most important of these was the learning curve in order to master the technique of access.

13.3 Why Urologist Is the Better Person Than Radiologist

Interventional radiologists have been traditionally employed to aid in the access since the beginnings of PCNL. They have either performed it in combination with the urologist in the operating room or in a staged procedure prior to the PCNL. A North American survey of general urologists carried out in 2003 has shown that 62% of the urologists treating stone with PCNL obtain access in the radiology department prior to the PCNL. Another 34% create access with the radiologist in the operating theatre, while only 16% perform access on their own or at times with a radiologist [1]. The reasons cited include the perception that percutaneous access was a radiological procedure which was better performed by the radiologist with better facilities available to them and lack of adequate training for the aspiring endourologist. However this trend has since changed. A more recent survey of endourologists rather than general urologists was performed in 2017, which showed that 82% of respondents obtained their own access [2]. Many studies have shown access-related complications were significantly lower when the urologist creates the access compared to the radiologist [3–5] (8.3% vs 27.8%). Majority of the complications related to access is bleeding. Clearly in the hands of the urologist, this is as low as 5%, whereas it was 16% when the radiologist performed it. In addition, the stone-free rates were significantly higher in this group where the urologist attained percutaneous access (86% vs 61%) [3]. It appears that the understanding of the pelvicalyceal system and the location of the stones result in a more appropriate placement of the access tract. Also, the need for multiple tracts in the PCNL for complex stones may only be determined during the surgery. Therefore, the skill for placing the tract as and when necessary is key to achieving better stone-free rates. This also avoids dependence on the skill and schedule of the radiologist for additional tract placement and allows greater flexibility in the procedure. In summary, it can be all done in the same setting in one location when the urologist performs the access, making the PCNL efficient.

13.4 Number of Cases Required to Learn Technique Well

The learning curve has been described by many authors. It is defined as the time taken to master the skills and expertise required to perform PCNL competently with minimal complications and excellent stone-free rates. There have been studies which determine the additional markers for competence in PCNL [6, 7]. They were operative time, fluoroscopic screening time and radiation dose. By following the progress of a novice surgeon, it was found that after 60 cases, the operative time reached a plateau, while after 115 cases, the fluoroscopy time and radiation dose also levelled off [6].

Training on percutaneous access has to start in residency. It has been investigated and found that trainees who had done significantly more procedures during their residency were more likely to continue with doing percutaneous renal surgery (24 vs 10) [8]. If the residency training was not possible, then a dedicated fellowship in endourology would be necessary.

The traditional method of training whereby theoretical knowledge are gained from books and journals and later apprenticeship under a mentor until one attains proficiency is vastly aided by the wealth of surgical videos available on the Internet. This can be supplemented by training models using animals and cadavers. Another modality is simulator training using inanimate models or virtual reality. This would enable the trainee to practise in an environment without having to worry about the patient outcome. Also, master class workshops present an opportunity to learn from the experts and hone their skills. These approaches should decrease the steep learning curve associated with PCNL. Once trained, it has been proposed that 14–16 cases need to be performed per year so as to maintain their skill levels [9].

13.4.1 Choice of Position: Prone and Supine

PCNL has been performed commonly in a prone position [10]. This was meant to enable access to a larger surgical field which will include an end on access to all posterior calyces, particularly those in the upper pole. Nephrostomy tract length is shorter as the access to the kidney is more direct [11]. In addition, this will allow a wider room for manoeuvring the instruments. This position places the renal pelvis in the dependent position which would allow the collecting system to distend well in order to have an optimal vision. It also had some drawbacks. Injuries specific to the placement of the patient into the prone position on turning have been described: corneal abrasion, hyperextension injuries to the cervical spine and brachial plexus injuries. Airway compromise has been reported, but techniques have been developed to ensure the endotracheal does not slip out. Ventilation has been difficult particularly in the obese patient as chest expansion is curtailed. Cardiac output was reported to decrease due to obstruction of the inferior vena cava and the consequent reduction in venous return. Hence caution has been advised when patients have poor cardiovascular reserve.

The supine position, which was first described in 1987 by Valdivia [12], has evolved over the years to allow endourologist similar capabilities in performing PCNL. The most important benefit has been to avoid the injuries associated with turning the patient. This may in some centres also save operating theatre time. In addition, several other advantages were suggested. Significantly, the supine position has been thought to ventilate the obese patient better as it allows for greater chest expansion compared to the same patient positioned in the prone position. This has been debated often and evidence has been contradictory. Smith and his colleagues in fact found that peak inspiratory pressures were not different between the two positions in obese (body mass index, BMI > 30 kg/m^2) or nonobese patients; however they found that obesity itself was the cause of higher peak pressures [13]. The higher peak pressures were found in obese patients both in supine and prone positions compared to the pressures seen in a patient of normal BMI. That is thought to be related to the reduced chest wall compliance and higher abdominal pressures.

Supine position is more ergonomic and preferable for the surgeon. It allows the surgeon to be seated during the surgery, and as a result the radiation dose to his hands is reduced as he is further away from the fluoroscopy. In addition, it may possibly even achieve better outcomes. Stone fragments preferentially drain out as the sheath is angled towards gravity throughout the procedure. Moreover, it permits for simultaneous antegrade and retrograde intervention. Some have also argued that the risk of colonic injury is less with the supine position [14].

Despite these proposed advantages, PCNL in the supine position remains less popular. The limited exposure of the flank results in poor access to all calyces particularly the upper pole. Kidney in the supine position is more mobile; hence puncture and dilatation may be challenging. The collecting system is often collapsed, so visualisation is difficult in some cases.

The recent meta-analysis on this controversy of prone or supine positioning in PCNL has yielded different results to the previous meta-analyses which stated that the stone-free rates were better in the prone position. Even though the operating time is indeed shorter in the supine PCNL, the stone-free rate is now comparable to that seen in prone PCNL [15]. This is a reflection of the evolution of the supine position to the variety of modified supine positions which has allowed it to overcome the difficulties stated above such as small area for puncture, limited access to the upper pole as well as small room for manipulation of the nephroscope. Furthermore, the combined percutaneous and ureteroscopic procedures improves stone-free rate considerably. The meta-analysis also showed comparable hospital stay and complication rate between the two PCNL positions [15]. However, the debate still remains on whether the treatment of the large stone burden such as complex staghorn stone would be as efficacious in either position.

13.4.2 Guidance for Percutaneous Access: Fluoroscopy, Ultrasound and CT Guidance

The C-arm fluoroscopy is very familiar to the urologist and easily available in most operating theatres. As such, it is preferred not only for percutaneous access but throughout the procedure including guidewire manipulation, tract dilatation, evaluation of residual stone fragment and nephrostogram at the end of the procedure. Though historically fluoroscopy-guided puncture was performed, ultrasound technology is increasingly used for percutaneous access as it avoids harmful radiation. Additionally, adjacent organs such as the spleen, liver and bowel can be visualised such that injury to these can be avoided. The depth of needle entry into the collecting system can be appreciated clearly. The colour Doppler mode can be utilised to avoid injury to large intrarenal vessels. It may be used in situations where the pelvicalyceal system cannot be opacified. This can be either due to inability to insert retrograde ureteric catheter in patients with complex ureteric reconstruction such as ileal conduits or where the stone is completely obstructing resulting in no contrast flowing proximal to the stone [16]. At present, few urologists exclusively use ultrasound alone for access and dilatation. Often they are complementary to each other. The initial access is created using ultrasound, while the tract dilatation is performed using fluoroscopic guidance. There was no difference found in terms of success of access, bleeding, operative time or hospital stay in a recent review [17].

When the access to the collecting system is difficult, even CT-guided percutaneous puncture may be necessary. It has been found to be useful in certain complex instances such as spinal deformities, morbid obesity, presence of retrorenal colon, abnormal renal anatomy such as multiple cysts or angiomyolipoma adjacent to the collecting system and malrotated ectopic kidney. It may also be preferred in a non-dilated pelvicalyceal system [18].

13.4.3 Preoperative Preparations

As preoperative preparation is already covered in the previous chapter, we will focus mainly on the prevention of infection as it is the most common complication related to stone surgery. The incidence of fever post PCNL is about 10%, whereas sepsis is rare (<0.01%) [19]. This can be explained by the release of bacteria during the manipulation of the collecting system and fragmentation of the stone in addition to the bacteria which may enter via the percutaneous tract created during the PCNL. When treating obstructed and infected systems, one has to drain it adequately with a ureteral stent or a nephrostomy tube before performing PCNL. The current recommendation from the International Consultation on Urological Diseases (ICUD) in preventing postoperative infection is a single dose of antibiotic which is as effective as multiple doses when the preoperative urine culture is negative [20]. This antibiotic is chosen according to the local antibiogram. In order to reduce the incidence of resistant bacteria, we need to be mindful and limit the use of antibiotics to those with the higher risk of infection.

Certain preoperative risk factors have been identified to predict for postoperative fever. These include female gender, hydronephrosis, presence of nephrostomy tube, complex stone burden, neurogenic bladder and diabetes mellitus. Furthermore, intraoperative conditions such as longer operative time, multiple access tracts, large volume of irrigation fluid and aspiration of purulent fluid on puncture result in increased rates of infection postoperatively. Hence other ICUD recommendations are to perform a urine culture and treat the positive culture prior to PCNL using culture-directed antibiotics. The duration of treatment can either be 1 week if giving orally or 24 h if administering intravenously prior to surgery [20]. A bladder urine culture which is negative, on the other hand, does not always exclude infection which is present in the pelvicalyceal system or in the stone [21].

13.4.4 Anatomy of Puncture Techniques Using Fluoroscopy

It is absolutely essential to understand the pelvicalyceal system and its relation to the adjacent vascular structures. The avascular Brodel's line lies between the anterior and posterior divisions of the renal artery. It is usually on this line that the posterior calyx is situated. Entry into this posterior calyx also enables the guidewire to manipulate easily into the ureter. The puncture should preferably be made through the papilla and not through the infundibulum or the renal pelvis. Sampaio showed that infundibular punctures result in interlobar vessel injury in 23% to 67% of the kidney endocast models; however in fornix punctures, venous injuries were less than 8%, and no arterial injuries were observed [22]. Direct entry into the renal pelvis must be avoided as large vessels which exist anterior and posterior to the renal pelvis are at risk of injury. This puncture may result in easy dislodgement of the access sheath or nephrostomy tube and prolonged urine leak.

The entry through the skin should be medial to the posterior axillary line. The colon is near the lower pole of the kidney and anterolateral to it. Moreover, one should not puncture too medially as it would be through the paraspinal muscles causing significant pain, and one should also avoid being too close to the ribs as intercostal neurovascular bundle lies on its inferior aspect. Ideal access through the papilla would align the calyx and infundibulum such that the rigid nephroscope can be easily manipulated inside the collecting system without much torque. This causes tears in the renal parenchyma resulting in bleeding.

13.4.5 Positioning

The patient is placed in lithotomy position, and a ureteric catheter is placed using a rigid cystoscope. This allows for retrograde instillation of diluted contrast for opacification of the pelvicalyceal system. An indwelling catheter is placed before turning the patient prone to lie on a padded operating table to prevent pressure injuries. Particular care should be taken to ensure the face, elbow, chest and hips are appropriately protected with foam padding. The feet must be elevated with a pillow to eliminate pressure on the toes. Ensure that the patient is secured to the table with a strap. There should also be consideration for maintenance of temperature using a warm air blanket [23].

Modification of the usual prone position called the prone-flexed position can also be used. The table is flexed 30 to 40 degrees with the patient renal angle placed at the table break. This would increase the availability of the puncture between the 12th rib and posterior iliac crest [24]. The authors found that the kidney is displaced inferiorly in this position; hence a supracostal puncture may be performed from an infracostal site.

Once the patient is in a prone position, the pelvicalyceal system is opacified and distended. The posterior calyces are less dense as the contrast medium is heavier which would preferentially flow into the anterior calyces which are more dense and darker. C-arm rotation towards the surgeon allows the calyces to be differentiated. Posterior calyces shorten and move towards the spine, while the anterior calyces do the converse [24]. Also, air pyelogram can delineate the posterior calyces. As air is lighter than contrast, it will fill the posterior calyces, while the anterior calyces remain filled with dense contrast. This is done by injecting 2–5 ml of air via the ureteric catheter. Currently two access techniques are well documented and presented below.

13.4.6 Triangulation Technique

Triangulation is defined as the use of two points in space to determine the third unknown point which is the targeted calyx. The first point is the point on the skin directly above the target calyx, while the second point is the skin puncture site which is a few centimetres lateral to the first point along the line of puncture, away from the ribs. The puncture line would be along the axis of the infundibulum towards the target calyx [25]. The progress of the needle is monitored with C-arm in 0 degrees (Fig. 13.1) until it reaches the target calyx (Fig. 13.2). Later we will place the C-arm at 30 degrees towards the surgeon. This allows the surgeon to assess the depth of the puncture. An accurate entry into the correct calyx would be confirmed when the fluoroscopic image at 30 degrees is the same as the image obtained at 0 degrees (Fig. 13.3).

It is important to understand that regardless of the depth of the needle puncture, the fluoroscopic image obtained with the C-arm at 0 degree would suggest the needle is in the desired calyx (Fig. 13.4). Only when the C-arm is rotated 30 degrees, the depth of the needle can be assessed. When the needle is seen to be away from the direction that the C-arm has moved, it is superficial in relation to the desired calyx. When the needle is seen closer to the direction that the C-arm has moved, the needle is deeper than the desired calyx (Fig. 13.5). If the needle is either

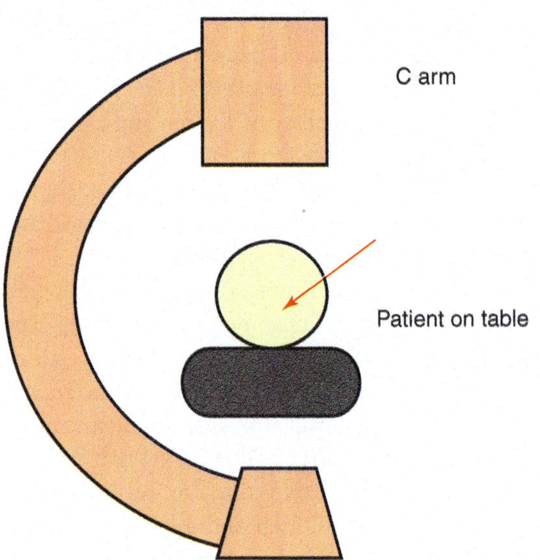

Fig. 13.1 Schematic cross-sectional diagram of the patient on the table and C-arm at 0 degrees. The red arrow represents needle entry into the kidney

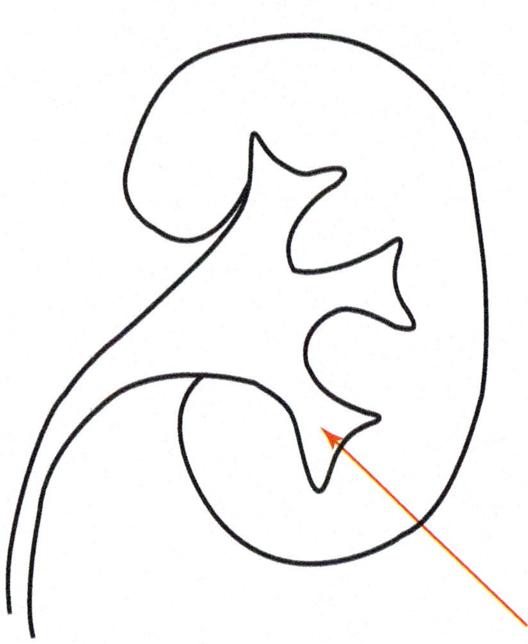

Fig. 13.2 Fluoroscopic image obtained with the C-arm at 0 degrees. The red arrow represents needle entry into the desired calyx

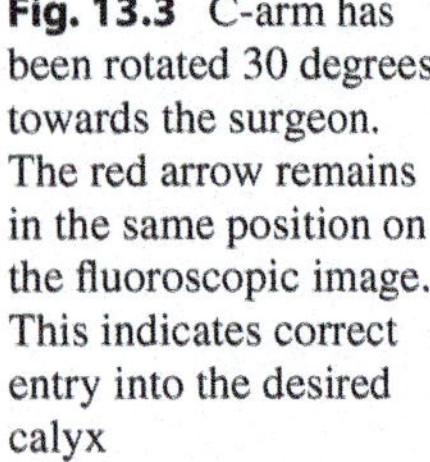

Fig. 13.3 C-arm has been rotated 30 degrees towards the surgeon. The red arrow remains in the same position on the fluoroscopic image. This indicates correct entry into the desired calyx

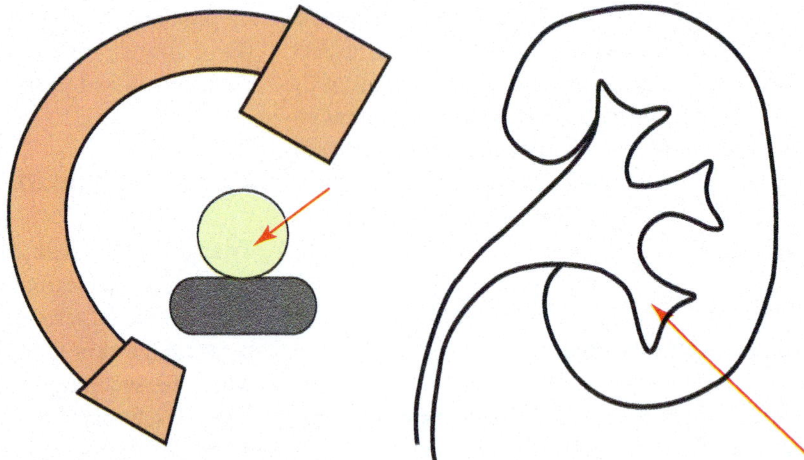

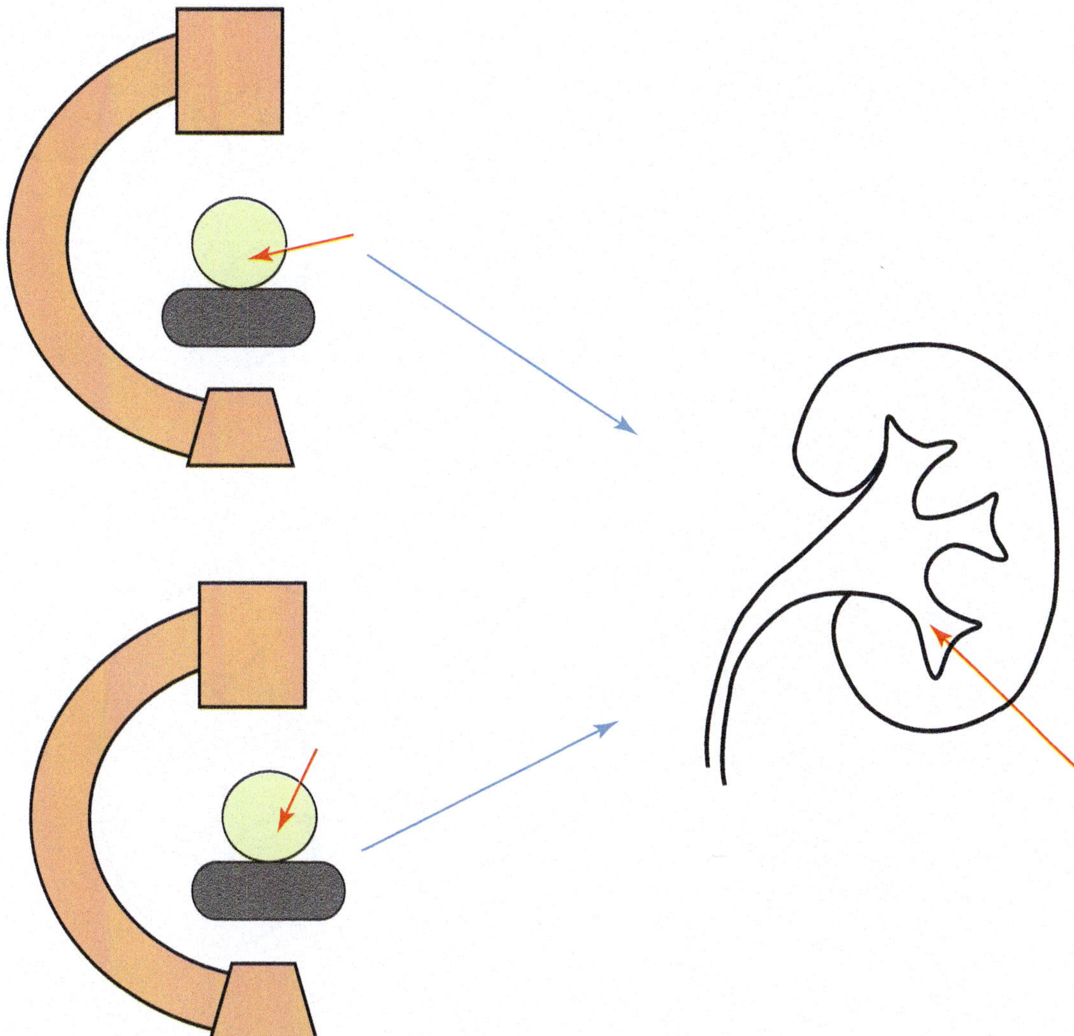

Fig. 13.4 C-arm is at 0 degrees. The red arrow represents needle entry into the kidney, and the top image is a superficial entry, while the bottom image is a deep entry. Despite the difference, the fluoroscopic image is the same despite the angle of entry

too deep or too superficial, the needle has to be pulled out of the renal capsule before adjusting the needle depth. The adjustment to the needle is made either by directing it more superficial or deeper depending on the earlier fluoroscopic image obtained in 30 degrees. Again the advancement of the needle is done only after the C-arm is moved back to 0 degrees. When the adjustment is made in one direction, it is essential not to change the orientation of the needle in the other direction. Ventilation is to be suspended in maximum expiration as the needle is advanced in the correct alignment towards the desired calyx [26].

The 30-degree rotation of the C-arm does not always need to be towards the surgeon. This rotation can also be done cranially or caudally depending on surgeon preference. The key concept here is that the needle is superficial when the image at 30 degrees is seen to have moved away from the direction of the C-arm movement (i.e. if the C-arm is rotated cranially, the needle moves caudally with reference to the calyx). Likewise, when the needle is deep, the needle is seen to have moved towards the direction of the C-arm movement (i.e. when the C-arm is rotated cranially, the needle moves cranially with reference to the calyx).

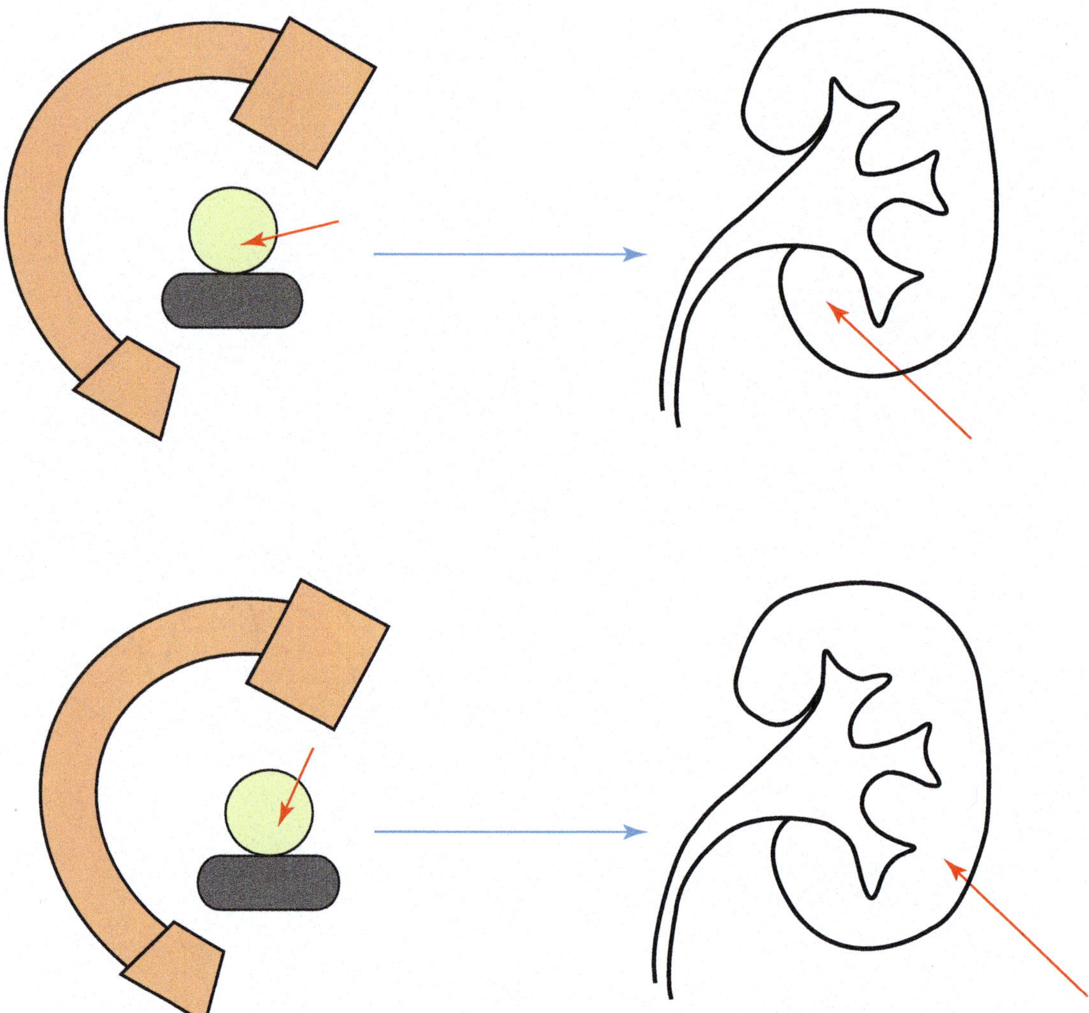

Fig. 13.5 C-arm has been rotated 30 degrees towards the surgeon. The top image is a superficial entry so at 30 degrees the fluoroscopic image shows the needle has moved in the opposite direction to the C-arm (away from the surgeon). The bottom image is a deep entry so at 30 degrees the fluoroscopic image shows the needle has moved in the same direction to the C-arm (towards the surgeon). This allows one to make the necessary adjustments to the needle entry

13.4.7 Bull's Eye Technique

C-arm is turned towards the surgeon in the 30-degree position. The 18-gauge needle is placed such that the targeted posterior calyx, needle tip and needle hub are all in line. For lower pole calyx, the C-arm should be tilted caudally by 10 degrees, while for upper pole calyx, the C-arm should be tilted cranially by the same extent. This gives it the bull's eye effect on the fluoroscopy screen. The needle is held by an artery forceps so as to reduce radiation to the surgeon's hand. The hand is stabilised, and the needle is advanced on continuous fluoroscopy to ensure the alignment is maintained. Once the needle is near the calyx, the C-arm is moved to 0-degree position to gauge the depth of the puncture [26].

13.4.8 Tract Dilatation and Access Sheath Placement

Once the needle enters the calyx, urine should flow freely. A hydrophilic guidewire is passed through the needle. The guidewire is manoeuvred towards the ureter; however if it does not pass down the ureter easily, it is coiled in the renal pelvis. Fascial dilator is passed over the guidewire, and later an angled catheter can be utilised to place the guidewire down the ureter. Some surgeons also exchange the hydrophilic guidewire for stiffer working wire prior to dilatation.

Having a secure guidewire down the ureter enables the subsequent dilatation to be carried out safely without the guidewire slipping out inadvertently. Additionally, some also prefer having second safety guidewire in place before proceeding with dilatation of the tract.

Dilatation may be accomplished using sequential Amplatz dilators, telescopic dilators or balloon dilators. Balloon dilatation which uses radial forces has been found to cause less trauma to the renal parenchyma as compared to serial dilators where shearing forces cause more damage and higher haemoglobin drop [27].

13.5 Conclusion

The technique using fluoroscopy to obtain percutaneous access remains the most preferred method. Once the perfect access is created, the PCNL naturally progresses without much difficulty. This understanding will go a long way in the training of the budding endourologist wanting to learn PCNL.

References

1. Bird VG, Fallon B, Winfield HN. Practice patterns in the treatment of large renal stones. J Endourol. 2003;17(6):355–63.
2. Ahmad AA, Alhunaidi O, Aziz M, et al. Current trends in percutaneous nephrolithotomy: an internet-based survey. Ther Adv Urol. 2017;9(9-10):219–26.
3. Watterson JD, Soon S, Jana K. Access related complications during percutaneous nephrolithotomy: urology versus radiology at a single academic institution. J Urol. 2006;176(1):142–5.
4. Aslam MZ, Thwaini A, Duggan B, et al. Urologists versus radiologists made PCNL tracts: the U.K. experience. Urol Res. 2011;39(3):217–21.
5. Speed JM, Wang Y, Leow JJ, et al. The effect of physician specialty obtaining access for percutaneous nephrolithotomy on perioperative costs and outcomes. J Endourol. 2017;31(11):1152–6.
6. Allen D, O'Brien T, Tiptaft R, Glass J. Defining the learning curve for percutaneous nephrolithotomy. J Endourol. 2005;19(3):279–82.
7. Tanriverdi O, Boylu U, Kendirci M, Kadihasanoglu M, Horasanli K, Miroglu C. The learning curve in the training of percutaneous nephrolithotomy. Eur Urol. 2007;52(1):206–11.
8. Lee CL, Anderson JK, Monga M. Residency training in percutaneous renal access: does it affect urological practice? J Urol. 2004;171(2 Pt 1):592–5.
9. de la Rosette JJ, Laguna MP, Rassweiler JJ, Conort P. Training in percutaneous nephrolithotomy—a critical review. Eur Urol. 2008;54(5):994–1001.
10. Valdivia JG, Scarpa RM, Duvdevani M, et al. Supine versus prone position during percutaneous nephrolithotomy: a report from the clinical research office of the endourological society percutaneous nephrolithotomy global study. J Endourol. 2011;25(10):1619–25.
11. Duty B, Waingankar N, Okhunov Z, Ben Levi E, Smith A, Okeke Z. Anatomical variation between the prone, supine, and supine oblique positions on computed tomography: implications for percutaneous nephrolithotomy access. Urology. 2012;79(1):67–71.
12. Valdivia JG, Valle J, Lopez JA, et al. Technique and complications of percutaneous nephroscopy: experience with 557 patients in the supine position. J Urol. 1998;160:1975.
13. Siev M, Motamedinia P, Leavitt D, et al. Does peak inspiratory pressure increase in the prone position? An analysis related to body mass index. J Urol. 2015;194(5):1302–6.
14. Tuttle DN, Yeh BM, Meng MV, Breiman RS, Stoller ML, Coakley FV. Risk of injury to adjacent organs with lower-pole fluoroscopically guided percutaneous nephrostomy: evaluation with prone, supine, and multiplanar reformatted CT. J Vasc Interv Radiol. 2005;16(11):1489–92.
15. Li J, Gao L, Li Q, Zhang Y, Jiang Q. Supine versus prone position for percutaneous nephrolithotripsy: a meta-analysis of randomized controlled trials. Int J Surg. 2019;66:62–71.
16. Lojanapiwat B. The ideal puncture approach for PCNL: fluoroscopy, ultrasound or endoscopy? Indian J Urol. 2013;29(3):208–13.
17. Corrales M, Doizi S, Barghouthy Y, Kamkoum H, Somani BK, Traxer O. Ultrasound or fluoroscopy for PCNL access, is there really a difference? J Endourol. 2021;35(3):241–8. https://doi.org/10.1089/end.2020.0672. Epub 2020 Aug 6

18. Ghani KR, Patel U, Anson K. Computed tomography for percutaneous renal access. J Endourol. 2009;23(10):1633–9.
19. Labate G, Modi P, Timoney A, et al. The percutaneous nephrolithotomy global study: classification of complications. J Endourol. 2011;25(8):1275–80.
20. Preminger G. Chapter 7 Stone disease: antibiotics and the handling and prevention of complications. In: Denstedt J, de la Rosette J, editors. Stone Disease. A Joint SIU-ICUD International Consultation. Glasgow, Scotland, October 12–15, 2014:400–4. Available from: http://www.siu-urology.org/society/siu-icud. Accessed 15 Aug 2020.
21. Korets R, Graversen JA, Kates M, et al. Post-percutaneous nephrolithotomy systemic inflammatory response: a prospective analysis of preoperative urine, renal pelvic urine and stone cultures. J Urol. 2011;186(5):1899–903.
22. Sampaio FJ. Renal anatomy. Endourologic considerations. Urol Clin North Am. 2000;27(4):585.
23. Ibrahim A, Wollin D, Preminger G, Andonian S. Technique of percutaneous nephrolithotomy. J Endourol. 2018;32(S1):S17–27.
24. Ray AA, Chung DG, Honey RJ. Percutaneous nephrolithotomy in the prone and prone-flexed positions: anatomic considerations. J Endourol. 2009;23(10):1607–14.
25. Sharma GR, Luitel B. Techniques for fluoroscopy-guided percutaneous renal access: an analytical review. Indian J Urol. 2019;35(4):259–66.
26. Miller NL, Matlaga BR, Lingeman JE. Techniques for fluoroscopic percutaneous renal access. J Urol. 2007;178(1):15–23.
27. Peng PX, Lai SC, Seery S, et al. Balloon versus Amplatz for tract dilation in fluoroscopically guided percutaneous nephrolithotomy: a systematic review and meta-analysis. BMJ Open. 2020;10(7):e035943.

14 How to Perform Renal Puncture: Ultrasound Approach

Kai-Yi Tzou, Shao-Wei Dong, and Chen-Hsun Ho

Abstract

Percutaneous nephrolithotomy (PCNL) is a common urologic surgery for large renal stone and staghorn stone. In this article, we summarized the tips and tricks of ultrasound-guided puncture PCNL from experienced endourologists covering the diagnostic or therapeutic use. We also discussed about the difference guided methods' and dilation methods' pros and cons.

Keywords

Percutaneous nephrolithotomy · Ultrasound Urolithiasis · Puncture · Dilation

14.1 Introduction

Percutaneous nephrolithotomy is a common urologic surgery for treating large renal stones or staghorn stones. Since it was published in 1976 [1], PCNL has evolved over the years into several different variances. The variances were noted almost on every step of whole procedure including patient position, access guidance, size of access tract and instrument, method of stone fragmentation, and nephrostomy wound management. Because of its diversity, it makes the young urologists difficult to learn this procedure. Percutaneous access to the collecting system could be achieved under the guidance of ultrasound, fluoroscopy, or CT [2]. Ultrasound (US) guided puncture is becoming more popular among urologists in Asian countries. However, the use of the US in PCNL had already been described for more than forty years [3]. The US-guided access has several advantages than fluoroscopic access including radiation-free, more convenient, safer, and cheaper. It also could reduce the risk of adjacent organ injury. Table 14.1

Table 14.1 Advantages and disadvantages of ultrasound-guided PCNL

Advantages
• No radiation exposure.
• More convenient and portable.
• Detecting radiolucent stone.
• Visualize surrounding tissue and organ.
• Depict renal vasculature and avoid injury.
• For special situation, e.g. spine deformity.
Disadvantages
• Difficult to access to the non-dilated collecting system.
• Poor visualization of guidewire, dilator, and sheath.

K.-Y. Tzou · S.-W. Dong
Department of Urology, Shuang Ho Hospital, Taipei Medical University, New Taipei City, Taiwan

C.-H. Ho (✉)
Division of Urology, Department of Surgery, Shin Kong Wu Ho-Su Memorial Hospital, Taipei, Taiwan

School of Medicine, College of Medicine, Fu Jen Catholic University, New Taipei City, Taiwan

A. C.F. Ng et al. (eds.), *Practical Management of Urinary Stone*,
https://doi.org/10.1007/978-981-16-4193-0_14

showed the advantages and disadvantages of radiation-free US-guided PCNL. However, few articles introduce this procedure step by step. Therefore, we had reviewed published literature and would like to share our experience of ultrasound-guided PCNL.

14.2 Patient Selection

The ideal patient for ultrasound-guided PCNL is non-staghorn stone and the presence of hydronephrosis [4]. That is because there is a sharp outline of the collecting system when the kidney is hydronephrotic. Moreover, it also creates a space between stone and calyx which could allow puncture needle to go through. Oppositely, staghorn stone is usually full of the collecting system and there is barely space for puncture needle and guidewire. Folding guidewire, losing direction, or false tract formation easily occurred in staghorn stone PCNL [4]. Besides, morbid obesity is not a good candidate. The kidney will be deeper away from the skin. When the ultrasound signal went through fatty tissue, there will be attenuation of the ultrasound image. The poor quality of the image makes puncture difficult [5]. Although obesity is not the absolute contraindication of ultrasound-guided access, there could be more complications. According to a multivariance regression study, more than 30% odds increase in severe Clavien–Dindo complications are related to a 5-unit increase in BMI [6]. Previous open kidney surgery is a risk of access failure although it is not the contraindication. More resistance would be met during tract dilation [7].

14.3 Preoperative Evaluation and Preparation

The routine hemogram including complete blood count with or without differential count, coagulation function (PT/APTT), and biochemistry test are performed before surgery. The uncorrected coagulopathy is an absolute contraindication to percutaneous surgery [2]. The preoperative routine urinalysis, urine culture, and sensitivities are also performed, and antibiotics should be used for 7 days if the urine culture is positive. To the assessment of stone size, location, and hydronephrosis grade, a preoperative image is necessary, including intravenous pyelography or computed tomography (CT) of the abdomen. But for ultrasound-guided PCNL, abdominal CT is highly recommended because it could provide more details including renal anatomy, stone characteristics, and caliceal axis. The general anesthesia with endotracheal intubation is favorite anesthesia for this procedure because of a decrease in the movement of the kidney.

14.4 Instruments

The following are essential instruments necessary for ultrasound-guided PCNL.

- Portable ultrasound unit.
- Cystoscopy tray.
- Cystoscope (rigid or flexible).
- Ureteral catheter.
- Occlusion balloon catheter.
- Puncture needle (Chiba needle if available).
- J-tip guidewire.
- 8-French fascial dilator
- Dilating system.
  - Metal telescopic dilators.
  - Balloon dilation system.
  - Amplatz dilation system.
- Working sheath.
- Nephroscopy (rigid or flexible).
- Lithoclast.
- Holmium YAG laser system.
- Double J ureteric stents.

14.5 Patient Position

The traditional position is the prone position. Because of the retroperitoneal location of the kidney, this position is thought easy to direct access to the calyx. But the supine position getting more popular because it is suited for morbidly obese, cardiovascular disease, and maintaining

Table 14.2 Comparing advantage and disadvantage between prone and supine position

Prone position	Supine position
Advantage	
Provides a broader surface area with a wider choice for needle access	Save time (skip the repositioning procedure)
Easy for manipulating the instrument	Better airway control
Easy for upper calyx puncture	Less Pulmonary and cardiovascular event
The visceral and bowel are drop-down, minimizing the risk of injury	Synchronous retrograde manipulation
Disadvantage	
Pulmonary and cardiovascular compromise	Small space for instruments
Difficult in severe obesity	The limited angle of puncture
Difficult airway maintenance	Increased risk of intraabdominal organ injury
Longer preparation time (reposition)	

good airway control. Radiation-free ultrasound-guided PCNL could be performed under either a prone position or supine position. It depends on surgeon preference and patient factors. Table 14.2 showed the advantage and disadvantages of both positions. Furthermore, Yuan et al. [8] reported a meta-analysis study including thirteen studies with a total of 6881 patients that showed a prone position is associated with a higher stone-free rate and less blood transfusion. But Li et al. [9] recently reported an updated meta-analysis including fifteen studies that revealed supine position had the shorter operative time and less postoperative fever whereas comparable stone-free rate and overall complication.

14.6 Procedural Steps

14.6.1 Step 1 Create Artificial Hydronephrosis

Non-dilated collecting system is not a good candidate for US-guided percutaneous access. The

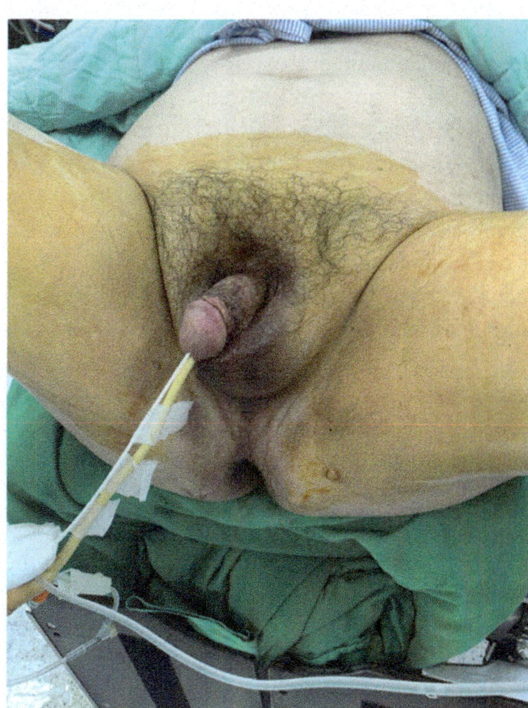

Fig. 14.1 The ureter catheter is fixed with a Foley catheter

renal calyx is usually difficult to differentiate from the renal pyramid if there is no presence of hydronephrosis. Therefore, creating artificial hydronephrosis for the renal stones without consequent hydronephrosis is important for ultrasound-guided access. Once artificial hydronephrosis had been created, the renal calyx can be more easily identified from renal parenchyma, which is often darker black. Li et al. [10] presented an effective method to create artificial hydronephrosis with a retrograde ureter catheter. In our experience, a 5 Fr open-ended ureteral catheter was inserted into the ipsilateral upper ureter or renal pelvis in retrograde fashion under rigid cystoscopy at the beginning of the procedure. The catheter is fixed with a Foley catheter to prevent migration (Fig. 14.1). Afterward, the saline is injected retrogradely through the ureteral catheter to collecting system with pressure pump or gravity flow of 40–50 cm high than kidney.

Sometimes, the patient was placed in a modified supine and the retrograde semirigid ureteroscopy was advanced up to renal pelvis to create hydronephrosis and guidewire retrieval [11]. To our experience, this method is very effective to make good hydronephrosis. Besides, some surgeons use an occlusion balloon catheter instead. The balloon near the tip is inflated to create an occlusion on the ureteropelvic junction to facilitate hydronephrosis [12]. Alternatively, Bai et al. [13] recently introduced a method to create artificial hydronephrosis by indwelling double J stent and reflux of bladder. In our experience, a 6-Fr double J stent was placed under cystoscopy rather than ureter catheter. Then an 18 or 20 Fr. three-way Foley catheter was placed within the bladder. The bladder is distended by occlusion of tube and saline solution filled the bladder with gravity flow. Artificial hydronephrosis could also be achieved by the reflux of the bladder.

Besides, some authors reported usage of diuretic administration for transiently dilatation of collecting system to facilitate the success of puncture [14]. To the best of our experience, the effect of the diuretic agent to create hydronephrosis is not good.

14.6.2 Step 2 Renal Ultrasonography

The linear or curve 3.5-MHz ultrasound transducer could be used by the surgeon's preference. But we prefer the curve transducer so that we could adjust the puncture angle easily. The area of skin entry point must be situated between 12th rib, iliac crest, paraspinal muscle, and posterior axillary line. Drawing posterior axillary line before surgery is suggested, especially in the supine position. Puncturing within this area that could avoid intraperitoneal organ injury and pleura injury. Preoperative computed tomography can provide much more information, such as the orientation of calyxes, relative location of stones, and the adjacent organs including colon, spleen, liver, and gallbladder. The appropriate depth of the ultrasound should be set to maximize the size of the kidney on the screen. The gain of ultrasound should be increased to differentiate the collecting system from renal parenchyma. At the initial of renal ultrasound, the whole kidney is scanned completely in longitudinal and transverse planes, from lateral to medial and superior to inferior, respectively, by sliding, swinging, fanning, and rotating. The renal parenchyma, pelvicalyceal system, hydronephrosis, stones, perirenal tissue, and surrounding organs are all visualized. If the image interferes with ribs, you could rotate the probe a little and try to make it parallel to the 11th rib. The proper skin access site to calyx is chosen according to your surgical design and stone location. In general, rigid nephroscope from upper pole calyx access could approach to renal pelvis, ureter, and most of lower pole calyx. But rigid nephroscope from lower pole calyx access could approach to the renal pelvis and few of upper pole calyx in few patients. Middle pole calyx access could approach to the renal pelvis and upper ureter in some cases. It is worth mentioning that puncturing should go through the calyceal fornix. The puncture direct into the renal pelvis should be avoided because there is a high risk of renal vessel injury. Although upper pole calyx could approach most calyx of the kidney, it usually needs a supracostal puncture that could cause pleura injury and sequential problems. Sometimes, color Doppler ultrasound images could be used to avoid large renal vessels which could result in severe hemorrhage [15]. The decision of target calyx is based on anatomic factor and the surgical goal that surgeon plan to accomplish. Good access to the ideal calyx system determines the success of subsequent procedure [16].

14.6.3 Step 3 Renal Puncture

After choosing optimal window and angle for access, a 20 cm puncture needle is inserted into skin. The Chiba needle is suggested to perform renal puncture because it had high echogenicity and visibility [17]. The optimal puncture angle needs to be parallel to the central axis of the infundibulum. But too oblique angle should be avoided because that can make subsequent steps more difficult [18]. Meanwhile, the ultrasound probe should be adjusted to the plane that targets calyx and renal pelvis could be seen at the same time. Consequently, severe bending could be avoided as entering renal pelvis from the calyx. The timing of puncture is important because the kidney is moving during respiration. It is more consistent at the end expiration [19].

14.6.3.1 Puncture with Guide

For the beginner, using a probe with puncture guide attachment is highly suggested, which can help direct the needle with fixing the angle of entry and keep the needle visualization in ultrasound image (Fig. 14.2). In addition, the electronic dotted line on the ultrasound screen predicts the path of the needle (Fig. 14.3). It could help manipulate the needle precisely and easily.

14.6.3.2 Puncture Without Guide (Freehand)

For a skilled surgeon, controlling the needle freehand is much more used. It means there is better flexibility of puncture angle as performing without a needle guide. It can be performed by either longitudinal insertion or transverse insertion [18]. For the longitudinal needle insertion, the needle can be placed on the cranial or caudal side of the probe, which is positioned along the longitudinal axis of the kidney (Fig. 14.4). For the transverse needle insertion, the needle is placed on either side of the ultrasound probe, which is positioned along the transverse axis of the kidney (Fig. 14.5). It can provide a greater range of entry angles and avert rib shadowing. To performing a free hand longitudinal puncture, the surgeon held the probe fixed by non-dominant hand with

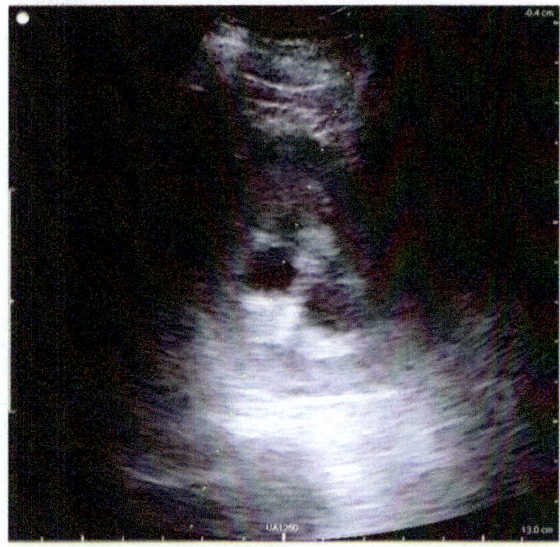

Fig. 14.3 The electronic dotted line on the screen will predict the path of the needle

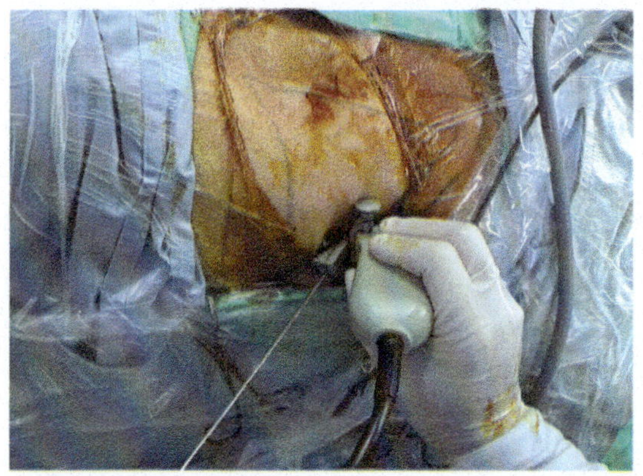

Fig. 14.2 Renal puncture is assisted by a probe with puncture guide attachment

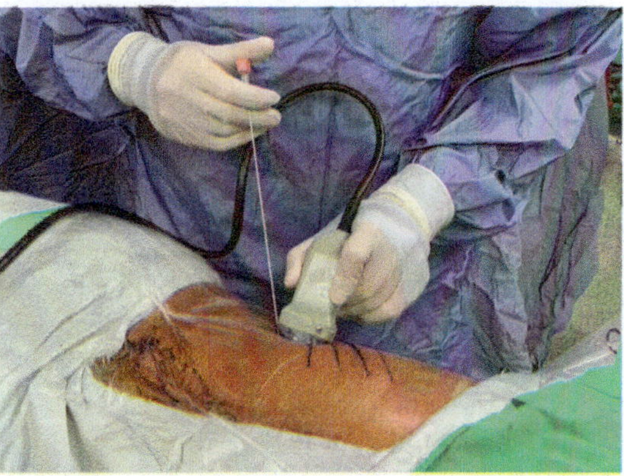

Fig. 14.4 The in-plane kidney puncture without adaptor (freehand)

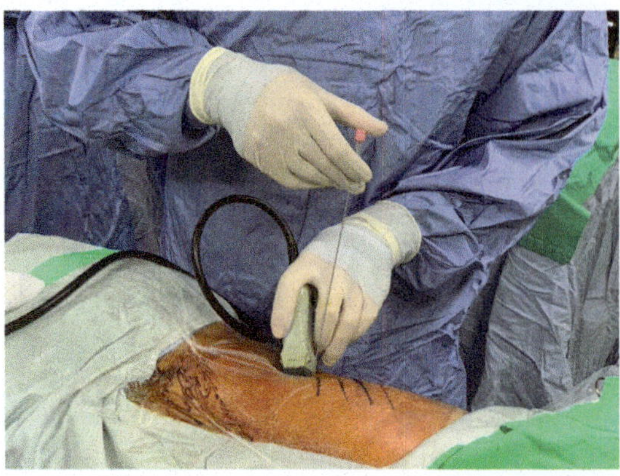

Fig. 14.5 The out-of-plane kidney puncture without adaptor (freehand)

securing it on patient body and held the needle by dominant hand. Bouncing the needle help to find needle tip then the needle was moved into the imaging plane. Keeping the needle parallel to the longitudinal plane of the probe is important to maintain visualized the needle. The needle retained under the soundbean of the probe will always emerge on the sonogram. It needs strict coordination between probe hand and needle hand.

For the freehand transverse puncture, the puncture needle is not on the imaging plane. The probe needs to be fanning back and forth to localize the needle tip and direct it into the desired calyx [18].

The entire procedure should be monitored in real-time by ultrasound especially the whole course of the needle. Sometimes the image of the needle tip is missing as advancing through the subcutaneous tissue. That is because it may not be on the same plane with the ultrasound transducer. At this moment, wiggling the needle gently or moving the probe back and forth will help the operator find the needle tip [19]. Sometimes, the localization of the needle could be determined by the movement of adjacent tissue. If the location of the needle could not still be identified, it should be pulled out and try again. Only the needle tip could be seen during the whole puncture, the needle could be brought to the calyx safely. After puncturing into the target calyx, needle stylet is removed. The efflux of clean urine through needle or aspiration of urine by using a 10 ml syringe could help confirm the success of target calyx access. Meanwhile, the depth of needle that means the length of the tract from skin to target calyx should be recorded and mark on dilators for subsequent dilation.

14.6.3.3 Ultrasound-Guided Needle Repositioning of Residual Stone

Chu et al. [18] had ever introduced the technique of repositioning of residual stone. It could help improve the stone-free rate without additional tracts. But to our experience, it could only be successfully performed in those cases with wide infundibulum and moderate hydronephrotic pelvis.

14.6.4 Step 4 Guidewire Access

J-tip made of a metal guidewire is preferable because it is stiff to resist kinking and bending and detected under the ultrasound. After needle puncture into the collecting system, we could remove the needle stylet and insert a coaxial 0.035-inch J-tip guidewire through the needle. Under the real-time vision of ultrasound, the surgeon could see the guidewire go into the renal pelvis and down the upper ureter. Sometimes guidewire cannot be put into the upper ureter and just curling within the renal pelvis. Once the guidewire is confirmed within the collecting system, the puncture needle can be removed. The beading on the wire could help confirm the collecting system deposition. Moving the guidewire must be gentle and stop if meeting resistance. Forceful insertion of the guidewire could cause renal pelvic perforation or kink of the guidewire. Then it could make subsequent steps difficult. Terumo guidewire is not suggested because it is too soft and invisible under ultrasound image.

14.6.5 Step 5 Tract Dilation

Before dilation, the skin incision should be made the wound wide along the guidewire. Moving the wire back and forth help locate where need to cut. The tract dilation is the most important step of ultrasound-guided PCNL. There are several dilation methods, including sequential rigid metal dilators [20], semirigid plastic dilation sets (Amplatz) [21], and balloon dilators [22]. The most popular method is the dilation balloon and Amplatz dilation system.

14.6.5.1 Rigid Metal Telescopic Dilators (MTD)

Rigid metal dilators are a series of coaxial dilators. It comprised eight metal rods that extended up from 9-Fr to 24-Fr at 3 Fr intervals. The first step of tract dilation is to advance an 8 Fr guide rod along the 0.035 guidewires until the depth of calyx. There is a ball tip on the guide rod that could prevent the following dilators go beyond the tip of the guide rod. Next, the second coaxial dilators are advanced along the guide rod. Then the subsequent coaxial dilators are passed through the former until the proper size of the tract.

14.6.5.2 Amplatz Dilator System

Amplatz dilator system is a semirigid plastic dilation system including a minimum of 10 dilators. The first step is dilating the wound by an 8 Fr fascial dilator along the guidewire until the depth of calyx. However, the dilator is not echogenic, and guidewire will disappear on ultrasound screen when dilator is passing over. Then the 8 Fr dilator was withdrawn and the guidewire was left in place. The subsequent dilation of 10 Fr and 12 Fr fascial dilator was achieved by the same method. After that, an 8-Fr PTFE guiding catheter was placed over the guidewire. The size of Amplatz dilators increasing by 2 French were used to dilate the tract along the guiding catheter one by one until the final size diameter is accomplished. The working sheath is placed over the final dilator. Then the final dilator and guiding catheter are removed, leaving the working sheath and guidewire in place. Sometimes, the dorsolumbar fascia is so dense that it is hard to dilate especially on male patients and secondary to previous renal surgery. In this instance, twisting dilator in a back-and-forth manner can help penetrate resistance and advance the dilator. Pushing too hard against the resistance could go beyond the proper depth and result in severe renal trauma. One important thing to remember while performing dilation is shallow is better than deep. Serial dilation one by one is time consuming, so some surgeons could skip some of size, e.g. the 16-Fr, 24-Fr. Moreover, Frattini et al. [23] ever present a modified one-step Amplatz dilation, named one-shot dilation that directly used only desired size Amplatz dilator (24–30 Fr). It had short fluoroscopy time and reduced radiation exposure [24]. But this benefit did not exist under ultrasound-guided access.

14.6.5.3 Balloon Dilator

The dilation with balloon dilator is a kind of one-step dilation method. It could save dilation time and reduce repetitive dilation that causes renal trauma [25]. The first step is to insert an 8-Fr fascial dilator along the guidewire under the real-time vision of ultrasound until the previously recorded depth. Then, a balloon dilator (Bard, USA) with preloaded working sheath was inserted until the distal tip is entering inside the target calyx. The balloon was inflated with saline at 20 ATM by pressure gun. The whole procedure should be monitored with ultrasound. The balloon usually moves outward along the wire during the inflation, so holding tightly to a secure location is needed. The balloon dilator was holding in the position for 3 min to facilitate tract hemostasis. Afterward, a working sheath was advanced into target calyx over the inflated balloon by spiral motion with one hand holding the balloon dilator in place. The exact length of sheath and balloon is matching. Advancement of the sheath is completed when the proximal edge of balloon dilator is seen. Then the balloon was deflated, and the dilator set was removed. The working sheath and guidewire were left in place for safety.

14.6.6 Step 6 Nephroscopy and Stone Fragmentation

Nephroscopy and stone fragmentation are same with fluorescent guided PCNL. Rigid nephroscopy is the basic instrument in standard PCNL. A basket or grasper can be used to facilitate stone removal. Stone fragmentation is performed by pneumatic lithotripter, ultrasonic lithotripter, laser lithotripter, or a combination. Lithoclast (Electromedical system, Kaufering, Germany) is a useful ballistic lithotripsy that provided a jackhammer-like effect on stones. Holmium laser lithotripsy is also a main method of lithotripsy especially mini-PCNL. Combining both methods seems to shorten operative time [26]. For a large renal stone (>20 mm) and hard stone (> 1000 HU), ballistic lithotripsy is used to fragmentize stone to less than 10 mm initially. The laser lithotripsy is then used to reduce stone size smaller enough to removal from the working sheath. With the advancement of a high-power laser system, laser lithotripsy could be more useful [27] for large and hard stones.

14.6.7 Step 7 Post-op Renal Drainage or Tubeless (Hemostasis)

After stone removal, a 6 Fr double J catheter is placed antegrade. Then the working sheath is removed. The management of wound could be left to open with a nephrostomy tube or closed with suture. The placement of a nephrostomy tube at the end of PCNL is originally designed to promote hemostasis and drain the pelvicalyceal system [28].

Depending on the surgeon's preference, there are three main methods for drainage of the collecting system including nephrostomy tube, ureteral stent, and tubeless. According to the degree of hematuria and amount of residual stone fragments, these methods could be used on the proper patients. In our experience, we routinely used 20 Fr. Council tube as a nephrostomy tube with a 6 Fr double J ureteral stent in conventional PCNL. The double J stent could be placed in an antegrade or retrograde fashion. At the end of this procedure, we left an 8-Fr PTFE guiding catheter in place. Then a 20 Fr council tube was advanced along this guiding catheter until reaching renal pelvis. For the small size of tract (< 18 Fr), we used an 8 Fr. pigtail tube as a nephrostomy tube, which is placed over a guidewire. In a prospective study of Maheshwari et al., a small size of nephrostomy tube reduces the need for analgesic agents and the duration of urinary leakage after tube removal significantly [29]. But according to a randomized study of Pietrow et al., small-bore nephrostomy seems to decrease postoperative pain score and analgesic agent dosage, but it did not reach a significant difference [30].

14.6.7.1 Tubeless PCNL (Only Double J Ureteral Stent Placement) and Total Tubeless PCNL

Sometimes the PCN tract was closed without leaving a nephrostomy tube, known as tubeless PCNL. Furthermore, some surgeons even placed neither a nephrostomy nor ureter stent, known as total tubeless PCNL. According to a systemic review and meta-analysis study, it could reduce pain, shorter hospital stay, and shorter time to return to normal activity [31]. But it should be used in the selected patient. In our experience, tubeless PCNL is only performed in that patients without obvious residual stones, severe hemorrhage, renal pelvis perforation, sepsis and the presence of any other intraoperative complications. In addition, the hemostasis agent including fibrin glue or sealants could be used to seal the tract and reducing bleeding from the tract additionally [32]. There is still no strong evidence or long-term data that support the benefit of using a hemostatic agent.

14.7 Which Is the Best Dilation Method?

The most effective dilation method remains still undetermined in ultrasound-guided access. The preference of the dilation method largely depends on the surgeon's training. In the literature review, the result of these dilation methods is diverse. Pakmanesh et al. [33] ever present the first randomized control trial comparing the Amplatz dilation and balloon dilation in ultrasound-guided PCNL. Due to the limited vision of dilator under ultrasound, short dilation could be the main concern, that means dilators push the kidney rather than a puncture into the calyx. Amplatz dilation had a higher short dilation rate than balloon dilation, especially in lower pole access although it is much cheaper than balloon dilator. The other parameters including access time, stone-free rate, hemoglobin drops, and overall complications are not significantly different between both. Moreover, Wu et al. [34] recently reported the meta-analysis study comparing these dilatation methods. Balloon dilation had reduced blood loss compared with Amplatz dilation, but the transfusion rate is similar. The balloon dilation can tamponade injured vessels by the balloon pressure. Dehong et al. [35] showed the efficacy and the safety of balloon are better than Amplatz dilatation. Beiko et al. [36] mentioned using balloon dilator can be guided by ultrasound more easily than Amplatz dilators. However, balloon dilator is thought to easily fail in patients with previous open kidney surgery [7]. That is because it is hard for balloon dilator to dilate the fibrotic scar of the kidney. In this instance, Amplatz dilation and MTD are more useful than balloon dilation [37]. Furthermore, how to choose between Amplatz and MTD? Ozok et al. [38] noted that MTD is better than Amplatz dilators in cases that the guidewire was not able to be placed through the collecting system due to obstruction of the infundibulum by stones.

14.8 Previous Literatures of Ultrasound-Guided PCNL

There are many literatures described about ultrasound-guided PCNL. Few article performed ultrasound-guided puncture with fluoroscopy guided dilation [6, 15, 39, 40]. Most articles performed with pure ultrasound-guided PCNL with difference dilation method [6, 36, 39, 41–44]. Table 14.3 listed the previously literary with ultrasound-guided PCNL and compared of tract successful rate, operative time, and stone-free rate (SFR).

14.9 Trouble Shooting in Ultrasound Access

Several previously published literatures showed on the feasibility and safety of the ultrasound-guided both renal tract access and dilatation [6, 49]. But there is still some troublesome challenge of renal puncture and dilation for beginner. A rarely mentioned but important aspect of trouble management during ultrasound-guided access is crucial for surgeons. Regarding to our surgical experience of ultrasound guidance access and literature review, the following Table 14.4 showed some useful troubleshooting for surgeons.

Table 14.3 Previous literatures of ultrasound-guided PCNL and comparison of tract successful rate, operative time, and stone-free rate

	Puncture	Dilation guided	Dilator	Tract successful rate	Op time (min)	SFR
Agarwal M [15]	Ultrasound	Fluoroscopy	Fascial	100%	(no show)	100%
Wei Z [40]	Ultrasound	Fluoroscopy	Fascial	96.60%	60.6 ± 32.9	55.10%
Ding X [45]	Ultrasound	Fluoroscopy	Balloon	95.80%	61.8	90.10%
Ding X [45]	Ultrasound	Ultrasound	Balloon	95.10%	58.3	88.60%
Manuel A [6]	Ultrasound	Fluoroscopy	Balloon	100%	138 ± 69	56%
Manuel A [6]	Ultrasound	Ultrasound	Balloon	94.93%	117 ± 42	57%
Zhou T [41]	Ultrasound	Ultrasound	Balloon	(no show)	82.2 ± 28.8	83.30%
Zhou T [41]	Ultrasound	Ultrasound	Balloon	(no show)	118.0 ± 24.6	88.60%
Beiko D [36]	Ultrasound	Ultrasound	Balloon	88.40%	73.1 ± 21.4	82.60%
Hosseini MM [42]	Ultrasound	Ultrasound	Alken	95.70%	(no show)	93.61%
Basiri A [46]	Ultrasound	Ultrasound	One-shot	93.50%	110.2	79%
Falahatkar S [44]	Ultrasound	Ultrasound	One-shot	(no show)	88.46 ± 39.49	88.50%
Karami H [47]	Ultrasound	Ultrasound	One-shot	100%	44.7 ± 6.4	86.70%
Wei S [48]	Ultrasound	Ultrasound	One-shot	(no show)	108.4 ± 31.7	79.10%
Usawachintachit M [43]	Ultrasound	Ultrasound	(no show)	65.60%	145.6 ± 48.0	77.40%

Table 14.4 The trouble shooting and management of ultrasound-guided access

Trouble	Management
Not be able to see the needle	– Using high frequency probe and increasing the gain of probe could help this situation. – Changing high echogenic needle also could overcome this difficulty.
No efflux of urine	Scenario 1: Complicated renal stone with infection sometimes could make the fluid viscous, or pus. It is sticky and thick and does not flow out easily. – Applying a syringe to aspirate it from needle help overcome this difficulty. Scenario 2: Not successful access into collecting system – Compression for hemostasis then repuncture
Fluid is mixed with blood	– Straining all fluid through gauze or filter paper to determine whether it is urine or blood.
Unable to passing a wire due to stone obstruction	– Use sensor guidewire [50] – Advance the needle into the stone and keep push stone forward after stylet is withdrawn. Try coiling of the wire tip around the limited calyceal space [51]
Short dilation	Short dilation is a common situation under ultrasound guide access. – Using small caliber nephroscope or ureteroscope and advancing along the guidewire until into collecting system; Then advancing working sheath along the endoscope.

References

1. Fernstrom I, Johansson B. Percutaneous pyelolithotomy. A new extraction technique. Scand J Urol Nephrol. 1976;10(3):257–9. https://doi.org/10.1080/21681805.1976.11882084.
2. Marcovich R, Smith AD. Percutaneous renal access: tips and tricks. BJU Int. 2005;95(Suppl 2):78–84. https://doi.org/10.1111/j.1464-410X.2005.05205.x.
3. Karamcheti A, O'Donnell WF. Percutaneous nephrolithotomy: an innovative extraction technique. J Urol. 1977;118(4):671–2. https://doi.org/10.1016/s0022-5347(17)58148-3.
4. Usawachintachit M, Tzou DT, Hu W, Li J, Chi T. X-ray-free ultrasound-guided percutaneous nephrolithotomy: how to select the right patient? Urology. 2017;100:38–44. https://doi.org/10.1016/j.urology.2016.09.031.
5. Wang S, Zhang Y, Zhang X, Tang Y, Xiao B, Hu W, et al. Tract dilation monitored by ultrasound in percutaneous nephrolithotomy: feasible and safe. World J Urol. 2020;38(6):1569–76. https://doi.org/10.1007/s00345-019-02876-7.
6. Armas-Phan M, Tzou DT, Bayne DB, Wiener SV, Stoller ML, Chi T. Ultrasound guidance can be used safely for renal tract dilatation during percutaneous nephrolithotomy. BJU Int. 2020;125(2):284–91. https://doi.org/10.1111/bju.14737.
7. Joel AB, Rubenstein JN, Hsieh MH, Chi T, Meng MV, Stoller ML. Failed percutaneous balloon dilation for renal access: incidence and risk factors. Urology. 2005;66(1):29–32. https://doi.org/10.1016/j.urology.2005.02.018.
8. Supine versus prone position in percutaneous nephrolithotomy for kidney calculi: a meta-analysis. J Endourol. 2016;30(7):754–763. https://doi.org/10.1089/end.2015.0402.
9. Li J, Gao L, Li Q, Zhang Y, Jiang Q. Supine versus prone position for percutaneous nephrolithotripsy: a meta-analysis of randomized controlled trials. Int J Surg. 2019;66:62–71. https://doi.org/10.1016/j.ijsu.2019.04.016.
10. Li JX, Tian XQ, Niu YN, Zhang X, Kang N. Percutaneous nephrolithotripsy with pneumatic and ultrasonic power under B-type ultrasound guidance for treatment of renal calculi in non-dilated collecting system. Zhonghua Wai Ke Za Zhi. 2006;44(6):386–8.
11. Khazaali M, Khazaeli D, Moombeini H, Jafari-Samim J. Supine ultrasound-guided percutaneous nephrolithotomy with retrograde semi-rigid ureteroscopic guidwire retrieval: description of an evolved technique. Urol J. 2017;14(6):5038–42. https://doi.org/10.22037/uj.v14i6.4080.
12. Shen CH, Cheng MC, Lin CT, Jou YC, Chen PC. Innovative metal dilators for percutaneous nephrostomy tract: report on 546 cases. Urology. 2007;70(3):418–421; discussion 21–2. https://doi.org/10.1016/j.urology.2007.03.083.
13. Bai FD, Wu HF, Zhang N, Chen JM, Wen JM. The feasibility, safety, and efficacy of the preemptive indwelling of double-J stents in percutaneous nephrolithotomy surgery: a randomized control trial. Urol J. 2020;17(3):232–6. https://doi.org/10.22037/uj.v0i0.4957.
14. Lojanapiwat B. The ideal puncture approach for PCNL: fluoroscopy, ultrasound or endoscopy? Indian J Urol. 2013;29(3):208–13. https://doi.org/10.4103/0970-1591.117284.
15. Agarwal M, Agrawal MS, Jaiswal A, Kumar D, Yadav H, Lavania P. Safety and efficacy of ultrasonography as an adjunct to fluoroscopy for renal access in percutaneous nephrolithotomy (PCNL). BJU Int. 2011;108(8):1346–9. https://doi.org/10.1111/j.1464-410X.2010.10002.x.
16. Wein AJ, Kavoussi LR, Partin AW, Peters C. Campbell-Walsh urology. 2016.

17. van de Berg NJ, Sanchez-Margallo JA, van Dijke AP, Lango T, van den Dobbelsteen JJ. A methodical quantification of needle visibility and echogenicity in ultrasound images. Ultrasound Med Biol. 2019;45(4):998–1009. https://doi.org/10.1016/j.ultrasmedbio.2018.10.004.
18. Chu C, Masic S, Usawachintachit M, Hu W, Yang W, Stoller M, et al. Ultrasound-guided renal access for percutaneous nephrolithotomy: a description of three novel ultrasound-guided needle techniques. J Endourol. 2016;30(2):153–8. https://doi.org/10.1089/end.2015.0185.
19. O'Neill WC. Renal relevant radiology: use of ultrasound in kidney disease and nephrology procedures. Clin J Am Soc Nephrol. 2014;9(2):373–81. https://doi.org/10.2215/CJN.03170313.
20. Alken P. The telescope dilators. World J Urol. 1985;3(1):7–10. https://doi.org/10.1007/BF00326880.
21. Rusnak B, Castaneda-Zuniga W, Kotula F, Herrera M, Amplatz K. An improved dilator system for percutaneous nephrostomies. Radiology. 1982;144(1):174. https://doi.org/10.1148/radiology.144.1.7089252.
22. Benway BM, Nakada SY. Balloon dilation of nephrostomy tracts. J Endourol. 2008;22(9):1875–6; discussion 87, 89. https://doi.org/10.1089/end.2008.9786.
23. Frattini A, Barbieri A, Salsi P, Sebastio N, Ferretti S, Bergamaschi E, et al. One shot: a novel method to dilate the nephrostomy access for percutaneous lithotripsy. J Endourol. 2001;15(9):919–23. https://doi.org/10.1089/089277901753284143.
24. Peng PX, Lai SC, Ding ZS, He YH, Zhou LH, Wang XM, et al. One-shot dilation versus serial dilation technique for access in percutaneous nephrolithotomy: a systematic review and meta-analysis. BMJ Open. 2019;9(4):e025871. https://doi.org/10.1136/bmjopen-2018-025871.
25. Davidoff R, Bellman GC. Influence of technique of percutaneous tract creation on incidence of renal hemorrhage. J Urol. 1997;157(4):1229–31.
26. Tangal S, Sanci A, Baklaci U, Babayigit M, Karaburun MC, Kubilay E, et al. What is the optimum lithotripsy method for high density stones during mini-PNL? Laser, ballistic or combination of both. Lasers Med Sci. 2020;35:1765–8. https://doi.org/10.1007/s10103-020-02971-x.
27. Pietropaolo A, Jones P, Whitehurst L, Somani BK. Role of 'dusting and pop-dusting' using a high-powered (100 W) laser machine in the treatment of large stones (>/= 15 mm): prospective outcomes over 16 months. Urolithiasis. 2019;47(4):391–4. https://doi.org/10.1007/s00240-018-1076-4.
28. Shoma AM, Elshal AM. Nephrostomy tube placement after percutaneous nephrolithotomy: critical evaluation through a prospective randomized study. Urology. 2012;79(4):771–6. https://doi.org/10.1016/j.urology.2011.09.042.
29. Maheshwari PN, Andankar MG, Bansal M. Nephrostomy tube after percutaneous nephrolithotomy: large-bore or pigtail catheter? J Endourol. 2000;14(9):735–737; discussion 7–8. https://doi.org/10.1089/end.2000.14.735.
30. Pietrow PK, Auge BK, Lallas CD, Santa-Cruz RW, Newman GE, Albala DM, et al. Pain after percutaneous nephrolithotomy: impact of nephrostomy tube size. J Endourol. 2003;17(6):411–4. https://doi.org/10.1089/089277903767923218.
31. Wang J, Zhao C, Zhang C, Fan X, Lin Y, Jiang Q. Tubeless vs standard percutaneous nephrolithotomy: a meta-analysis. BJU Int. 2012;109(6):918–24. https://doi.org/10.1111/j.1464-410X.2011.10463.x.
32. Merinov DS, Gurbanov SS, Artemov AV, Arustamov LD, Epishov VA. Prevention of bleeding during tubeless percutaneous nephrolithotomy. Urologiia. 2019;4:38–43.
33. Pakmanesh H, Daneshpajooh A, Mirzaei M, Shahesmaeili A, Hashemian M, Alinejad M, et al. Amplatz versus balloon for tract dilation in ultrasonographically guided percutaneous nephrolithotomy: a randomized clinical trial. Biomed Res Int. 2019;2019:3428123. https://doi.org/10.1155/2019/3428123.
34. Wu Y, Xun Y, Lu Y, Hu H, Qin B, Wang S. Effectiveness and safety of four tract dilation methods of percutaneous nephrolithotomy: a meta-analysis. Exp Ther Med. 2020;19(4):2661–71. https://doi.org/10.3892/etm.2020.8486.
35. Dehong C, Liangren L, Huawei L, Qiang W. A comparison among four tract dilation methods of percutaneous nephrolithotomy: a systematic review and meta-analysis. Urolithiasis. 2013;41(6):523–30. https://doi.org/10.1007/s00240-013-0598-z.
36. Beiko D, Razvi H, Bhojani N, Bjazevic J, Bayne DB, Tzou DT, et al. Techniques – ultrasound-guided percutaneous nephrolithotomy: how we do it. Can Urol Assoc J. 2020;14(3):E104–E10. https://doi.org/10.5489/cuaj.6076.
37. Safak M, Gogus C, Soygur T. Nephrostomy tract dilation using a balloon dilator in percutaneous renal surgery: experience with 95 cases and comparison with the fascial dilator system. Urol Int. 2003;71(4):382–4. https://doi.org/10.1159/000074090.
38. Hakki Ugur Ozok LS, Senturk AB, Karakoyunlu N, Topaloglu H, Ersoy H. A comparison of metal telescopic dilators and amplatz dilators for nephrostomy tract dilation in percutaneous nephrolithotomy. J Endourol. 2012;26(6):630–4. https://doi.org/10.1089/end.2011.0291.
39. Ding X, Hao Y, Jia Y, Hou Y, Wang C, Wang Y. 3-dimensional ultrasound-guided percutaneous nephrolithotomy: total free versus partial fluoroscopy. World J Urol. 2019;38(9):2295–300. https://doi.org/10.1007/s00345-019-03007-y.
40. Zhu W, Li J, Yuan J, Liu Y, Wan SP, Liu G, et al. A prospective and randomised trial comparing fluoroscopic, total ultrasonographic, and combined guidance for renal access in mini-percutaneous nephrolithotomy. BJU Int. 2017;119(4):612–8. https://doi.org/10.1111/bju.13703.

41. Zhou T, Chen G, Gao X, Zhang W, Xu C, Li L, et al. 'X-ray'-free balloon dilation for totally ultrasound-guided percutaneous nephrolithotomy. Urolithiasis. 2015;43(2):189–95. https://doi.org/10.1007/s00240-015-0755-7.
42. Hosseini MM, Hassanpour A, Farzan R, Yousefi A, Afrasiabi MA. Ultrasonography-guided percutaneous nephrolithotomy. J Endourol. 2009;23(4):603–7. https://doi.org/10.1089/end.2007.0213.
43. Usawachintachit M, Masic S, Chang HC, Allen IE, Chi T. Ultrasound guidance to assist percutaneous nephrolithotomy reduces radiation exposure in obese patients. Urology. 2016;98:32–8. https://doi.org/10.1016/j.urology.2016.04.012.
44. Falahatkar S, Allahkhah A, Kazemzadeh M, Enshaei A, Shakiba M, Moghaddas F. Complete supine PCNL: ultrasound vs. fluoroscopic guided: a randomized clinical trial. Int Braz J Urol. 2016;42(4):710–6. https://doi.org/10.1590/S1677-5538.IBJU.2014.0291.
45. Ding X, Hao Y, Jia Y, Hou Y, Wang C, Wang Y. 3-dimensional ultrasound-guided percutaneous nephrolithotomy: total free versus partial fluoroscopy. World J Urol. 2020;38(9):2295–300. https://doi.org/10.1007/s00345-019-03007-y.
46. Basiri A, Mirjalili MA, Kardoust Parizi M, Moosa Nejad NA. Supplementary X-ray for ultrasound-guided percutaneous nephrolithotomy in supine position versus standard technique: a randomized controlled trial. Urol Int. 2013;90(4):399–404. https://doi.org/10.1159/000345796.
47. Karami H, Rezaei A, Mohammadhosseini M, Javanmard B, Mazloomfard M, Lotfi B. Ultrasonography-guided percutaneous nephrolithotomy in the flank position versus fluoroscopy-guided percutaneous nephrolithotomy in the prone position: a comparative study. J Endourol. 2010;24(8):1357–61. https://doi.org/10.1089/end.2009.0099.
48. Sun W, Liu MN, Yang ZW, Wang Q, Xu Y. Ultrasound-guided percutaneous nephrolithotomy for the treatment in patients with kidney stones. Medicine (Baltimore). 2017;96(51):e9232. https://doi.org/10.1097/MD.0000000000009232.
49. Beiko D, Razvi H, Bhojani N, Bjazevic J, Bayne DB, Tzou DT, et al. Techniques – Ultrasound-guided percutaneous nephrolithotomy: How we do it. Can Urol Assoc J. 2019;14(3):E104–E10. https://doi.org/10.5489/cuaj.6076.
50. Khanna R, Monga M. Instrumentation in endourology. Ther Adv Urol. 2011;3(3):119–26. https://doi.org/10.1177/1756287211403190.
51. Rais-Bahrami S, Friedlander JI, Duty BD, Okeke Z, Smith AD. Difficulties with access in percutaneous renal surgery. Ther Adv Urol. 2011;3(2):59–68. https://doi.org/10.1177/1756287211400661.

Tips and Tricks of Supine PCNL

15

Suriaraj Karppaya, Wei Lun Tam, Li Yi Lim,
and Noor Ashani Md Yusoff

Abstract

Supine percutaneous nephrolithotomy (PCNL) is easy to perform and has many advantages over traditional prone PCNL. It enables the procedure to be carried out in a single position, as such reduces operative time and removes the risks of inadvertent injuries during repositioning. Moreover, anaesthetic risk is lower in supine position as it eliminates cardiac and respiratory encumbrance associated with prone position. Supine position also has the additional advantage to perform synchronous retrograde intrarenal surgery.

This chapter described the patients' position and techniques of supine PCNL, with emphasis to the tips and tricks for successful supine PCNL. Furthermore, we detailed the advantages and disadvantages of supine PCNL and compared the outcome of supine and prone PCNL.

Keywords

Nephrolithotomy percutaneous · Kidney calculi · Urolithiasis · Patient positioning Supine

15.1 Introduction

Percutaneous nephrolithotomy (PCNL) is the gold standard in treatment of large and complex renal stones. This procedure, however, associated with many morbidities. In particularly, its classic prone position posts high anaesthesia risk. The introduction of supine PCNL by Valdivia et al. in 1987 has addressed the high anaesthesia risk associated with prone PCNL [1]. Over the years, supine PCNL has evolved remarkably and resulted in variants of patient positions and techniques to facilitate the success of this procedure.

15.2 Supine Versus Prone PCNL

PCNL was first described in prone position due to concerns of inadvertent colon injury during access if procedure is performed in other positions. It is important, however, to note that intravenous pyelography was the standard imaging modality for stone assessment at the time PCNL was introduced. Computed tomography (CT) was not widely used. With CT readily available, sur-

S. Karppaya · W. L. Tam · N. A. M. Yusoff (✉)
Hospital Kuala Lumpur, Jalan Pahang,
Kuala Lumpur, Wilayah Persekutuan Kuala Lumpur,
Malaysia

L. Y. Lim
Hospital Canselor Tuanku Muhriz UKM, Jalan
Yaacob Latif, Bandar Tun Razak,
Kuala Lumpur, Wilayah Persekutuan Kuala Lumpur,
Malaysia

A. C.F. Ng et al. (eds.), *Practical Management of Urinary Stone*,
https://doi.org/10.1007/978-981-16-4193-0_15

geons have a good pre-operative understanding of the peri-renal anatomy, thus lower the risk of inadvertent colon perforation. Moreover, studies have showed that risk of colon perforation is less in supine, with the incidence of retro-renal colon position being 1.9% in supine position and up to 10% in prone position [2].

Supine PCNL has many advantages over pone PCNL. It enables the procedure to be carried out in a single position, as such reduces operative time and removes the risks of inadvertent injuries during repositioning. Moreover, anaesthetic risk is lower in supine position as it eliminates cardiac and respiratory encumbrance associated with prone position. Supine position also has the additional advantage to perform synchronous retrograde intrarenal surgery. This "endoscopic combined intrarenal surgery" (ECIRS) is an effective approach for large or complex stones. Supine PCNL also has superior ergonomic for the surgeon. Surgeon can operate comfortably in sitting position and avoiding stress on the back.

While supine PCNL has many advantages over prone PCNL, it has few significant drawbacks. In supine position, the flank is not fully exposed, thus limiting the operative field and reduces the possibility of multiple access when needed. Furthermore, it is difficult to achieve upper pole puncture in supine position. Even though study has shown that it is more likely to access upper calyx through lower pole puncture when patient is in supine position than in prone position (80% versus 20%) [3], supine PCNL may not be ideal for large upper calyceal stone or staghorn calculi. In addition, kidney is more mobile when in supine position, making the access and navigation of instrument towards the kidney more challenging.

Supine PCNL has similar intraoperative and post-operative outcome as prone PCNL.

i. Operative Time

   One of the main advantages of supine PCNL is omission of the need and time spend for repositioning of patient. Meta-analyses have shown that mean operative time was statistically shorter in supine PCNL by 18.27 to 24.84 mins [4–8].

ii. Stone free rate

   Studies have shown conflicting results on stone free rate of supine versus prone PCNL. While there are few meta-analyses that demonstrated superior stone free rate with prone PCNL [6, 7, 9], others showed similar stone free rate between these two positions [4, 10]. In a recent meta-analysis of Li et al., which included 1474 patients from 15 randomised controlled trials, showed no statistically significant difference in stone free rate of prone and supine PCNL [8].

iii. Complications

   Supine PCNL has similar complication rate to prone PCNL [4, 6, 10]. The rate of inadvertent colonic injury and pleural injury is comparable to prone PCNL (0.5% and 0%, respectively) [8]. Two meta-analyses noted lower incidence of blood transfusion associated with supine PCNL [7, 10] and one meta-analysis found lower fever rate in supine group [10].

iv. Length of hospital stay

   Data from all the meta-analyses have consistently showed no difference in length of hospital stays after supine and prone PCNL [5–8, 10] (Fig. 15.1, Table 15.1).

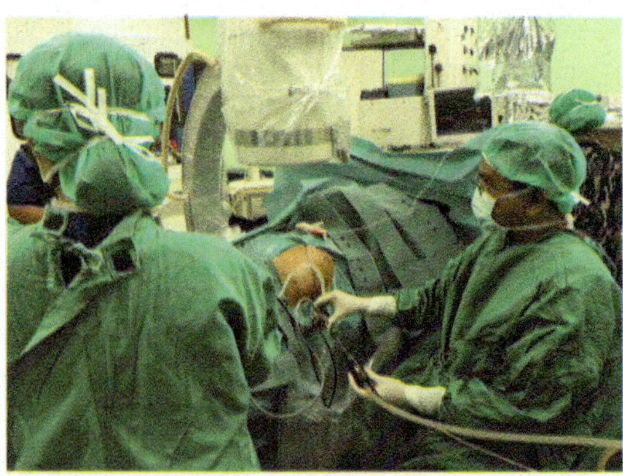

Fig. 15.1 Surgeon performs supine PCNL in a comfortable sitting position

Table 15.1 Advantages and disadvantages of supine and prone PCNL

	Prone	Supine
Advantages	Larger operative field and possibility of multiple punctures Easy puncture as kidney is fixed and easier identification of calyx Wider space for instrument manipulation	No patient repositioning Allows endoscopic combined intrarenal surgery Better calyceal drainage Superior ergonomic for surgeons
Disadvantages	Injuries associated with positioning • Cervical spine, skeletal, and ocular injuries. Cardiac and respiratory encumbrance	Hypermobility of kidney Small operating field Difficult upper pole puncture or multiple punctures Long percutaneous tract limits movement and stone clearance

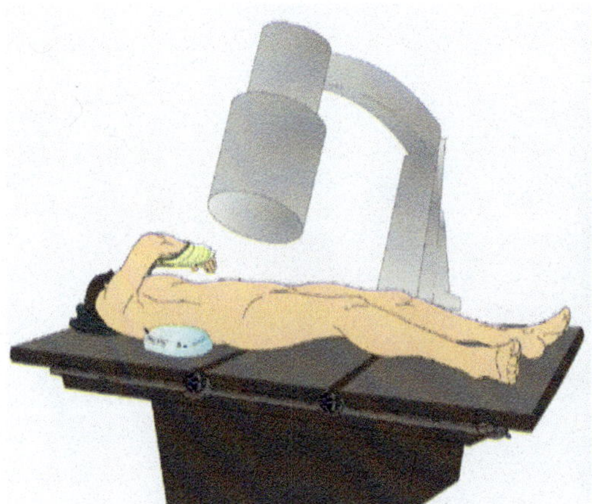
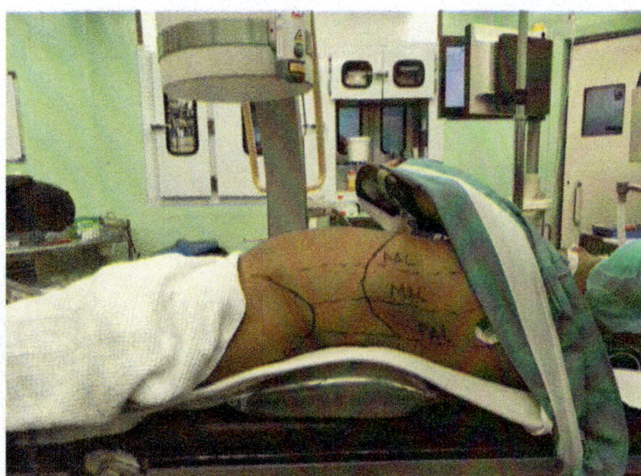

Fig. 15.2 Valdivia position for supine PCNL

15.3 Patient Positioning

The original supine PCNL as described by Valdivia et al. is supine position with 3-litre saline bag to elevate the ipsilateral flank (Fig. 15.2) [1].

Subsequently there are many modifications to the initial Valdivia position. In one of the modified Valdivia position, patients' both legs are flexed with ipsilateral leg slightly more elevated to facilitate synchronous ureteroscopy (Fig. 15.3).

In 2007, Galdakao further modified the Valdivia position and soon become the position of choice for many surgeons [11]. For this "modified Galdakao-Valdivia position", patient is supine with slight rotation to the contralateral side. The ipsilateral flank is elevated by 20–25°. Patient's ipsilateral arm is placed over the chest, high enough to make sure it does not interfere with C-arm and enables proper flank exposure. Patient's ipsilateral leg is extended and contralateral leg is flexed to provide substantial room for second surgeon to perform simultaneous retrograde intrarenal surgery (RIRS) should the need arises (Fig. 15.4). By leaving the ipsilateral leg extended, there is an additional advantage of ease of instrument mobilisation especially when trying to reach the upper calyx through lower pole access, as instruments will no longer collide with the leg or the stirrup-holder.

Another popular variation of Valdivia position is "Barts flank-free modified supine position" [12]. This position is similar to the modified Galdakao-Valdivia position, patient is in slight lateral position, with ipsilateral arm is placed over the chest, ipsilateral leg extended, and contralateral leg abducted. The main difference is

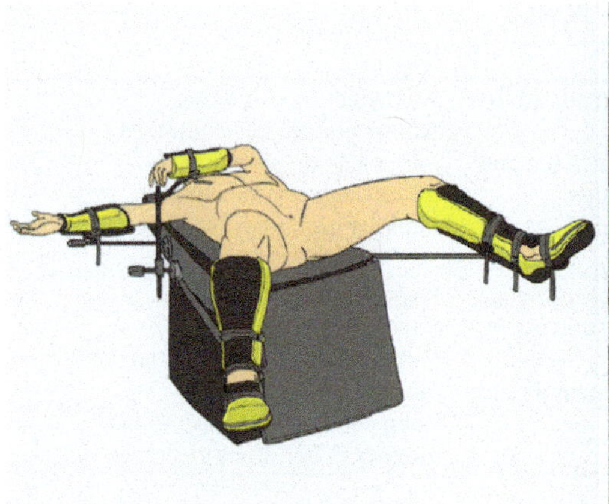

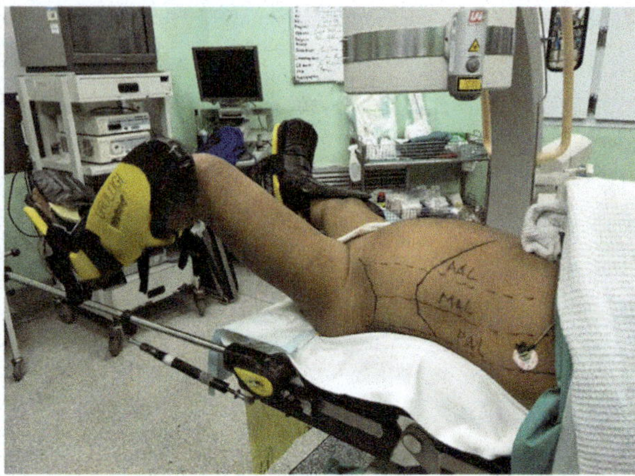

Fig. 15.3 Modified Valdivia position

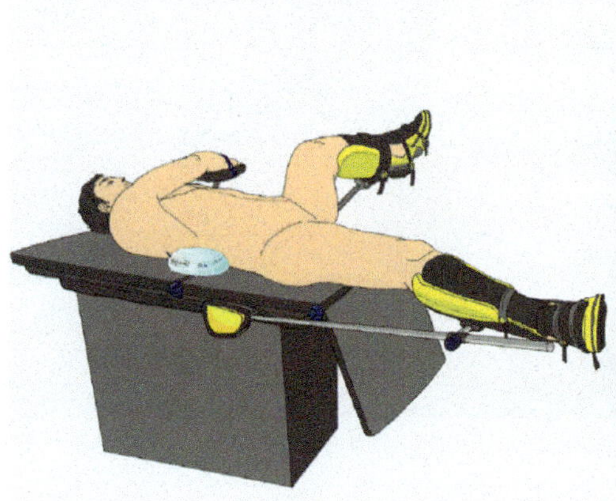

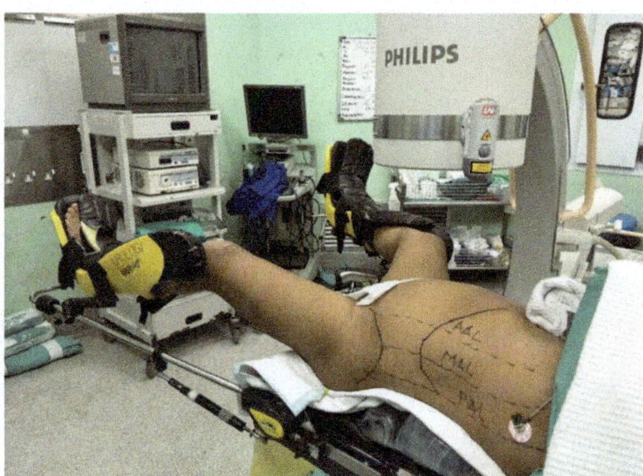

Fig. 15.4 Modified Galdakao-Valdivia position for supine PCNL

patient is tilted 15° by using 3-L saline bag under the ipsilateral rib cage and a small gel pad under ipsilateral pelvis. There is no support under the loin thus allowing more space for renal access (Fig. 15.5).

15.4 Technique of Puncturing

In supine PCNL, the puncture must be within the safety area that is borders superiorly by 12th rib, inferiorly by iliac crest, and anteriorly by posterior axillary line (surface landmark for posterior peritoneum reflection). It is important to draw these safety landmarks when patient in supine position to avoid lines displacement during positioning.

Puncture in supine PCNL can be carried out via the following methods:

i. Fluoroscopy guidance.
ii. Ultrasound guidance.
iii. Combined fluoroscopy-ultrasound guidance.
iv. Ureteroscopy guidance.

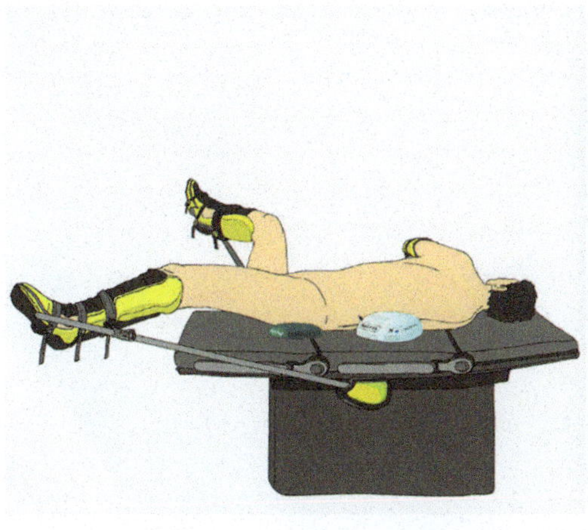

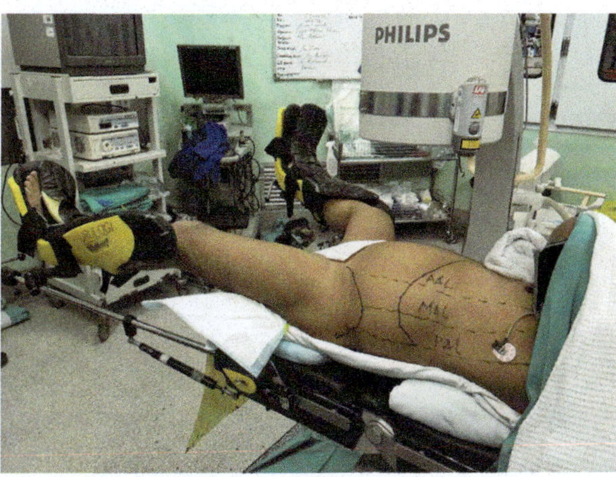

Fig. 15.5 Barts flank-free modified supine position

The table below explained the techniques and advantages of each technique.

Technique	Description	Advantages
Fluoroscopy guidance	Retrograde pyelogram is performed to identify the target calyx for puncture. Needle advanced under real-time fluoroscopy guidance. The depth of puncture can be confirmed by rotating the C-arm cephalad.	Clear visualisation of calyceal system. In correct trajectory, indentation of calyx can be seen when needle entered the desired calyx.
Ultrasound guidance	Establishment of access tract can be performed by radiologist before the procedure or by urologist in the theatre.	Radiation free Clear visualisation of surrounding structures during puncture to avoid inadvertent injuries
Combined fluoroscopy-ultrasound guidance	Establishment of access tract with ultrasound Antegrade pyelogram via access tract or retrograde pyelogram via angio-catheter to facilitate dilatation with fluoroscopy guidance	Minimal radiation exposure Safe puncture with ultrasound guidance Guided dilatation under fluoroscopy
Ureteroscopic guidance	Puncture of target calyx either with ultrasound or retrograde nephrostomy puncture wire via flexible ureteroscopy. Dilatation and sheath insertion under direct vision of ureteroscopy to confirm the placement.	Radiation free Continuous visualisation from puncture to PCNL. Any complications can be easily identified

15.5 Tips and Tricks During Supine PCNL

i. Patient selection

   As with all the PCNL, at the beginning of learning curve it is best to select patient with dilated system. Supine PCNL is best suited for lower pole access, as such patients with calculi that required upper pole puncture or large staghorn calculi are not ideal candidates for supine PCNL.

ii. Positioning of patient close to the edge of operating table

   It is pertinent to position patient closer to the edge of operating table (6 cm away from the edge of table to avoid the radiopaque edge of the operating bed) to prevent collision of

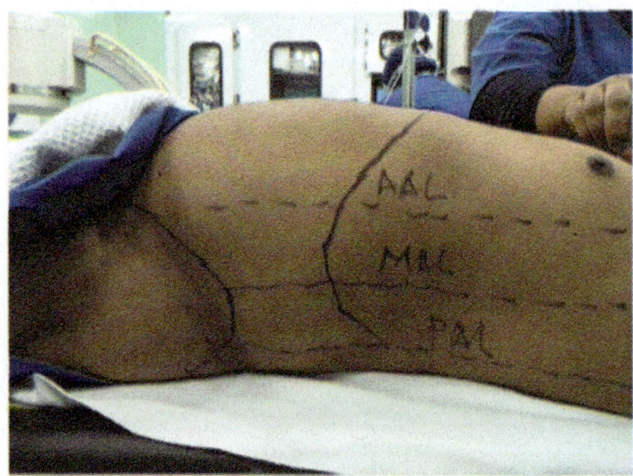

Fig. 15.6 Marking of safety landmarks before positioning

instruments with the bed, thus improves manoeuvrability of the instruments.

iii. Marking of safety landmarks

It is important to mark the three safety landmarks for puncture (posterior axillary line, inferior edge of 12th ribs, and iliac crest) when patient in supine position to maintain the orientation after patient positioning and draping (Fig. 15.6).

iv. Preparation of long scope and sheath

Percutaneous tract in supine PCNL is longer than prone PCNL due to pliable and thick anterior abdominal wall, especially for obese patients. Furthermore, the puncture is more lateral. Hence, it is important to prepare long access sheath and nephroscope.

v. Secure access sheath

Longer percutaneous tract increases the risk of inadvertent migration of sheath into the tract, hence it is important to secure the access sheath to the skin (Fig. 15.7).

vi. Antegrade insertion of guidewire into bladder to fix kidney

Kidney tends to be more mobile in supine position as compared to prone position due to loss of weight and rigidity of posterior abdominal wall against the operating table. Excess movement of kidney increases the difficulty during puncture and dilatation and increases the risk of losing the tract.

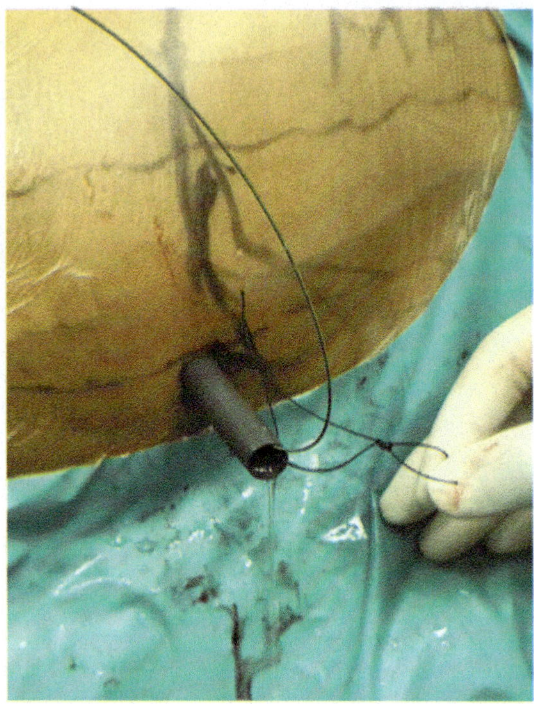

Fig. 15.7 Access sheath secured with suture to prevent migration

Abdominal compression with assistant's hand during puncture can aid to stabilise the kidney. Alternatively, antegrade insertion of guidewire through ureter into bladder allows some fixation to the mobile kidney and facilitates dilatation.

15.6 Our Experiences

Our centre starts to perform supine PCNL since year 2010. Prone PCNL, however, remains the default due to familiarity of the procedures by surgeons, as well as for the training of young urologists. Our patient's selection mainly for patient with medical conditions that preclude a safe prone PCNL such as morbid obesity and cardiopulmonary conditions. We exclude patients that require upper pole puncture or full staghorn calculi.

We performed all cases in modified Galdakao-Valdivia position (Fig. 15.8). For patients with

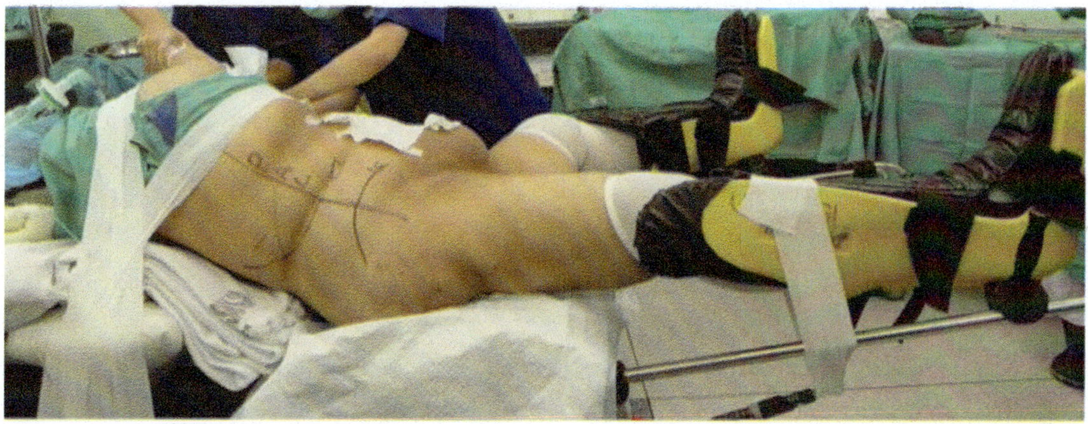

Fig. 15.8 Supine PCNL for a lady with BMI of 47 kg/m^2. Modified Galdakao-Valdivia position with flank elevated using blankets. Safety landmarks (posterior axillary line (PAL), inferior margin of 12th rib, and iliac crest) are marked before positioning

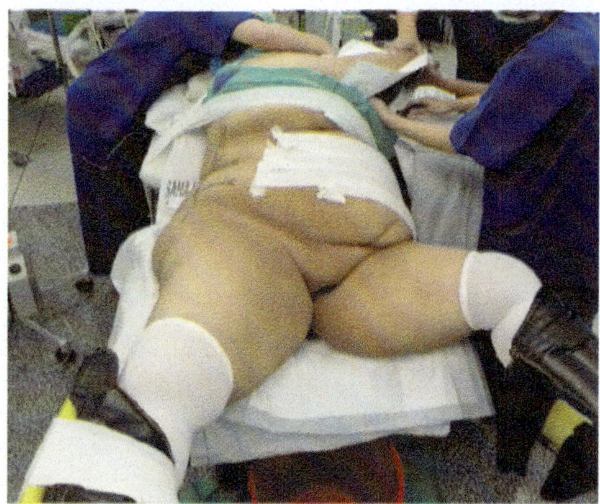

Fig. 15.9 Abdominal fat is strapped away by adhesive tape to increase exposure of flank region

floppy anterior abdominal wall, we strapped away the abdominal fat to open up the flank region (Fig. 15.9). In vast majority of cases, we gained access with ultrasound and performed dilatation under fluoroscopy guidance. We prefer combined fluoroscopy-ultrasound guided access as it avoids inadvertent puncture of adjacent organs, lower the radiation exposure as compared to pure fluoroscopic guided technique but retains the safety profile of dilatation with fluoroscopy guidance. With this technique, we able to achieve safe access and so far, there is no inadvertent injury.

Our experiences show that supine PCNL is safe with comparable stone clearance rate as prone PCNL.

References

1. Valdivia Uría JG, Lachares Santamaría E, Villarroya Rodríguez S, Taberner Llop J, Abril Baquero G, Aranda Lassa JM. Percutaneous nephrolithectomy: simplified technic (preliminary report). Arch Esp Urol. 1987;40(3):177–80.
2. Hopper KD, Sherman JL, Luethke JM, et al. The retrorenal colon in the supine and prone patient. Radiology. 1987;162:443–6.
3. Sofer M, Giusti G, Proietti S, Mintz I, Kabha M, Matzkin H, Aviram G. Upper calyx approachability through a lower calyx access for prone versus supine percutaneous nephrolithotomy. J Urol. 2016;195(2):377–82.
4. Liu L, Zheng S, Xu Y, Wei Q. Systematic review and meta-analysis of percutaneous nephrolithotomy for patients in the supine versus prone position. J Endourol. 2010;24(12):1941–6.
5. Wu P, Wang L, Wang K. Supine versus prone position in percutaneous nephrolithotomy for kidney calculi: a meta-analysis. Int Urol Nephrol. 2011;43(1):67–77.
6. Zhang X, Xia L, Xu T, Wang X, Zhong S, Shen Z. Is the supine position superior to the prone position for percutaneous nephrolithotomy (PCNL)? Urolithiasis. 2014;42(1):87–93.
7. Yuan D, Liu Y, Rao H, et al. Supine versus prone position in percutaneous nephrolithotomy for kidney calculi: a meta-analysis. J Endourol. 2016;30(7):754–63.

8. Li J, Gao L, Li Q, Zhang Y, Jiang Q. Supine versus prone position for percutaneous nephrolithotripsy: a meta-analysis of randomized controlled trials. Int J Surg. 2019;66:62–71.
9. Birowo P, Tendi W, Widyahening IS, Rasyid N, Atmoko W. Supine versus prone position in percutaneous nephrolithotomy: a systematic review and meta-analysis. F1000Research. 2020;9:231.
10. Falahatkar S, Mokhtari G, Teimoori M. An update on supine versus prone percutaneous nephrolithotomy: a meta-analysis. Urol J. 2016;13(5):2814–22.
11. Ibarluzea G, Scoffone CM, Cracco CM, et al. Supine Valdivia and modified lithotomy position for simultaneous anterograde and retrograde endourological access. BJU Int. 2007;100:233–6.
12. Bach C, Goyal A, Kumar P, et al. The Barts 'flank-free' modified supine position for percutaneous nephrolithotomy. Urol Int. 2012;89:365–8.

Mini-PCNL

16

Ravindra Sabnis, Abhishek Singh,
and Michael Y.C. Wong

Abstract

Miniaturization of PCNL aims at decreasing morbidity and increasing stone clearance. Miniaturized PCNL has different classifications and nomenclatures and there is a need to understand these. In this chapter we try to explain the different instrumentations that are used in mini PCNL. As the tract size decreases the energy source also need to be modified and modern energy sources like lasers, Shock-pulse, and Triology need to be understood. Lastly, which miniaturized tool to use when is very important to understand and when to use standard PCNL is a critical decision that urologist need to make.

16.1 Introduction

Ever since the introduction of PCNL (percutaneous nephrolithotomy) in 1976 [1], the endeavor has been to achieve complete clearance of stone with minimal possible morbidity. PCNL have revolutionized stone management, but it is associated with its own sets of challenges and complications. Access and tract size are determinants of complications in PCNL [2].

Analysis of complications and better understanding of anatomy and physiology have led to the development of modern instrumentation which include scopes, sheaths, and ancillary equipment. Lasers are now the most important energy source and have practically become the workhorse for all these procedures. Challenges associated with fragmentation, retrieval, and vision have increased with the upsurge of miniaturization of instruments [3].

Amidst the various tract sizes available, dilemma still remains which tract size and scope to be used. Newer nomenclature of mini PCNL is heterogeneous and there is lot of confusion surrounding the newer names. All innovators and manufacturers have named their instruments and procedures differently, making the classification difficult. Schilling et al. have tried to bring all the different instruments under one umbrella, this is based on the outer tract size diameter. The tracts have been classified as XL(>25 fr), L (20–25 fr), M (15–20 fr), S(10–15 fr), XS (5–10 fr), and XXS (<5 fr) [4].

R. Sabnis · A. Singh
Department of Urology, Muljibhai Patel Urological Hospital, Nadiad, India

M. Y.C. Wong (✉)
International Urology, Fertility and Gynecology Centre, Mount Elizabeth Hospital,
Singapore, Singapore
e-mail: email@drmichaelwong.com;
http://www.singaporeurology.com

A. C.F. Ng et al. (eds.), *Practical Management of Urinary Stone*,
https://doi.org/10.1007/978-981-16-4193-0_16

16.2 What Is the Importance of Tract Size and Does It Make a Difference in Stone Management?

Tract size is very important and it does make a difference in management of stone disease. For example, the larger the tract size, the more blood loss was observed [2]. Also, the incidence of prolonged urinary leak from the nephrostomy site increases. VAS scores for pain are higher in patients with nephrostomy tube. Larger tract size is associated with longer hospital stay [5].

On the other hand, smaller tracts are associated with decreased blood loss and decreased length of stay [5]. Tubeless procedures are associated with decreased pain and are more likely with smaller tracts [5]. But in infected system smaller tract can potentially increase the intra pelvic pressure and potentially lead to increased chances of sepsis. Also, in a closed outflow system of any miniaturized PCNL, the chances of infection can be high. Therefore, in the following text, we will understand the details of the technicalities of various modifications of PCNL's.

16.3 Mini PCNL

Mini PCNL was first described by Helal et al. and they performed this procedure on a 2-year-old female child. In this case, sequential dilation to 16 fr was done followed by use of a 15 F vascular peel away sheath [6]. Nephroscopy was using a 10 F pediatric cystoscope and small grasper was used to remove the stones.

The term mini PCNL has been coined by Jackman et al. In their initial description, sheath size of <22 fr was defined as mini PCNL [7]. In the present time a tract size of <20 fr is considered mini PCNL. In many parts of the world, Udo Nagele's description of MIP (minimally invasive PCNL), which was initially a 16.5 fr became representative of mini PCNL [8].

In the coming paragraphs mini PCNL will be described in terms of tract size, instrumentations used, and unsolved problems.

During the evolution of mini PCNL, the tract size between 12 fr and 20 fr was considered a mini PCNL. For practical purpose, it can be considered the "M" from shillings classification, though there are still sheaths of 12–14 fr which were considered a part of miniaturized PCNL spectrum.

The instrumentation and systems available for Mini PCNL are as follows:

1. MIP-M by Karl Storz™ (Tuttlingen, Germany): This system is developed by Karl Storz™. Two sheath sizes which encompass the definition of mini PCNL include 15/16 fr and 16.5/17.5 fr (Fig. 16.1a–d). A metallic dilator is available with the metallic sheath and a third larger size sheath of 21/22 fr size is also available. So, after passing a wire into the pelvicalyceal system, fascial dilatation is done, following which dilator of the MIP system is introduced on which MIP Sheath can be passed [9].

   These metallic sheaths are radio opaque. A fiberoptic scope (Karl Storz™) which is 12 fr scope is size is available and can be used with this system. The length of the scope is 22 cm and it has a 6.7 fr working channel, which can accommodate a 5 fr instrument.

   Mechanism of stone extraction: The metallic sheath described above has a hydrodynamic action. This phenomenon is called the Vacuum cleaner effect [9]. The jet of water passes through the scope into the pelvicalyceal system (PCS) and the stone fragments come out as the surgeon withdraws the scope out of the sheath. Once the stone is fragmented, with each withdrawal of scope multiple fragments come out. With this system there is no need to increase the irrigation pressure or add suction.
2. *Richard Wolf™ system:* For Mini PCNL a 12 fr, Richard Wolf™ scope is available commercially. It can be purchased along with two continuous irrigation sheaths of 15 and 18 fr [10]. Both the sheaths are available with single step dilator for performing mini PCNL. This system has been developed by Lahme et al.
3. *Boston scientific system:* A 16 fr Amplatz sheath has been developed which can be used in mini PCNL's.

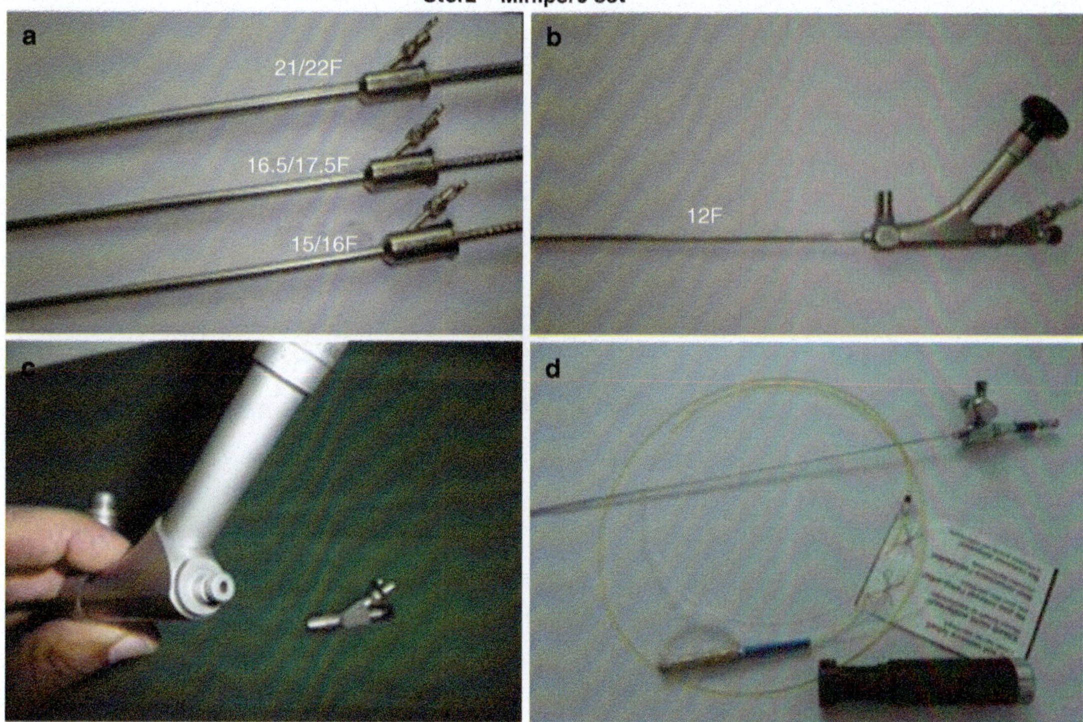

Fig. 16.1 (**a–d**) Panel 1a showing MIP-M sheaths, 1b showing 12 fr Karl Storz™, MIP-M scope, 1c 6.7 fr working channel for MIP-M scope, 1d laser fiber and lithoclast burr for MIP-M

Efficacy of mini PCNL: It causes decreased blood loss [5]. Smaller systems have increased maneuverability in the PCS. This may potentially decrease the need for number of tracts and use of the flexible nephroscope. Decrease in the pain due to decrease in the size of tract. Decreased hospital stay has been reported in many series.

16.4 Variations of Miniaturized PCNL

Modification in the instrumentations and in the techniques has been described by various authors to make fragmentation and retrieval more efficient.

16.4.1 Use of Laser with Suction

Laser with suction device is a prototype manufactured by EMS™ (Electro Medical Systems, Nyon, Switzerland). It is a 4.5 fr hollow metallic suction tube which houses another small metallic channel (Fig. 16.2a–b) [11]. Through the metallic channel a 365-micron fiber can pass. The suction is controlled by a hand-held clutch. This device enables continuous fragmentation and suction. Fragments as large as 1 mm can be sucked out and the device can pass through working channel of a 12 fr scope. The instrument also stabilizes the tip of the laser fiber [12].

16.4.2 Suction Attached to the Sheath

These devices have suction directly to sheath making fragment extraction more efficient. In PCNL the suction is attached to a closed irrigation system and various mini PCNL systems having the suction attached to sheath have been described.

(a) Super mini perc:

This technology has been described by Zeng et al. [13]. The system consists of a

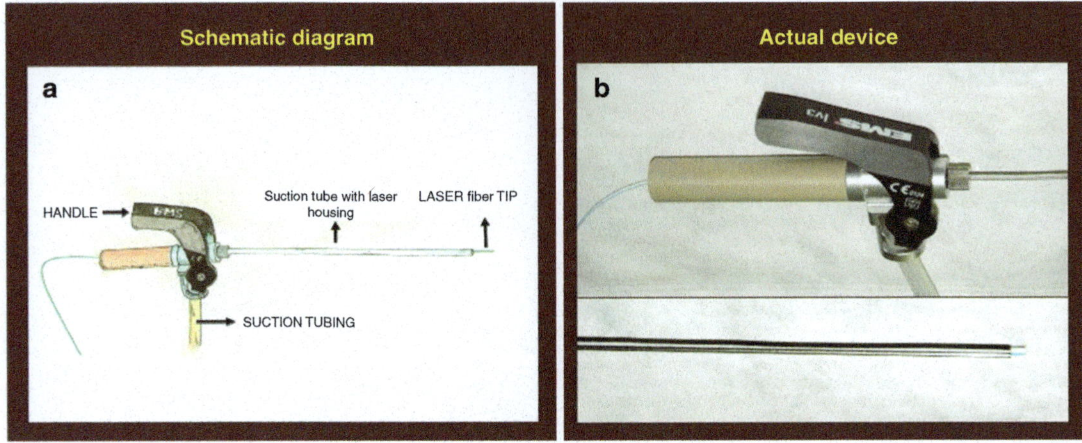

Fig. 16.2 (**a**) Schematic representation of laser with suction device, (**b**) Actual laser with suction device

10–14 fr access sheath with a suction evacuation function. The sheath has a handle with a straight and offset channel. The straight channel is covered by a rubber cork which allows passage of 7 fr nephroscope and at the same time forming a water seal around the scope. The offset channel is connected to a suction device and has a pressure vent. The suction can be activated by occluding the pressure vent. Suction can be controlled by the surgeon by partially or completely occluding the pressure vent.

(b) Super perc:

Multiple sheaths are available with this technology, i.e. 10 fr, 12 fr, and 15 fr. The sheath has been innovated by Shah et al. and the length of the sheath may vary from 8–20 cm (Fig. 16.3) [14]. The key feature of this technology is that the master suction is attached to the sheath rather than the scope and this channel is at right angles to the sheath. The authors described used of a multi-hole ureteric catheter for retrograde irrigation while using this sheath. The ureteric catheter has holes at every 10 cm allowing a free retrograde flow of saline. Enabling a better irritant flow even with suction. The suction tubing is attached to the outlet of the superperc sheath. The suction is controlled using a suction port which is finger controlled, on occlusion of port with finger suction gets activated. It allows larger fragment size retrieval. A short ureteroscope can be used as nephroscope with this sheath for mini PCNL's as described by the author and other nephroscopes compatible with the size of the sheaths can also be used. Microperc telescope, micro nephroscope from Apple life sciences, UMP (ultra mini perc) telescope with inner sheath or Karl Storz™ nephroscope can be all used with 10 and 12 F sheath. Miniperc nephroscope from Karl Storz™, Olympus™, or Richard Wolf™ can be used with 15 F sheath size.

(c) Petra sheath:

Clear sheath was popularized by the Welllead group. The sheath is a 12, 14, 16, and 18 fr sheath with its own dilator (Fig. 16.4) [15]. After tract dilatation with fascial dilator, the sheath with its dilator is introduced into the PCS. The sheath has a large offset channel where suction can be attached. It can suck out fragments as large as 3 mm. The transparent suction channel and the terminal sheath allow visualization of the fragments being sucked out as the scope is withdrawn. The suction channel is an offset channel making a smoother passage for the stone out once it is sucked. Any 12 fr or 14 fr scope can be used with this sheath.

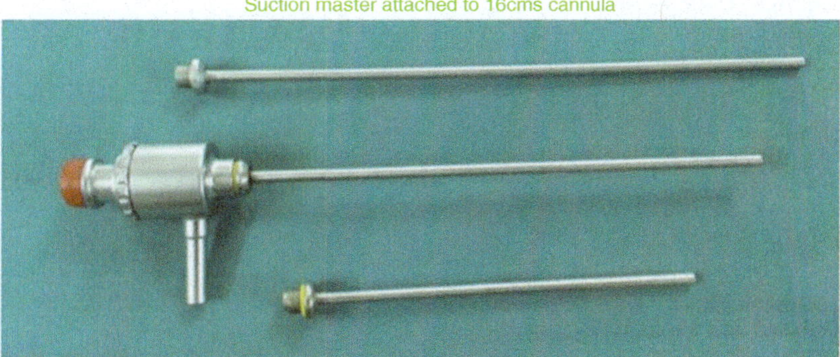

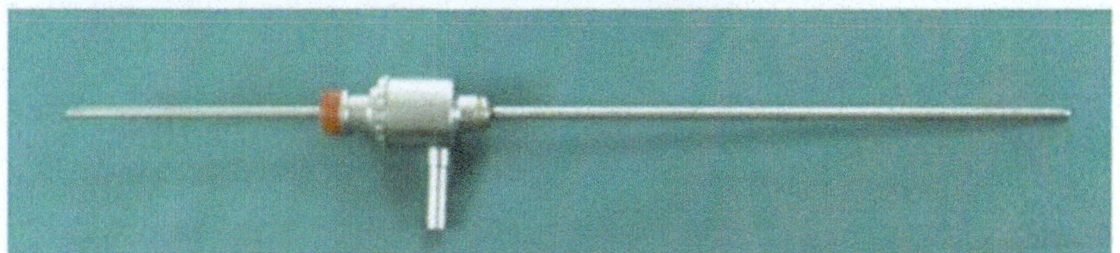

Fig. 16.3 Shah's Superc sheath

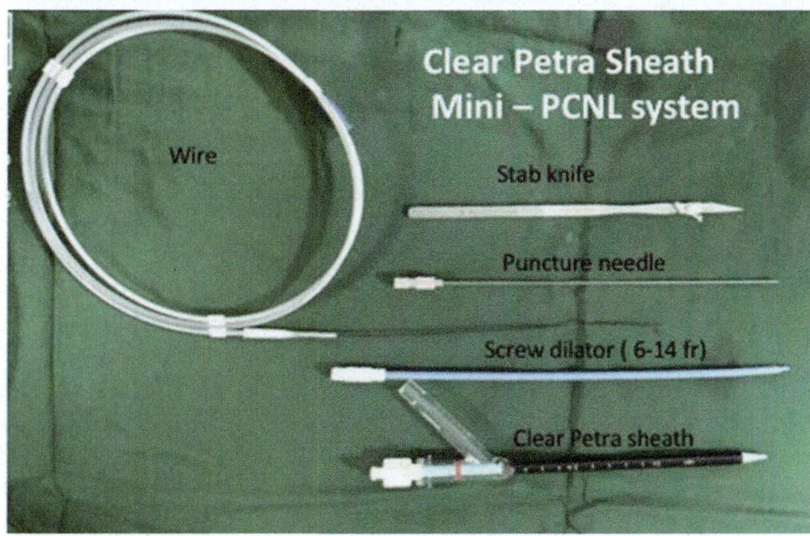

Fig. 16.4 Clear petra sheath

16.4.3 PCNL with Tract Size <15 fr and >5 fr

(a) Ultra mini perc:

Ultra miniperc (UMP) is a further miniaturization of the tract size for PCNL. UMP™ (LUT Germany) system has a 7.5 fr nephroscope sheath which has three channels [15]. First one is for a 1 mm telescope to pass, second one is dedicated for saline irrigation, and the third one allows a 365-micron laser fiber to pass. The metallic cannula is available in two sizes, i.e. 11 fr and 13 fr (Fig. 16.5). These cannulas serve as the outer sheath during the procedure [16].

After stone is fragmented using laser there is spontaneous expulsion of stones by water jet effect. In principle this technology works on the eddy currents which are developed by the jet of water going through the nephroscope into the PCS and these currents return

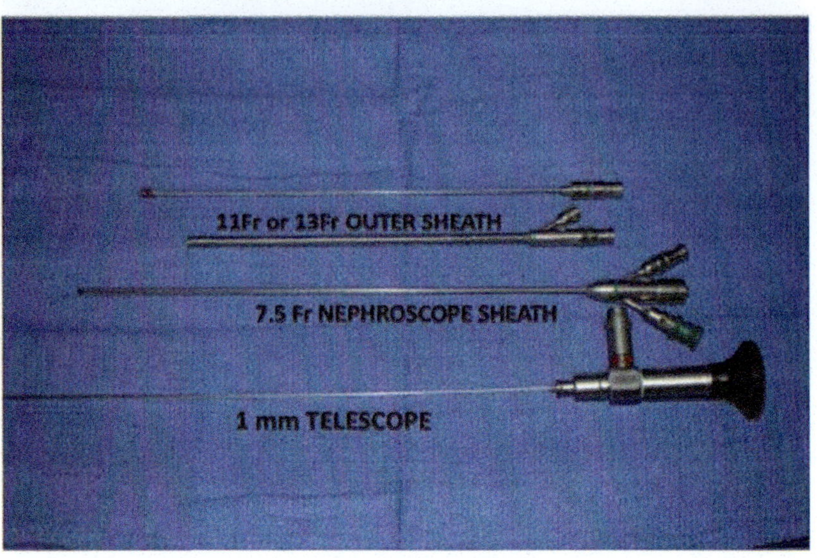

Fig. 16.5 UMP Sheath

to the sheath when the scope is withdrawn and along with irrigant it gets along the stone fragments.

Various phenomenon's, namely Whirlpool effect, water jet effect, eddy current effect, vacuum cleaner effect, or the Bernoulli's effect have been used to describe the mechanism of spontaneous stone extraction using a water jet entering the PCS from nephroscope and returning back with stone fragments.

Design and construction of the outer sheath is a major determinant of the above effect development. With the sheath size of less than 10 fr and more than 22 fr, the impact of this currents fades away.

(b) MIP S/XS:

This system developed by Karl Storz™, consists of a 7.5 fr fiber optic telescope and its sheath (Fig. 16.6). The scope is 24 cm in length, has 2 fr working channel and a 3 fr irrigation channel. In its description by Nagele et al. to maintain the intra renal pressures and to ensure visualization pressurized irrigation was used and at the same time a suction was attached to the ureteric catheter. The suction and irrigation was maintained by same device in the original description (UROMAT™ Karl Storz).

There are two different sheaths available with the system, i.e. 8.5/9.5 fr and 11/12 fr size [16]. The length of the sheath is 15 cm, which is designed for prone PCNL, a longer sheath of 18 cm length is available for PCNL in supine position. Sable et al. have shown the efficacy of this system in stone clearance to be 100% at one month [17].

(c) Micro perc:

Microperc uses a 4.5 fr "all seeing needle" or a needloscope [18]. This concept was developed by Brader et al., the philosophy was visualization as you puncture.

The microperc needle is a 16-gauge three-part needle (Fig. 16.7), the three parts consist of an outer hollow sheath, inner stylet, and inner sheath. After a successful puncture, a three-way Tuohy Borst adapter is connected to the outer sheath and from the central channel the fiber optic telescope is introduced. Form one of the lateral channels the laser fiber is introduced and from the other channel irrigation is connected. Fiber optic scope is 0.9 mm in diameter and has a resolution of 10,000 pixels (Fig. 16.8) [18]. The scope is connected to a fiber optic cable which in turn is connected to a light cable through a light pillar on the hub, also this hub allows con-

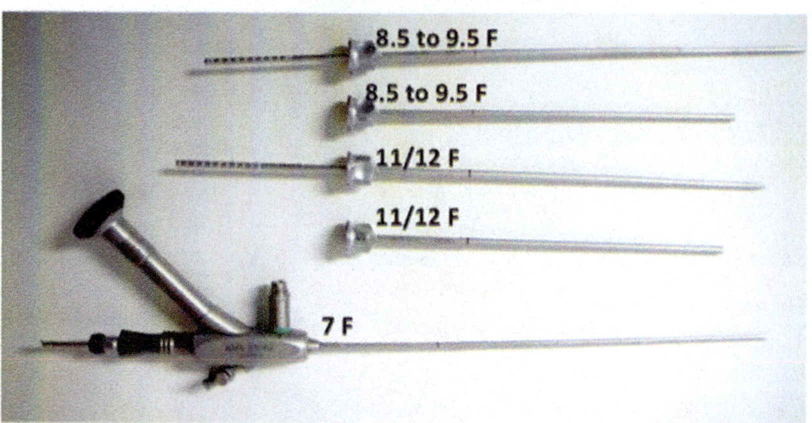

Fig. 16.6 MIP XS system

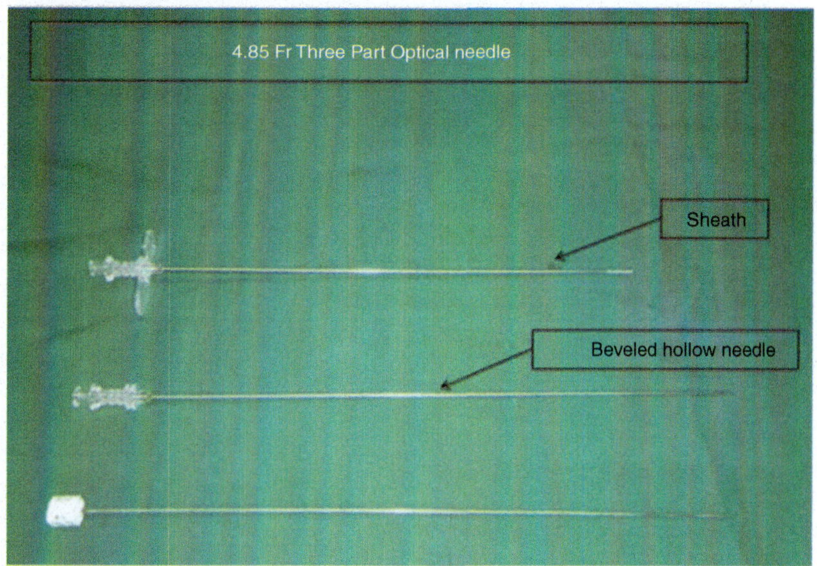

Fig. 16.7 Microperc needle

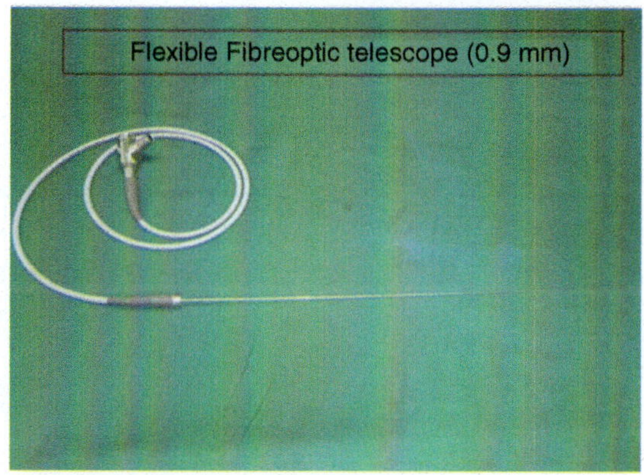

Fig. 16.8 Microperc scope

nection with the conventional camera head. The flow of irrigant through the third channel is kept at 100 ml/min on an intermittent mode using a pump.

A 7 fr multi-hole ureteric catheter, with multiple holes in the distal 5 cm of the ureteric catheter is introduced in the PCS [18, 19]. The PCS is distended with saline, and punctured under ultrasound guidance. On completion of the puncture the stylet is withdrawn and on efflux of urine, the inner sheath is also withdrawn and the outer sheath is connected to Tuohy Borst adapter.

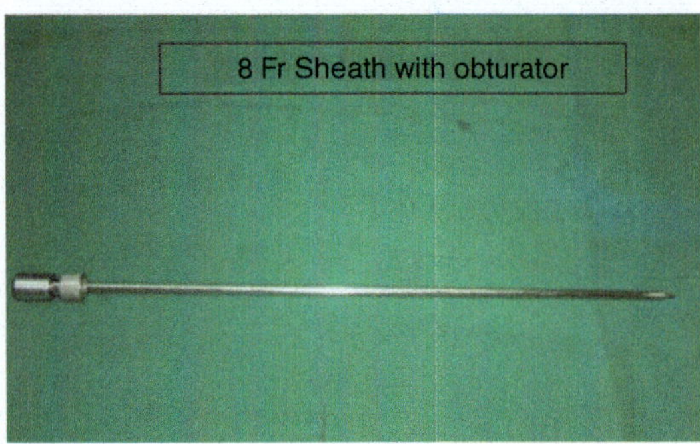

Fig. 16.9 Mini-Micro sheath

(d) Mini-Micro PCNL:

Since the microperc scope is flexible it may bend inside the PCS decreasing the visualization. Also, excessive mobilization using outer sheath of the needle may lead to PCS injury. In view of these problems mini-micro PCNL was developed. It basically using the same instrumentation of micro perc with an 8 fr metallic sheath (Fig. 16.9) [19]. After a puncture using three-part needle, wire is passed and tract is dilated to 8 fr using facial dilators and 8 fr sheath with its dilator is introduced. This sheath is connected to a Tuohy Borst adapter and the unit is used as it was done in micro perc.

Efficacy of micro perc ranges between 85% and 93%. In a randomized control trail comparing microperc with RIRS published by Sabnis et al. the clearance rate for micro perc was 97.1% [20].

16.5 Standard PCNL

Standard PCNL is defined as a tract size >20 fr used for carrying out PCNL's. In the era of miniaturization surgeons should not forget the utility of standard PCNL.

Advantages of standard PCNL:

1. Procedure is quick and time efficient [5].
2. Larger tract with Amplatz sheath acting as an open system does not allow the intra renal pressure to increase.
3. Larger tract, so larger fragments can be retrieved [5].
4. Through the larger tracts, larger nephroscopes can be introduced, thereby providing irrigation and vision.
5. In infected systems, larger tract does not allow the pressure to rise, decreases the pyelolymphatic back flow, and decreases the chances of sepsis.
6. Large stone sizes are better managed by larger tracts.
7. All the modern energy sources work best with standard PCNL's.

Standard PCNL, in an era of miniaturization still holds its position as there are situations where mini PCNL will just not be able to provide an efficient solution. A stone size >3–3.5 cm can only be efficiently managed using standard PCNL.

Efficacy of standard PCNL is around 95% in many series. The problems include increased blood loss; increased hospital stay, and PCS injury [5].

Considering various types of PCNL, which one to be used in which situation is the most important aspect of understanding mini PCNL. Horses for courses philosophy make each of these technologies useful.

Using the size criteria, the stones can be grouped in 4 categories:

1. < 1 cm
2. 1–1.5 cm
3. 1.5–2.5 cm
4. >2.5 cm.

Using the tract size criteria given by Schilling the tract can be divided as:

1. XL – >25 fr.
2. L – 20–25 fr.
3. M – 15–20 fr.
4. S – 10–15 fr.
5. XS – 5–10 fr.
6. XXS – <5 fr.

Various devices and tract sizes can be summarized as follows:

Tract size	Schillings classification	Nomenclature as per the developer	Ideally suited for stone size	Fragmentation device	Accessory	Scope size	Working Channel
>25 fr	XL	Standard PCNL	Staghorn larger than 4 cm	Ballistic, Ultrasound, Combined	Forceps	20 fr or more	10–11 fr
20–25 fr	L	Standard PCNL	2.5–4 cm	Ballistic, Ultrasound, Combined	Forceps	18–20 fr	9–10 fr
15–20 fr	M	MIP-M, Mini PCNL,	1.5–2.5 cm	Ballistic, Ultrasound,	Forceps, basket	12 fr	6 fr
		Super mini perc, Superperc, Clear Petra		Combined, laser	Forceps, basket	7 fr to 12 fr scope	–
10–15 fr	S	MIP-S,	1–1.5 cm	Laser	Basket	7.5 fr	2 fr
		UMP,	1–1.5 cm	Laser	Basket	7.5 fr	–
		Clear Petra (12/14 fr)	1–1.5 cm	Laser	Basket	12 fr/7.5 fr	
		Superperc (10 fr/12 fr)	1–1.5 cm	Laser	Basket		
5–10 fr	XS	MIP XS	1–1.5 cm	Laser	Basket	7.5	2 fr
		Mini Micro	1–1.5 cm	Laser	–	8 fr	–

16.6 Conclusion

It is important to understand that all tract sizes have relevance in modern endourology. Stone size is the single most important determinant of deciding the tract size. The other determinants include infection, duration of procedure, and expected blood loss. Advancement in the energy sources will help us achieve quicker stone clearance from the smallest possible tract. Uniformity of classification will help us better understand the different types of minimally invasive PCNL's.

References

1. Fernström I, Johansson B. Percutaneous pyelolithotomy. A new extraction technique. Scand J Urol Nephrol. 1976 Dec;10(3):257–9.
2. Kukreja R, Desai M, Patel S, Bapat S, Desai M. First prize: factors affecting blood loss during percutaneous nephrolithotomy: Prospective Study. J Endourol. 2004 Oct 1;18(8):715–22.
3. Proietti S, Giusti G, Desai M, Ganpule AP. A critical review of miniaturised percutaneous nephrolithotomy: is smaller better? Eur Urol Focus. 2017 Feb 1;3(1):56–61.
4. Schilling D, Hüsch T, Bader M, Herrmann TR, Nagele U. Training and research in urological surgery and technology group. Nomenclature in PCNL or the tower of Babel: a proposal for a uniform terminology. World J Urol. 2015;33:1905–7.
5. Mishra S, Sharma R, Garg C, Kurien A, Sabnis R, Desai M. Prospective comparative study of miniperc and standard PNL for treatment of 1 to 2 cm size renal stone. BJU Int. 2011 Sep 1;108(6):896–900.
6. Helal M, Black T, Lockhart J, Figueroa TE. The Hickman peel-away sheath: alternative for pediatric percutaneous nephrolithotomy. J Endourol. 1997 Jun;11(3):171–2.
7. Jackman SV, Docimo SG, Cadeddu JA, Bishoff JT, Kavoussi LR, Jarrett TW. The "mini-perc" technique: a less invasive alternative to per-cutaneous nephrolithotomy. World J Urol. 1998;16:371–4.
8. Nagele U, Schilling D, Anastasiadis AG, et al. Minimally invasive percutaneous nephrolitholapaxy (MIP). Urologe A. 2008;47:1068–73.
9. Nagele U, Nicklas A. Vacuum cleaner effect, purging effect, active and passive wash out: a new terminology in hydrodynamic stone retrieval is arising-does it affect our endourologic routine? World J Urol. 2016;34:143–4.
10. Lahme S. Miniaturisation of PCNL. Urolithiasis. 2018 Feb 1;46(1):99–106.
11. D'Souza N, Paul S. Mini percutaneous nephrolithotomy for renal calculi in paediatric patients: a review of twenty cases. Urol Ann. 2016 Jan;8(1):16.
12. Singh A, Jairath A, Chhabra J, Mishra S, Ganpule A, Sabnis R, Desai M. Laser with suction as an energy

source in mini percutaneous nephrolithotomy: muljibhai patel urological hospital experience. J Endourol Videourol. 2016 Jul;30(5).
13. Zeng G, Wan S, Zhao Z, Zhu J, Tuerxun A, Song C, Zhong L, Liu M, Xu K, Li H, Jiang Z. Super-mini percutaneous nephrolithotomy (SMP): a new concept in technique and instrumentation. BJU Int. 2016 Apr;117(4):655–61.
14. Shah K, Agrawal MS, Mishra DK. Superperc: a new technique in minimally-invasive percutaneous nephrolithotomy. Indian J Urol. 2017 Jan;33(1):48.
15. Zanetti SP, Sampogna G, Fontana M, De Lorenzis E, Gallioli A, Boeri L, Palmisano F, Sabatini I, Albo G, Longo F, Montanari E. Innovations in PCNL: a closed circuit mini-perc system. Eur Urol Suppl. 2018 May 31;17(4):e2121.
16. Desai J, Solanki R. Ultra-mini percutaneous nephrolithotomy (UMP): one more armamentarium. BJU Int. 2013 Nov;112(7):1046–9.
17. Sabale V, Pramanik P, Mane D, Satav V, Shah AS, Chaudari N, Kandari A. Our experience with Miniperc XS in the management of renal stones. Urol Sci. 2019;30:36–9.
18. Desai MR, Sharma R, Mishra S, Sabnis RB, Stief C, Bader M. Single-step percutaneous nephrolithotomy (microperc): the initial clinical report. J Urol. 2011;186:140–5.
19. Sabnis RB, Ganesamoni R, Ganpule AP, Mishra S, Vyas J, Jagtap J, Desai M. Current role of microperc in the management of small renal calculi. Indian J Urol. 2013 Jul;29(3):214.
20. Sabnis RB, Ganesamoni R, Doshi A, Ganpule AP, Jagtap J, Desai MR. Micropercutaneous nephrolithotomy (microperc) vs retrograde intrarenal surgery for the management of small renal calculi: a randomized controlled trial. BJU Int. 2013;112:355–61.

Recent Development of Endoscopic Intrarenal Stone Surgery: Approaches and Surgical Tips

17

Min Soo Choo and Sung Yong Cho

Abstract

Recent development of technology allows us to provide tailored management for patients with urolithiasis. Not only it significantly reduces rates of mortality and morbidity but also it increases surgical outcomes. In the era of flexible ureteroscopy and nephroscopy, urologists have shown the expanding indications of minimally invasive surgical therapy for managing complicated renal and ureteral stones. Combined approach of antegrade and retrograde manners for removal of complicated renal stones has been widely accepted to urologists over the last several decades. Endoluminal endourology contains endoscopic management of urinary stone, ureteral stricture, benign prostatic hyperplasia, and urothelial carcinoma. We will hereby review the indications and treatment modalities according to each approach in the field of endoluminal endourology.

Keywords

Urolithiasis · Urinary Calculi · Nephrolithotomy · Percutaneous · Ureteroscopy Minimally Invasive Surgical Procedures

17.1 Introduction

Urologists have been performing endourological procedures such as percutaneous nephrolithotomy (PCNL) in an antegrade manner and ureteroscopic surgery (URS) in a retrograde manner. When we choose the type of surgery, the patient's status and needs, renal function, patients' quality of life, and cost-effectiveness should be evaluated. Recently, many urologists recognized the importance of combined approach of antegrade and retrograde manners to increase surgical outcomes for patients with complicated renal and ureteral stones as shown in Fig. 17.1.

17.2 Indications for Combined Approaches

To determine the approach to the target lesion, the burden and location of the stones are the main important factors [1]. CT scan is essential

M. S. Choo
Department of Urology, SMG-SNU Boramae Medical Center, Seoul, South Korea
e-mail: mschoo@snu.ac.kr

S. Y. Cho (✉)
Department of Urology, Seoul National University, College of Medicine, Seoul National University Hospital, Seoul, South Korea

Specialized Endoluminal Endourology-Stone (SEES) Center & Usability Test Center in SNUH Innovative Medical Technology Research Institute, Seoul National University Hospital, Seoul, South Korea
e-mail: moretry@snuh.org

A. C.F. Ng et al. (eds.), *Practical Management of Urinary Stone*,
https://doi.org/10.1007/978-981-16-4193-0_17

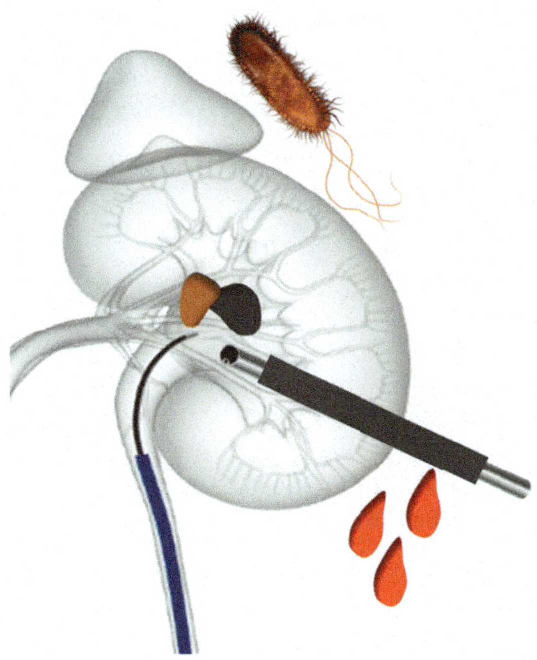

Fig. 17.1 Combined approach of antegrade and retrograde manners for patients with renal and ureteral stone

to determine the stone burden and location, and low dose CT protocol is recently available without sacrificing the diagnostic value significantly [2].

For renal stones larger than 20 mm, an antegrade approach should be considered as first-line therapy [3]. The antegrade approach is relatively contraindicated in pregnant women but may be an acceptable option in pediatric patients over 20 mm in size [3]. For lower pole stones over 10 mm, an antegrade approach has a higher stone-free rate, but greater morbidity than a retrograde approach [4]. The antegrade approach is preferred for patients with renal stones and a history of urinary diversion or transplanted kidney [3]. On the other hand, the retrograde approach should be considered as first-line therapy in patients with a tendency to bleed or unable to discontinue anticoagulant/antiplatelets [2]. Performing flexible nephroscopy at the end of PCNL procedures is essentially recommended to find possible small remnant stone fragments, and it is recently reported that a retrograde approach was more successful than an antegrade approach [5, 6].

There is a consensus that combined approach, performed with a modified supine position, is a safe and effective surgical method, and the indications have been continuously expanded over the last several decades [7, 8]. This combined approach in modified supine position may offer urological benefits such as reduction of X-ray exposure, possibility to avoid multiple percutaneous accesses, anesthesiologic advantages, and optimal drainage of stone fragments with vacuum cleaner effect [5, 9].

17.2.1 Indications for Combined Approaches to the Kidney or Ureter Stones

Selection of combined approach depends on the status of the renal and ureteral stones such as location, size, or presence of ureteral strictures. An antegrade approach remains the gold treatment option for large renal stones, staghorn stones, stones in the nephrocalcinosis, large renal and concomitant ureteral stones or contralateral small-to-medium renal stones, stones for patients with ileal conduit, and the impacted ureteropelvic junction stones with complete obstruction. We can consider ancillary procedures to increase surgical outcomes [3, 4]. PCNL can be considered when the infundibulopelvic angle is acute or the infundibulum is narrow even the lower pole stone is smaller than 2 cm. In this situation, additional small stones in the upper or midpole calyces can be removed by flexible URS [7].

Some congenital anomalies may need combined approach and we can maximize the stone-free rates with acceptable safety profiles. Retrograde approach to the orifice of ileal conduit with flexible URS, cystoscopy, or semi-rigid URS can be feasible and concomitant antegrade insertion of flexible URS or ureteral catheter would be necessary to check the direction to the ureter [10]. In case of a diverticular stone, combined approach can improve the stone-free rates, reduce postoperative complications, and prevent damage to the flexible scope [11]. Percutaneous antegrade approach to the upper pole calyx is helpful for patients with horseshoe kidneys because the flexible URS is not available to remove the stones in some cases when the renal stones are located in the lower pole next to the isthmus [12]. The flexible URS can be inserted to remove these stones through an antegrade approach [8].

17.3 Combined Approach

17.3.1 Optimal Set-up of Operating Room

Development of modified supine position has tried to achieve more working space, less stress to the spine, less rotation of the torso, and less mobility of the kidney with stones [9]. The leg should be split to acquire enough space for surgeons. When the first main surgeon moves to the place between the stirrups near the lower extremity after PCNL procedures, repositioning and mobilizing the knees and legs is helpful for acquiring enough space for flexible URS. However, specific care should be taken because oversplit legs can have risk of nerve palsy. The laser machine should be located as close to the operating table next to the surgeons when we consider limitation of the length of laser fibers.

17.3.2 Surgical Techniques

When surgeons consider combined approach to the target, percutaneous puncture can be performed by a ureteral catheter, a dual-lumen catheter, or an occlusion catheter. While the first surgeon performs PCNL, the second surgeon can perform flexible URS simultaneously or assist the first surgeon by ureteroscopic movement. Small fragmented stone segments can move to the ureter during PCNL procedures and this may obstruct the ureter. As a result, additional flexible URS may be necessary. Simultaneous flexible URS by the second surgeon may prevent this situation. Use of an occlusion catheter, a dual-lumen catheter, or a safety guidewire can help to avoid passage of fragmented small stones into the ureter during PCNL procedures.

The flexible URS can be used as guidance for puncture, and the guidewire can be drawn to the ureter by the flexible URS. This through-and-through technique may guarantee the stability of the percutaneous tract with acceptable safety issues.

The larger the size of the access sheath, the easier it is to irrigate and to remove larger stones, but the higher the risk of ureteral injury. Using ureteral access sheaths facilitates insertion of flexible URS, maintenance of lower intrarenal pressure, increased stone-free rates, and drainage of fragmented stone particles from the renal pelvis and the upper collecting system during PCNL procedures although long-term follow-up results are still lacking on what problems these ureteral injuries may cause after surgery.

Basically, 550 nm fibers can be applied to PCNL procedures with nephroscopes. The size of 275 to 365 nm fibers is appropriate for the use of flexible nephroscopes. If the tract size is small and frequent in-and-out movement is not available, dusting or pop-dusting technique might be a good option. This technique is also helpful to reduce the risk of scope damage.

17.3.3 Handling Ureter Lesions

Advancement of the flexible URS through a percutaneous puncture into the level of the mid ureter or below can be challenging. The puncture should be made through the upper pole or the midpole at least to reduce excessive movement of nephroscopes. Excessive torque with the rigid nephroscope may cause massive damage to the kidney. The size of percutaneous tract of 18 Fr to 20 Fr is recommended to reduce damage of outer surface of flexible URS during back and forth movement and the most fragile portion of f-URS is the medial side of working channel when deflected. Larger bore tracts may lead to a large space for flexible URS. However, at the same time, bleeding and poor vision even with high speed irrigation. The use of a disposable URS is strongly recommendable in an antegrade manner.

When surgeons consider combined approach for incision of ureteral stricture, the narrow seg-

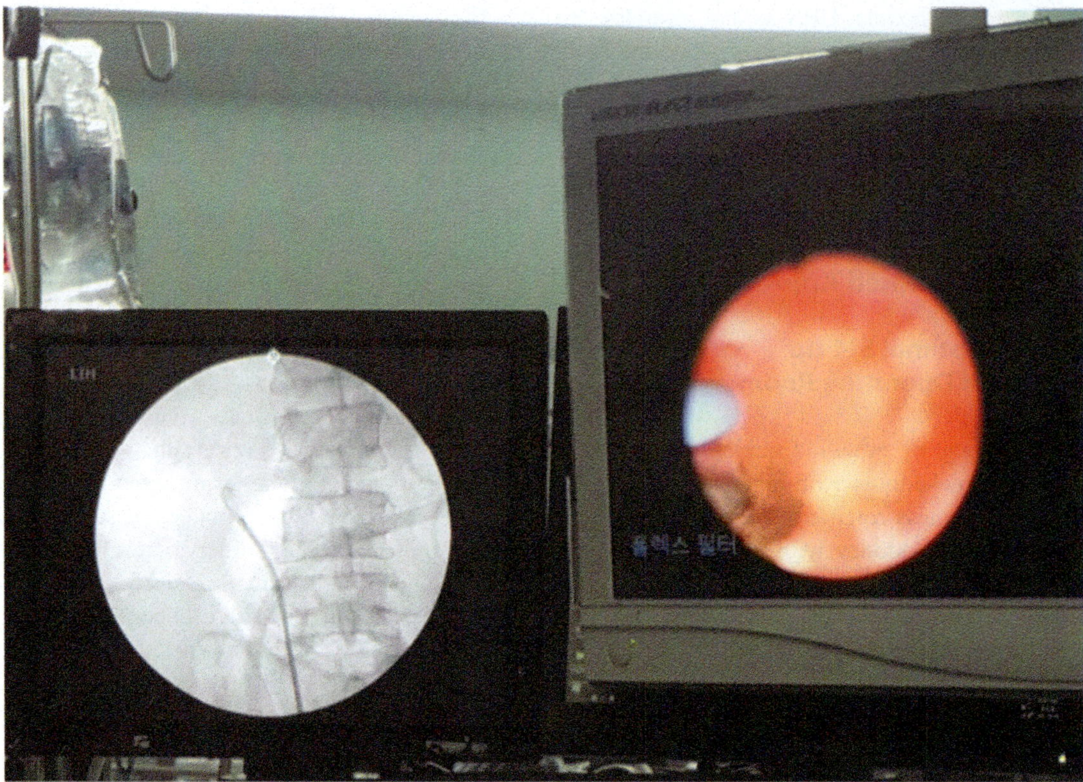

Fig. 17.2 Incision of the stricture site with laser

ment should be shorter than 5 mm if we want to significantly increase the success rates. Antegrade incision can increase the accuracy due to the straightforward direction and enough space of the upper ureter compared to retrograde incision. When we incise the lesion, we need to trace yellow-colored fibrotic part to go through the center of the stricture site as shown in Fig. 17.2. Indigo carmine or light in a retrograde approach can be helpful to find the right place for channeling the stricture site.

17.4 Summary

Tailored management for renal stones should be considered to manage renal and ureteral stones and stricture lesions to increase surgical outcomes and to reduce morbidity rates. In the age of flexible URS and miniaturized PCNL, the devices can be chosen on a case-by-case basis. Combined approach can be selected in proper cases and cost-effectiveness should be considered together in daily practice.

Acknowledgments This work was supported by a grant (No. 2019R1C1C1008339) of the National Research Foundation (NRF) grant funded by the Korean government (MSIT).

References

1. Desai M, Sun Y, Buchholz N, Fuller A, Matsuda T, Matlaga B, et al. Treatment selection for urolithiasis: percutaneous nephrolithotomy, ureteroscopy, shock wave lithotripsy, and active monitoring. World J Urol. 2017;35(9):1395–9.
2. Assimos D, Krambeck A, Miller NL, Monga M, Murad MH, Nelson CP, et al. Surgical management of stones: American Urological Association/Endourological Society Guideline, Part I. J Urol. 2016;196(4):1153–60.
3. European Association U. European Association of Urology Pocket Guidelines. 2020 Edition. Arnhem,

The Netherlands: European Association of Urology Guidelines Office; 2020.
4. Assimos D, Krambeck A, Miller NL, Monga M, Murad MH, Nelson CP, et al. Surgical management of stones: American Urological Association/Endourological Society Guideline, Part II. J Urol. 2016;196(4):1161–9.
5. Keller EX, De Coninck V, Doizi S, Traxer O. The role of ureteroscopy for treatment of staghorn calculi: a systematic review. Asian J Urol. 2020;7(2):110–5.
6. Gökce M, Gülpinar O, Ibiş A, Karaburun M, Kubilay E, Süer E. Retrograde vs. antegrade flexible nephroscopy for detection of residual fragments following PNL: a prospective study with computerized tomography control. Int Braz J Urol. 2019;45(3):581–7.
7. Cracco CM, Scoffone CM. Endoscopic combined intrarenal surgery (ECIRS) – tips and tricks to improve outcomes: a systematic review. Turk J Urol. 2020;
8. Jung HD, Kim JC, Ahn HK, Kwon JH, Han K, Han WK, et al. Real-time simultaneous endoscopic combined intrarenal surgery with intermediate-supine position: washout mechanism and transport technique. Investig Clin Urol. 2018;59(5):348–54.
9. Scoffone CM, Cracco CM. Invited review: the tale of ECIRS (Endoscopic Combined IntraRenal Surgery) in the Galdakao-modified supine Valdivia position. Urolithiasis. 2018;46(1):115–23.
10. Olson L, Satherley H, Cleaveland P, Zelhof B, Mokete M, Neilson D, et al. Retrograde endourological management of upper urinary tract abnormalities in patients with ileal conduit urinary diversion: a dual-center experience. J Endourol. 2017;31(9):841–6.
11. Patodia M, Sinha RJ, Singh S, Singh V. Management of renal caliceal diverticular stones: a decade of experience. Urol Ann. 2017;9(2):145–9.
12. Singh AG, Jairath A, Balaji SS, Tak G, Ganpule AP, Vijayakumar M, et al. Changing trends in the endourological management of urolithiasis in anomalous kidneys. BJU Int. 2019;123(2):318–27.

Percutaneous Nephrolithotomy: Management of Complications

18

Srinath Chandrasekera

Keywords

PCNL · Percutaneous nephrolithotomy
Renal stones · Kidney · Complications
Haemorrhage · Sepsis · Urine extravasation
Bowel injury · Pleural injury · Morbidity

"Primum Non Nocere" (first do no harm): Hippocrates 460 BC

18.1 Introduction

Percutaneous Nephrolithotomy (PCNL), the pivotal technique for treating larger renal stones, has seen major advancements and acceptance globally in the past decade. Data from numerous large-escale studies across several continents have provided a better understanding of complications associated with PCNL. The Modified Clavien-Dindo grading system is useful in analysing the severity of complications for comparative purposes. Common complications associated with PCNL are summarized in Information Box 18.1 and discussed for a clearer understanding of their management.

Information Box 18.1 Common complications of PCNL

- Fever/sepsis
- Bleeding
- Perforation of pelvicalyceal system/ extravasation
- Pleural injury
- Bowel injury
- Failure to complete procedure

Large studies estimate the overall rate of complications following PCNL at around 14% [1]. Of these, the majority are Clavien grade 1 due to infection, minor bleeding and urinary extravasation. The more serious morbidities include sepsis, haemorrhage requiring transfusion and/or intervention, injury or perforation of the pelvicalyceal system causing extravasation and visceral injury.

18.2 Infection and Sepsis

Infection and sepsis are the commonest complications associated with PCNL, with a reported incidence ranging from 0.3% to 7.7% in different studies [2, 3]. Post-PCNL sepsis is the leading cause of mortality following PCNL [4].

The common risk factors for sepsis following PCNL are summarized in Information Box 18.2.

S. Chandrasekera (✉)
Faculty of Medical Sciences, University of Sri Jayewardenepura, Nugegoda, Sri Lanka

A. C.F. Ng et al. (eds.), *Practical Management of Urinary Stone*,
https://doi.org/10.1007/978-981-16-4193-0_18

Information Box 18.2 Risk factors for sepsis following PCNL

- Past upper tract infection
- Infection (struvite) stones
- Prolonged procedures
- Large stones >25 mm
- Multitrack PCNL
- Need for blood transfusion
- Poorly controlled diabetes
- Distal obstruction
- Perinephric collection
- Undiagnosed visceral injury

Positive preoperative urine cultures, positive stone culture, the number of tracts used for access, blood transfusions, staghorn stones and poorly controlled diabetes are frequently associated with post-PCNL sepsis [4, 5]. The causal relationship between positive urine cultures and stone is obvious. However, the link between the number of tracts, blood transfusions and sepsis are likely reflections of the association between the complexity of the procedure and sepsis. Staghorn stones were known to be associated with infection in earlier studies stone composition revealed triple phosphate (struvite stones) that was a common cause of chronic urinary infection. More recent literature reveals that the incidence of struvite stones is on the decline and that a larger proportion of staghorn is composed of oxalate and or uric acid [6]. Age, gender, body mass index and positive renal pelvis culture have not been associated with a higher risk of sepsis in most larger scale studies [5].

Diagnosis of infection and sepsis requires a high degree of clinical suspicion. In high-risk patients and where the infection is suspected during surgery, the exit strategy should essentially include insertion of a stent and/or nephrostomy to ensure continuous drainage. "Tubeless" PCNL should not be performed in such instances. These patients are best managed in a high dependency unit with close monitoring and use of broad-spectrum intravenous antibiotics. De-escalation antibiotic therapy is preferred due to the potential severity of the consequences of urosepsis.

Common causes of unanticipated urinary sepsis include distal obstruction due to dislodged stone fragments/clots or perinephric collections the following extravasation. Computed tomography is useful to diagnose such causes. If the obstruction is diagnosed, urgent decompression should be carried out with a ureteric stent or perinephric drain. Placement of a percutaneous nephrostomy (PCN) immediately following PCNL can be challenging, as post-operative changes in the retroperitoneum limit ultrasonographic clarity. Another probable reason for sepsis in low-risk patients is an inadvertent breach of sterility, which is possible during an operative procedure requiring "multiple steps."

The incidence of inadvertent bowel puncture during access is likely under-diagnosed (see below under visceral injury). In the absence of dilation of a tract, these injuries may often be self-limiting. However, translocation of bowel pathogens to the retroperitoneum may follow such injuries giving rise to post-operative fever or sepsis. With antibiotic therapy and close observation, the majority of such cases settle without further sequelae.

18.2.1 Prevention

Routine use of antibiotics in all patients undergoing PCNL has demonstrated a reduction of post-PCNL sepsis irrespective of preoperative cultures [5]. Interestingly, the stone-free rate in this group too has been shown to be higher than those operated without antibiotics. If the infection is detected preoperatively, PCNL should be deferred until the infection is treated and confirmed by negative cultures. The general recommendation is for antibiotic therapy for at least for several days prior to surgery in such patients. Treatment should be continued on an appropriate prophylactic or therapeutic regime of antibiotics until PCNL is completed in these patients [7]. If the infection is suspected in association with obstruction, prompt drainage should be performed by appropriate means (percutaneous nephrostomy or stent). No significant difference has been demonstrated between the outcome following stent or nephrostomy. Therefore, the choice of a nephrostomy or stent may depend largely on the patient's cardiovascular stability and local logistics. The likelihood of overt infection in the upper tract remains high in previously treated patients and may flare up despite negative cultures after antibiotic therapy. In such patients, routine use of broad-spectrum therapeutic antibiotics is a safe practice.

Tubeless procedures should be avoided in those at risk of sepsis [7]. Mitigating the build up of intrarenal pressure (target less than 30 mm Hg) is another useful measure to prevent sepsis [8]. In the authors' experience, usage of low-pressure irrigation, allowing a wide space between the nephroscope and access sheath to facilitate free drainage of irrigation are practical steps to minimize chances of unduly increased intrarenal pressure. The use of suction systems is an alternative which may be with special access sheaths (e.g: Clearpetra[R]) or specially designed nephroscopes such as the super mini[R] PCNL system. When infection is suspected, stone fragmentation time should be minimized, and the particle size should be as large as possible. Techniques of stone dusting and popcorning are best avoided in such instances. At the end of the procedure, the pelvicalyceal system should be "clean" and free of residual stone or stone dust to minimize infective foci remaining within the system. Use of "Midi" 20–24f tracts as opposed to smaller tracts and the use of lithoclast, instead of lasers, and ultrasonic devices are steps useful to achieve the above objectives, although significant differences between the type of intracorporeal lithotripsy and infective outcomes have not been proven [5].

In instances where an apparently routine or uncomplicated case escalates to a high-risk situation (e.g. the stone appearing to be "infected," need for additional tracts, extravasation of irrigation, perforation of the renal pelvis or lengthy procedure), exit strategy should essentially include adequate tube drainage along with broad-spectrum therapeutic antibiotics and close observation.

Occasionally surgeons come across cases where frank pus or "infected looking" urine is noted during access despite negative cultures. The inflammatory markers are often equivocal in these patients. Such cases may often be due to chronic obstruction of calyces and may not necessarily reflect ongoing infection. However, it is best that appropriate drainage is carried out (stent/PCN) in such instances and PCNL be performed later as a general principle for safety. However, the surgeon may, on occasion, individualize decisions regarding tube drainage based on clinical judgement. Practical steps to avoid infection and sepsis following PCNL are summarized in Information Box 18.3.

Information Box 18.3 Practical measures to prevent sepsis following PCNL

- All patients to have antibiotics
- Preoperatively diagnosed infection should be treated until cultures are negative
- Drain infected systems preoperatively even if there is no overt sepsis
- Control diabetes before surgery
- Avoid residual stones: they may carry infection
- Avoid tubeless PCNL in high-risk patients
- Minimize build up of excessive intrarenal pressure at PCNL
- Try to avoid dusting and popcorning in cases at higher risk of infection

18.3 Bleeding

Bleeding is a frequent complication following PCNL. Clinically insignificant minor bleeding is frequent after PCNL and settles within a day or so without any further intervention. However, more significant bleeding at PCNL can cause serious morbidity, compromising haemodynamic stability and threatening life. The reported incidence of blood transfusion rates following PCNL vary from 5% to 18% [9].

Bleeding associated with PCNL can either be arterial or venous, the latter being more frequent.

Arterial injury could be due to leaking false aneurysms or arterio-venous fistulae with a reported incidence of 0.3–1.7% [10]. Arterial injuries almost always require intervention, whereas the majority of venous injuries settle with conservative measures. There are several factors that may precipitate haemorrhage during different stages of PCNL. These include tract dilatation and access, stone fragmentation and retrieval. Bleeding may also occur as a delayed post-operative event.

It is now established that the size of the tract (and therefore the access sheath) has a significant impact on the risk of haemorrhage during PCNL. Yamaguchi et al. demonstrated the risk of haemorrhage with an 18F or smaller tract is four times less than with a 24–26F tract. Conversely, the risk increases almost threefold when tract size increases from 24–26F to over 30F [11] Information Box 18.4. This study also challenges the established wisdom of balloon dilators, increasing the risk of bleeding compared to Alken dilators. Irrespective of tract size or type of dilatation, overly aggressive dilatation is one of the key reasons for bleeding during this stage of PCNL. Whilst the findings of this study emphasize the importance of using smaller tracts to minimize bleeding, the choice of tract size is often determined by other factors, including stone size, calyceal anatomy, availability of miniaturized instruments and indeed, the method each surgeon has adopted over a period of time. It is recommended through personal experience that miniaturized PCNL (<18F) are best for stones less than 2 cm and larger stones; even staghorn be managed using 24F sized sheaths in most instances.

Information Box 18.4 Relationship of tract size to bleeding

Tract size (F)	Bleeding
<18	1.1%
24–26	4.8%
27–30	5.9%
>32	12.1%

Ref: Yamaguchi et al. J Endourol 25(6):933–939

Significant bleeding may be encountered during the next stage of access due to several reasons. When access is attempted into calyces packed with stones, immediate positioning of the access sheath within the calyx may not be possible. Therefore, the operator has to start the procedure with some the renal parenchyma directly exposed without the tamponade effect of the sheath. This can lead to bleeding from the exposed parenchyma. With experience, the operator learns to increase fluid pressure to maintain visibility during this stage and perform brisk but careful fragmentation and retrieval of some of the stones packed within the calyx. Such a manoeuvre enables the advancement of the sheath into the calyx. The access sheath has an excellent tamponade effect and, once advanced into the calyx, contains parenchymal bleeding promptly. Occasionally, the puncture may result in injury to a segmental artery or vessels around the calyceal neck, which is more challenging to control (Fig. 18.1c).

Secondly, if the dilatation "overshoots" the calyx, there may be an injury to parenchyma on the contralateral calyceal wall, which is more difficult to resolve. Acute angulation or shearing of

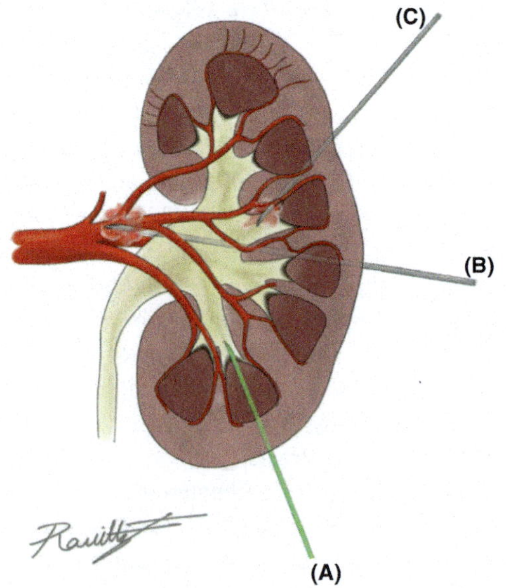

Fig. 18.1 Renal access: Ideal puncture and vascular complications due to suboptimal puncture. (**a**) Ideal puncture (**b**) Deep puncture leading to major vascular injury (**c**) Puncture through calyceal neck resulting in vascular injury

the sheath against the parenchyma is an important and preventable cause of tearing. The commonest reason for this is poorly planned punctures at an acute angle with the main axis of the calyx. Here the operator will be compelled to turn the sheath acutely immediately after entering the calyx, which carries a high risk of tearing (Fig. 18.2). Further, such angulation compromises the ability to navigate through the calyceal system, which is crucial with PCNL for larger stones and also risks damage to the scope due to shearing. Aggressive manipulation of access sheath across tight calyceal necks and resultant tearing of vessels around it is another reason for bleeding during PCNL. Narrow calyceal necks are easily seen on contrast CT images or retrograde studies, and when encountered, sheath size should be chosen appropriately. Use of excessive fluid pressure, especially with a snuggly fitting nephroscope, aggressive handling of lithoclast or stones fragments are other common causes of bleeding from the mucosa. EAU guidelines recommend an irrigation pressure of less than 30 mmHg during PCNL [7]. Lithotripsy should be carried out as gently as possible avoiding injury to the calyceal lining. Clear visualization of the stone prior to fragmentation and a gentle technique is important to avoid undue injury.

With increasing experience, the operator learns to carry out PCNL with mild or moderate bleed-

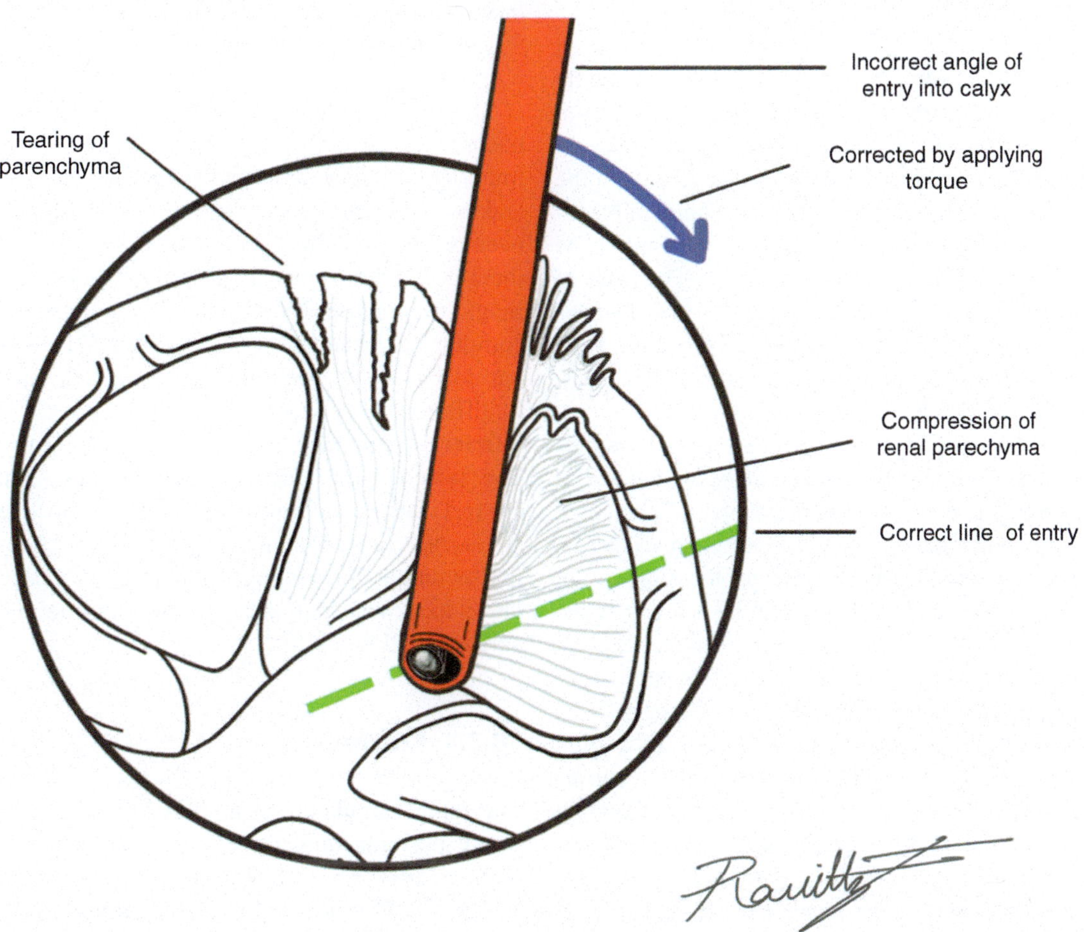

Fig. 18.2 Entry at an acute angle to the calyx requires additional shearing, which may result in parenchymal tearing

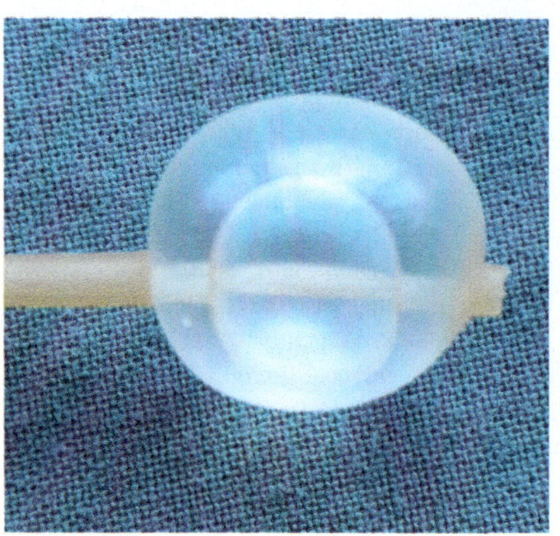

Image 18.1 Foley catheter improvized as a tamponade balloon

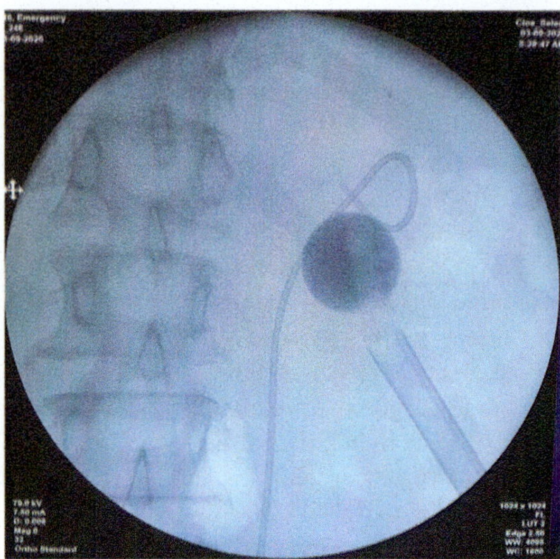

Image 18.2 Use of dilute contrast enables accurate positioning of the tamponade catheter

ing by increasing the flow of irrigation and gentle manipulation of the axis of surgery away from bleeding sites, maintaining visibility and progression. Advancement of the sheath further into the calyceal system and away from the point of bleeding facilitates better visibility until the tamponade effect contains the haemorrhage. The use of tranexamic acid has been found to reduce the incidence of blood transfusions [12]. However, such use is not routinely practiced and is instead limited to situations with excessive bleeding.

If bleeding is excessive and/or threat to hemodynamic stability, PCNL should be abandoned. It is safe practice to exit with a tamponade catheter. A suitably sized (16–18F) Foley catheter can be improvized with the tip beyond the balloon cut off to make a "Zero Tip" tamponade tube (Image 18.1). Dilute contrast is used to inflate the balloon under fluoroscopy, which allows proper placement and adequate inflation (Image 18.2). These patients should be managed in a high dependency setting as renal haemorrhage can be life threatening. In the vast majority, bleeding settles with balloon tamponade. A relook PCNL can be performed few days later (48–72 h) using the same tract with much clearer visibility. If bleeding continues, the arterial injury should be suspected, and urgent selective angiography/embolization carried out.

Occasionally patients develop significant haematuria several days after surgery. It is important to note that arterio-venous fistulae, leaking false aneurysms as well as secondary haemorrhage manifest during this period. It is, therefore, safer to consider all significant hemorrhagic events after 48 h or later as an "arterial complication" until proven otherwise. CT angiography is a non-invasive diagnostic technique to differentiate between the above causes. CT is inferior in accuracy to selective angiography. The selection of imaging should be based on clinical judgement and availability. Selective angiography and embolization is a highly effective technique for treating vascular injury within the kidney with high success rate and minimal parenchymal loss [13].

18.3.1 Prevention

The renal vasculature is arranged in a manner where the branching vessels divide into a network of arterioles and venules around the calyceal necks. Puncture and tract dilatation through calyceal necks therefore increases the risk of vascular injury (Fig. 18.1c). Inadvertent dilatation deeper into the parenchyma as a result of suboptimal localization technique can also cause injury to larger segmental arteries, which can result in major haemorrhage (Fig. 18.1b). On the contrary, the calyceal fornix is less vascular and puncture through the fornix facilitates relatively bloodless access. More significantly, puncture through the fornix is invariably in line with the long axis of the calyx (Fig. 18.1a). An access tract that is in line with the calyx is ideal as it prevents shearing of the parenchyma and tearing in addition to limiting several vascular complications already enumerated. The entry point should be laterally placed, appreciating the natural angles of the calyces. In the case of the lower calyx, the angle is often 30 degrees outwards and posteriorly. Careful perusal of contrast CT images in axial cuts helps to plan the desired calyx and the angle of puncture in most instances.

The use of smaller-sized tracts to reduce the risk of bleeding has already been discussed. Miniaturized versions of PCNL (Mini,Ultra Mini, Super Mini, and Micro PCNL) may be most advantageous in the reduction of haemorrhagic complications. However, the use of miniaturized PCNL is by large limited to small and moderately sized stones [14]. Therefore, the surgeon should choose the optimal tract/sheath size considering multiple factors such as calyceal anatomy, stone bulk and the availability of instruments. Important preventable causes of bleeding associated with PCNL are summarized in Information Box 18.5.

Information Box 18.5 Preventable causes of bleeding at PCNL

- Puncture through calyceal necks
- "Over shooting" of the tract beyond the calyx
- Over dilatation/large tracts
- Acute angulation of tract/sheath at the point of entry to the calyx
- Use of disproportionately large sheaths across calyceal necks
- Overdistention of PC system with high irrigation pressure
- Aggressive lithotripsy and stone retrieval

18.4 Visceral Injury

Kidneys lie in close proximity to other viscera in the abdomen and thorax (Fig. 18.3). Each of these organs is at risk of injury if the relationship of these organs to the point of access is not fully appreciated. The reported overall incidence of visceral injury at PCNL is up to 12% [14]. Of these, colon and pleura are the most frequently injured. Injury to the viscera may occur due to a misdirected tract or as a through and through injury whilst having reached the target calyx accurately (Figs. 18.4 and 18.5). The latter is frequent with pleural injury.

18.5 Pleural Injury

The anatomical relationship of the lower thorax and pleura to the kidney renders the former vulnerable to injury, especially during access to the upper pole of the kidney. The incidence may range between 3.5% and 12.5% with upper pole access [9, 14]. Pleural perforation could result in hydrothorax, pneumothorax, haemothorax, or a combination of these. With delayed manifestations, pneumonia, and pyothorax is also a possibility. Of the above, hydrothorax is the commonest manifestation. The access sheath, in most instances, delays full-blown manifestation of pleural injury during PCNL as the access sheath acts as a splint preventing extravasation of fluid

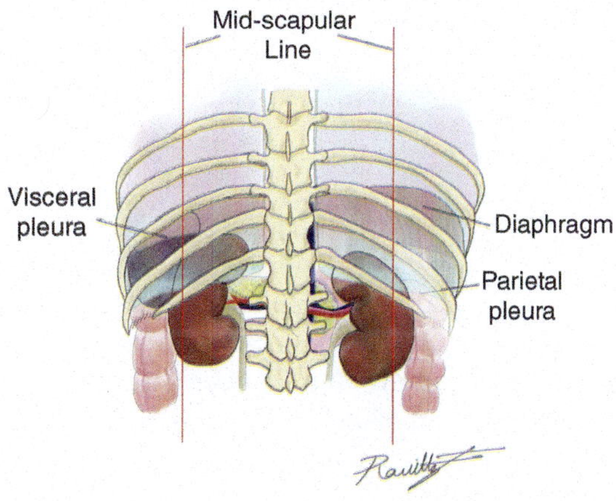

Fig. 18.3 Viscera surrounding the kidneys which are at risk of injury

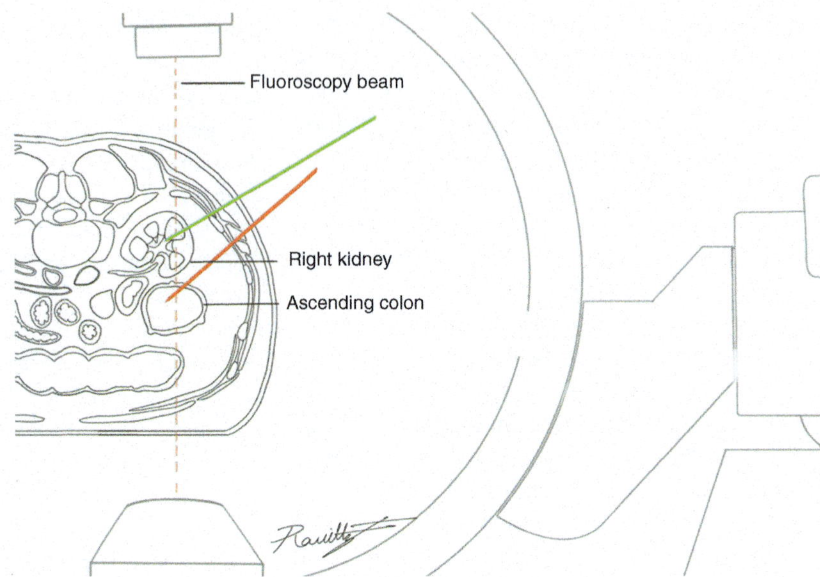

Fig. 18.4 Visceral injury due to misdirected tract

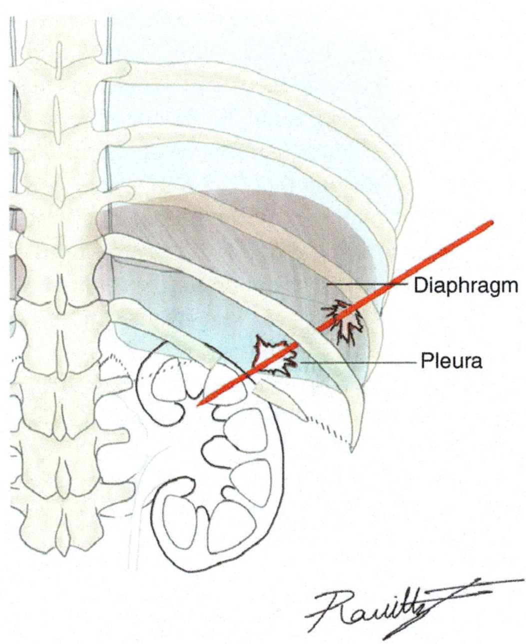

Fig. 18.5 "Through and through" visceral injury

into the pleura. The irrigation fluid/urine or air gets sucked into the pleura when the access sheath is removed. On rare occasions, the visceral pleura of the lung may get injured, causing a bronchopleural fistula.

There may be minimal signs of pleural injury during surgery. A high degree of clinical suspicion is needed for early diagnosis. Chest pain, respiratory distress and reduced air entry, evidence of fluid or air on auscultation of the affected side should raise concerns regarding a possible breach of the pleura, especially with "high" punctures. On-table ultrasonography demonstrates fluid in the costophrenic angle when significant (>50 ml). Fluoroscopy will reveal effusion or pneumothorax. If suspected during the immediate post-operative period, a chest X-ray is useful in the diagnosis. It is safe practice to adopt clinical and radiological assessments to exclude pleural injury "on-table" in all upper pole punctures prior to recovery from anaesthesia. A chest X-ray should also be performed after removal of nephrostomy tubes in those who have had supra costal puncture as air or fluid can get sucked into the breached pleural space after removal of nephrostomy.

Small effusions or pneumothorax in a stable patient with minimal symptoms could be aspirated or managed conservatively with close observation and antibiotic therapy. In such instances, serial radiological assessment is required to ascertain resolution. If clinically manifest or large, an intercostal tube drain should be inserted promptly. All such patients should have a ureteric stent and an indwelling bladder catheter for a few days allowing the puncture tract and pleural fistula to heal. The addition of an anticholinergic has been recommended by some in order to reduce bladder spasm and resultant reflux through the stent [14] If a nephrostomy is needed, the route should be below the costal margin avoiding the pleura to ensure healing and closure of the fistula. If this is not feasible, a perinephric drain can be inserted. When both nephrostomy and intercostal tube are inserted, the nephrostomy should be removed first, and the patient observed to ensure that there is no re-accumulation of fluid in the pleural space before the intercostal tube is removed. Late manifestations of pleural injury may present as a pyothorax. Tube drainage per se may not be sufficient in such a situation, and further interventions such as video-assisted thoracoscopy may be necessary to decorticate encysted collections.

18.5.1 Prevention

The visceral pleura is at a higher level than the parietal pleura and moves with respiration. In order to minimize risks of lung injury, upper pole puncture should be made while the patient is in expiration. The lower boarder of the parietal pleura curves upwards from a medial to the lateral direction. Generally, a puncture made as lateral as possible to the mid-scapular line and below the tenth rib avoids the visceral pleura in supra costal punctures.

Arguably, the best way to avoid pleural injury is to stay below the costal margin. The anatomical relationship of the kidney to the diaphragm and thorax is such that the upper calyces are frequently above the costal margin. The concept of accessing the lower (infra costal) calyces and using flexible or narrower instruments to access the upper pole is a practical solution to reduce pleural injuries. The availability of high-powered laser renders this option even more effective as relatively larger stones can effectively be fragmented using a high-powered laser. Endoscopic Combined Retrograde Intra Renal Surgery (ECIRS) is another useful alternative adopting the same principle to avoid high punctures and associated complications [15]. Although the likely stone-free rates with ECIRS may be lower when compared to PCNL, judicious selection of this option, especially to prevent a significant complication, is worthwhile. Mechanically manipulating the upper pole of the kidney below the costal margin (torqueing) as a measure to avoid supra costal puncture can be effective in selected cases. Here a needle puncture to the Gerota facia facilitates the kidney to be levered down several centimetres. On many occasions, this manoeuvre helps to convert a "would have been" supra costal to a subcostal.

18.6 Colonic Injury

The close anatomical relationship of the colon to the kidneys renders the former vulnerable to injury during PCNL. The reported incidence is up to 1% [9]. Rarely the colon may lie behind the kidney (retro renal colon), increasing the risk of injury. Retro renal colon has a reported prevalence of 0.3–11% [16]. Previous open renal surgery, megacolon, gross hydronephrosis and horseshoe kidney are often cited as risk factors for colonic injury during PCNL. Colonic injuries are reported more frequently on the left side and are mostly associated with lower calyceal punctures. This is likely to be due to the differential anatomical relations of the kidneys to the colon between the two sides and upper/lower poles.

Manifestation of colonic injury could be during surgery or in the early post-operative period. At surgery, contrast extravasation into the bowel (seen on fluoroscopy), emission of faecal odour or gas, passage of faeces or food particles through the PCNL tract may suggest bowel perforation. Delayed manifestation includes excessive pain and tenderness of the loin, fever, sepsis, discharge of faecal material or gas through the nephrostomy or puncture site or perinephric abscess. Almost all these injuries are retroperitoneal.

If the colonic injury is detected during surgery, the access sheath can be advanced to the colon, and a "percutaneous colostomy" is created using a balloon catheter. A wide bore Foley catheter can be used for this purpose. Gentle traction should be maintained on the catheter, tugging the colon closer to the abdominal wall in order to render the management of a possible enterocutaneous fistula relatively easier. An indwelling ureteric stent should also be inserted through the retrograde route. The patient should be treated with broad-spectrum antibiotics, including anaerobic cover and observed closely for sepsis. Bowels should be rested, and parenteral nutritional support commenced. The vast majority of colonic injuries can be contained by such conservative measures as they heal without the need for surgical repair [17]. Occasionally colonic injuries present late with sepsis and abscess formation requiring drainage, exteriorization of the bowel, followed by delayed repair of the colon.

Injury to other viscera are very rare and may require individualized treatment plans based on the specific scenario.

18.6.1 Prevention

As with all other complications, prevention plays a major role in bowel injury. Good understanding of the anatomical relationship of the kidney to other viscera and appreciation of the limitations of two-dimensional fluoroscopy to access the pelvicalyceal system, which has varying degrees of anatomical complexity, is vital. Careful scrutiny of preoperative images helps to strategize an optimal puncture and tract. With complexed stones/anatomy and redo surgery, a contrast CT with composite images and a retrograde study during ureteric catheterization helps the surgeon to plan the best possible access strategy. Placing the puncture behind the posterior axillary line is a time tested and simple step to avoid the colon, as in the vast majority, the colon is placed anterior to the posterior axillary line most often (Fig. 18.6). There has not been a significant difference in the incidence of colonic injury between prone and supine positions [18].

It may well be that inadvertent puncture of most viscera occurs more frequently than those that are clinically apparent. Most such injuries are self-limiting, as needle puncture per se may not result in major consequences apart from postoperative fever, paralytic ileus and pain. However, dilatation of tracts into the viscera does cause major injury. Therefore, the key step in preventing clinically significant visceral injury is to avoid dilatation of a tract unless the surgeon is absolutely confident that the puncture is safely within the collecting system of the kidney. Signs of success include free flow of retrogradely injected "blue" and confirmation of the position of the needle tip at least in two dimensions. Occasionally at puncture, the needle tip appears to be in the right place on two conventional views (0° and 30°) without the flow of "blue." This is when the needle tip is a millimetre close but not within the calyx. In such situations "biplanar" views at 0° and 90° are useful to confirm the exact position of the needle tip (Fig. 18.7). The use of ultrasound and fluoroscopy has become increasingly popular to increase the accuracy of access. Ultrasound also helps to determine the

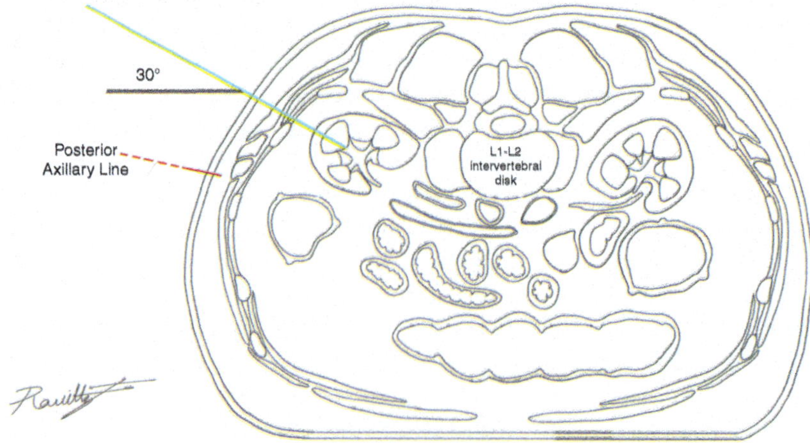

Fig. 18.6 Relationship of the colon to the posterior axillary line

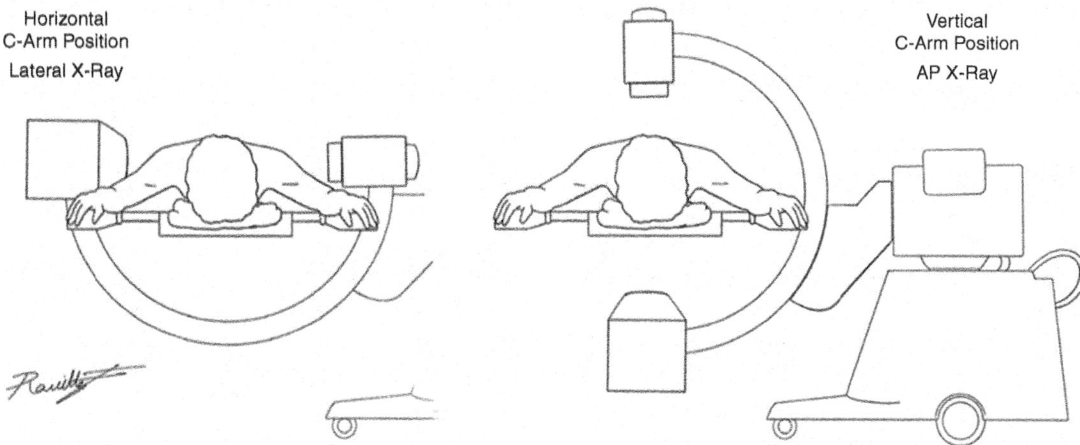

Fig. 18.7 Biplanar imaging using a fluoroscopic C-arm

relationship of bowel and other viscera to the kidney, which minimizes the risks of visceral injury.

Visceral injury evokes immense anxiety in patients and the surgical team. Such injuries may require complex interventions, significantly higher costs and a protracted recovery. Preoperative counselling and informed consent regarding the rare but possible chance of visceral injury is therefore important, especially in cases with higher risk.

18.7 Complications Associated with Positioning

In the CROES PCNL global study, the majority of patients were operated on in the prone position [5]. However, in the decade since this study, the popularity of supine PCNL has grown substantially. Whilst the perceived view is that supine position is more advantageous to reduce adverse events related to surgical position such as airway and respiratory embarrassment, skeletal and nerve injuries, there has been no convincing evidence to substantiate this view [19]. In fact, the preference for PCNL appeared to be the prone position for patients with high body mass index, possibly due to the longer tracts needed. Overall, the reported incidence of complications between different surgical positions does not seem to differ significantly [5], although the operating time in the supine position has been longer [5]. Within a subgroup analysis for staghorns, the stone-free rates have been noted to be higher in the prone position than supine [20]. The choice of surgical position appears to be due to several patient and surgeon-related factors and should ideally remain an individualized choice. Although there are no published reports, the possibility of injury to the anesthetized patient during positioning, especially prone position, should never be underestimated in centres particularly where new PCNL programmes are being initiated.

18.8 Failed Procedure

The reported incidence of failed access is rare in contemporary literature. There are several reasons that may lead to a failed PCNL procedure, amongst which failed access is common. In a practical scenario, complexed anatomy, including aberrations, body habitus and experience of the surgeon, may contribute to failure. The evidence available to analyse the relationship of each of these factors to failed access and morbidity is sparse. However, in the CROES Global PCNL study, there were no significant differences in the overall outcomes of patients with increasing BMI and anatomically aberrant kidneys [5]. The choice of imaging modality too has been shown to influence the success rate of access; the use of ultrasound has demonstrated superiority over fluoroscopy with a higher rate of success and shorter procedure time [21].

18.9 Extravasation

Urinary extravasation following PCNL may occur due to several reasons, of which leakage through the tract is commonest. Breach or perforation of the pelvicalyceal system and the use of excessive irrigation pressure may also result in fluid extravasation around the kidney. In the absence of distal obstruction, most such cases settle spontaneously within a short period of time. If fluid extravasation persists beyond a few days, distal obstruction must be suspected. In such a situation, appropriate imaging (CT) followed by insertion of an indwelling stent usually resolves leakage. In cases where a stent is inserted primarily or as a secondary procedure, an indwelling catheter should be left in situ for a few days after leakage settles as bladder contractions cause urine to reflux through the stent resulting in persistence of extravasation. Anticholinergics may be added on an individualized basis [14]. Occasionally when there is a significant perinephric collection, percutaneous drainage may be necessary for addition to placement of the stent. All patients who develop urinary extravasation should be treated with therapeutic antibiotics and observed for sepsis.

18.9.1 Prevention

The key step in preventing extravasation apart from avoiding the above causative factors is to plan the exit strategy following PCNL carefully. There is a clear trend towards performing tubeless and totally tubeless PCNL in the last decade. However, the safe default option for PCNL should always be with tube drainage, and patients should be consented accordingly. In the absence of contraindications (Information Box 18.6) at the end of the procedure, the surgeon may, at that point, decide on a tubeless PCNL. It is important to note that the operating surgeon may well decide to insert a drain irrespective of criteria [7].

Information Box 18.6 Contraindications for tubeless PCNL

- Distal obstruction
- Significant bleeding
- Infection
- Renal impairment
- Residual stones
- Need for relook PCNL
- Single (functioning) kidney
- Complex anatomy

18.10 Other Factors Contributing to Complications

The relationship between surgical case load and outcomes following PCNL are well documented. The ideal case load for peak performance has been postulated around 120 per annum, where the incidence of complications, stone-free rates and operating time were optimized [22]. This fits a normal distribution with a decline in outcomes both with lower as well has higher case numbers.

The CROES Global PCNL study, which analysed over 5000 cases across all continents, shed light on many interesting facets. The key factors proven to be associated and more importantly, not associated with significant differences in outcomes according to this seminal study are summarized in Information Box 18.7. PCNL has now established its place as a safe and effective technique for staghorn stones and those with complex anatomy, contrary to traditional opinion. Similarly, renal anomalies such as horseshoe kidney, imaging modality and the type of lithotripsy technique have not been associated with differences in outcome. Increase body mass index (BMI) over 40, solitary kidney and chronic kidney disease, however, have resulted in higher morbidity rates [23–25].

Information Box 18.7

Antibiotic prophylaxis	Reduces incidence of sepsis and complications
Positioning	No overall difference between different positions
Staghorn stones	Prone position higher stone-free rates Safe for PCNL
Imaging and lithotrite technique	No influence on complications
Renal anomalies	No difference in stone-free rates compared to normal kidneys
Solitary kidney	Lower stone-free rate
BMI >40 CKD Age > 70	Higher complication rates

Summary of the findings of CROES PCNL Study
Ref: Kemphius et al. world J Urol (2015) 33:223.

There will be little argument that the key to a successful PCNL is well-planned access and a tract with access to relevant areas of the pelvicalyceal system. An optimal renal puncture is the first step towards this objective. A suboptimal puncture could lead to a cascade of events leading to numerous complications already enumerated. Time spent on planning access for PCNL is THE key investment to ensure a successful procedure. Review of the images, particularly the composite CT images, appreciation of the colon in relation to the site of access, pelvicalyceal anatomy to ensure safe access are important steps. The entire team should participate in this exercise and more experienced opinions sought in difficult cases. Access for PCNL may be performed either by a radiologist or the surgeon him/herself. While there seem to be differing protocols in different countries, it is generally considered that the tract created by the surgeon him/herself may lead to a more favourable outcome, provided the surgeon has achieved necessary levels of proficiency [26].

During preoperative planning, the team should ideally agree on the anticipated outcomes following PCNL. With complex stone burden or anatomy, removal of all stones may not be practical in a single session. The patient should always be counselled regarding such outcomes preoperatively in order to avoid undue expectations and disappointment. In the absence of such preplanned strategies, perseverance to clear large and complex stone bulk may result in unnecessary morbidity. Sometimes a second look at PCNL is necessary to remove all stones safely. As with most other complicated surgical procedures, the principle of relook surgery is invaluable to ensure maximum safety.

The age-old preaching of Hippocrates is fundamental to PCNL, where the principle of “first do no harm” should be foremost in the minds of all surgeons. PCNL is almost always an elective surgical procedure and frequently in minimally symptomatic patients. The operation to remove the stone, therefore, should not make the patient more symptomatic than they were and certainly not cause more harm than the stone would have. Awareness of achievable goals, adequate planning and expert assistance when necessary in complex scenarios are all important steps to ensure optimum outcomes.

Acknowledgements Ramith Fonseka (rfonseka97@gmail.com): Illustrations.

Nithesh Ranasinha (nithesh.ranasinha@gmail.com): Formatting and editing.

References

1. Tyson MD 2nd, Humphreys MR. Postoperative complications after percutaneous nephrolithotomy: a contemporary analysis by insurance status in the United States. J Endourol. 2014 Mar;28(3):291–7.
2. Olvera-Posada D, Tailly T, Alenezi H, Violette PD, Nott L, Denstedt JD, et al. Risk factors for postoperative complications of percutaneous nephrolithotomy at a tertiary referral center. J Urol. 2015 Dec;194(6):1646–51.
3. Bootsma AMJ, Laguna Pes MP, Geerlings SE, Goossens A. Antibiotic prophylaxis in urologic procedures: a systematic review. Eur Urol. 2008 Dec;54(6):1270–86.
4. Lai WS, Assimos D. Factors associated with postoperative infection after percutaneous nephrolithotomy. Rev Urol. 2018;20(1):7–11.
5. Kamphuis GM, Baard J, Westendarp M, de la Rosette JJMCH. Lessons learned from the CROES percutane-

ous nephrolithotomy global study. World J Urol. 2015 Feb;33(2):223–33.
6. Viprakasit DP, Sawyer MD, Herrell SD, Miller NL. Changing composition of staghorn calculi. J Urol [Internet]. 2011;186(6):2285–2290.
7. Türk C, Petřík A, Sarica K, Seitz C, Skolarikos A, Straub M, et al. EAU guidelines on diagnosis and conservative management of urolithiasis. Eur Urol. 2016 Mar;69(3):468–74.
8. Wu C, Hua L-X, Zhang J-Z, Zhou X-R, Zhong W, Ni H-D. Comparison of renal pelvic pressure and postoperative fever incidence between standard- and mini-tract percutaneous nephrolithotomy. Kaohsiung J Med Sci. 2017 Jan;33(1):36–43.
9. Michel MS, Trojan L, Rassweiler JJ. Complications in Percutaneous Nephrolithotomy. Eur Urol [Internet]. 2007;51(4):899–906.
10. Sacha K, Szewczyk W, Bar K. Massive haemorrhage presenting as a complication after percutaneous nephrolithotomy (PCNL). Int Urol Nephrol [Internet]. 1996;28(3):315–8.
11. Yamaguchi A, Skolarikos A, Buchholz N-PN, Chomón GB, Grasso M, Saba P, et al. Operating times and bleeding complications in percutaneous nephrolithotomy: a comparison of tract dilation methods in 5,537 patients in the Clinical Research Office of the Endourological Society Percutaneous Nephrolithotomy Global Study. J Endourol. 2011 Jun;25(6):933–9.
12. Bansal A, Arora A. A double-blind, placebo-controlled randomized clinical trial to evaluate the efficacy of tranexamic acid in irrigant solution on blood loss during percutaneous nephrolithotomy: a pilot study from tertiary care center of North India. World J Urol. 2017 Aug;35(8):1233–40.
13. Güneyli S, Gök M, Bozkaya H, Çınar C, Tizro A, Korkmaz M, et al. Endovascular management of iatrogenic renal arterial lesions and clinical outcomes. Diagn Interv Radiol [Internet]. 2015;21(3):229–234.
14. Maheshwari PN, Mane DA, Pathak AB. Management of pleural injury after percutaneous renal surgery. J Endourol. 2009 Oct;23(10):1769–72.
15. Zengin K, Tanik S, Karakoyunlu N, Sener NC, Albayrak S, Tuygun C, et al. Retrograde intrarenal surgery versus percutaneous lithotripsy to treat renal stones 2–3 cm in diameter. Thamilselvan S, editor. Biomed Res Int [Internet]. 2015;2015:914231.
16. Balasar M, Kandemir A, Poyraz N, Unal Y, Ozturk A. Incidence of retrorenal colon during percutaneous nephrolithotomy. Int Braz J Urol [Internet]. 2015;41(2):274–278.
17. Öztürk H. Treatment of colonic injury during percutaneous nephrolithotomy. Rev Urol [Internet]. 2015;17(3):194–201.
18. Liu L, Zheng S, Xu Y, Wei Q. Systematic review and meta-analysis of percutaneous nephrolithotomy for patients in the supine versus prone position. J Endourol. 2010 Dec;24(12):1941–6.
19. Mourmouris P, Berdempes M, Markopoulos T, Lazarou L, Tzelves L, Skolarikos A. Patient positioning during percutaneous nephrolithotomy: what is the current best practice? Res reports Urol [Internet]. 2018 Oct 30;10:189–93.
20. Astroza G, Lipkin M, Neisius A, Preminger G, De Sio M, Sodha H, et al. Effect of supine vs prone position on outcomes of percutaneous nephrolithotomy in staghorn calculi: results from the Clinical Research Office of the Endourology Society Study. Urology. 2013 Dec;82(6):1240–4.
21. Andonian S, Scoffone CM, Louie MK, Gross AJ, Grabe M, Daels FPJ, et al. Does imaging modality used for percutaneous renal access make a difference? A matched case analysis. J Endourol [Internet]. 2012 Jul 26;27(1):24–8.
22. Opondo D, Tefekli A, Esen T, Labate G, Sangam K, De Lisa A, et al. Impact of case volumes on the outcomes of percutaneous nephrolithotomy. Eur Urol [Internet]. 2012;62(6):1181–1187.
23. Okeke Z, Smith AD, Labate G, D'Addessi A, Venkatesh R, Assimos D, et al. Prospective comparison of outcomes of percutaneous nephrolithotomy in elderly patients versus younger patients. J Endourol. 2012 Aug;26(8):996–1001.
24. Fuller A, Razvi H, Denstedt JD, Nott L, Pearle M, Cauda F, et al. The CROES percutaneous nephrolithotomy global study: the influence of body mass index on outcome. J Urol. 2012 Jul;188(1):138–44.
25. Sairam K, Scoffone CM, Alken P, Turna B, Sodha HS, Rioja J, et al. Percutaneous nephrolithotomy and chronic kidney disease: results from the CROES PCNL Global Study. J Urol. 2012 Oct;188(4):1195–200.
26. Armitage JN, Withington J, Fowler S, Finch WJG, Burgess NA, Irving SO, et al. Percutaneous nephrolithotomy access by urologist or interventional radiologist: practice and outcomes in the UK. BJU Int. 2017 Jun;119(6):913–8.

Part V

Other Approaches

19 Principles of Modern ESWL and Best Lithotripsy Practice

David Leung and Anthony C.F. Ng

19.1 Introduction

Extracorporeal shockwave lithotripsy (SWL) represents a prevalent treatment modality for renal and ureteric stones. This technology is a composite of shockwave generation, a coupling system for transmission, a focusing system and imaging for monitoring. Over the past three decades, there has been evolving improvement in not only the machine design and settings but also better understanding of factors that can predict outcomes. Therefore, proper application of ESWL on carefully selected patients would deploy its full advantages in the modern practice of urology.

19.2 Patient Selection

In order to achieve satisfactory outcomes, the first step is to select the most suitable candidates for SWL. In this regard, there are stone factors, anatomical factors and patient factors that should be taken into consideration.

A meta-analysis by Lingeman et al. suggested that stone-free rates (SFR) for SWL were inversely correlated to the stone burden treated [1]. While ESWL is recommended for stones less than 2 cm [2], stone size larger than 2 cm is associated with lower success rates. Low mean stone density (average Hounsfield units <1000) was found to predict better SFR for SWL [3]. Brushite, calcium oxalate monohydrate, and cystine stones are known to be resistant to SWL.

Furthermore, Sahinkanat et al. reported lower SFR for lower pole stones (60%) as compared to upper and middle pole stones (80–90%) [4]. There are several anatomical factors to consider before treating lower pole stones with ESWL. Unfavorable factors include steep infundibulopelvic angle, narrow infundibulum and long infundibular length [5–7]. Lower pole stones of 1–2 cm with the above unfavorable factors should be treated primarily with retrograde intrarenal surgery (RIRS) or percutaneous nephrolithotomy (PCNL), according to European Association of Urology 2020 [2].

Modern diagnosis of urinary tract stone disease relies heavily on non-contrast computed tomography (NCCT), in addition to X-ray and ultrasound. Besides its high sensitivity and specificity of over 90%, researchers have shown that several NCCT parameters can predict the success of ESWL. Pareek et al. were the first to report

D. Leung
SH Ho Urology Centre, Department of Surgery, The Chinese University of Hong Kong, Hong Kong SAR, People's Republic of China

A. C.F. Ng (✉)
Department of Surgery, Chinese University of Hong Kong, Hong Kong, Hong Kong
e-mail: ngcf@surgery.cuhk.edu.hk

A. C.F. Ng et al. (eds.), *Practical Management of Urinary Stone*,
https://doi.org/10.1007/978-981-16-4193-0_19

that skin-to-stone distance (SSD) greater than 10 cm was associated with failure for SWL of lower pole stones [8]. A study by Ng et al. on 94 patients with proximal ureteric stones [3], for stones with these three factors (stone density < 593 Hounsfield units, stone volume <0.2 cc and SSD <9.2 cm) would have almost 100% SWL success rates at 3 months after one section of treatment. Tran et al. also described three similar favorable factors grouped as the "Triple-D score" (stone volume <150 μl, stone density <600 Hounsfield units, and SSD <12 cm) [9]. It was found that the more favorable factors, the higher the SWL success rates (21.4% for score 0, 41.3% for score 1, 78.7% for score 2 and 96.1% for score 3).

With respect to patient factors affecting SWL, practitioners need to assess their age and body habitus. Ng et al. showed that age above 60 is an unfavorable predictor for SWL of renal stones but not ureteric stones [10]. Moreover, a thicker renal cortex (larger cortical thickness) was associated with better SFR at three months after SWL [11]. One possible mechanism is that the kidneys with thinner cortical thickness have undergone sclerotic changes with aging and renal insults, which increase the acoustic impedance and hinder the transmission of shockwaves. A high body mass index (above 30 kg/m^2) was also reported to negatively predict SWL success in a study for renal stones less than 2.5 cm in size [12]. Since the majority of lithotripters have the focal length of around 15 cm, excessive body thickness would affect the positioning of the target stone into the focal zone (F2).

Before subjecting patients to SWL, the following contraindications need to be excluded. These include pregnancy, uncontrolled urinary tract infections, bleeding diatheses, adjacent arterial aneurysms, severe skeletal malformations, severe obesity and distal anatomical obstruction [2].

19.3 Preparation for SWL

In preparation for SWL, practitioners should review the X-ray and CT films (if any) taken close to the SWL session. This confirms the visibility of the target stones and excludes stone passage prior to SWL.

Urinalysis and blood tests should be undertaken to exclude active urinary treat infections and bleeding tendency as reflected by thrombocytopenia or coagulopathy. The indication, risk and alternative options should be clearly explained to patients. After obtaining informed consent and ruling out contraindications, SWL can proceed.

Antibiotic prophylaxis is not routinely recommended for patients with sterile urine before SWL [13, 14]. For patients with urinary tract infection symptoms or positive urine culture, a complete course of antibiotics should be administered before SWL.

19.4 Periprocedural Monitoring

In general, patients undergoing SWL require monitoring of their blood pressure, pulse, and oxygen saturation. Respiratory monitoring becomes more relevant when it comes to patients sedated with opioids to detect any respiratory depression.

The presence of an implantable cardioverter defibrillator requires the adjustment of modes before SWL [2]. Cardiac monitoring is recommended for patients with underlying heart disease or dysrhythmia, according to a prospective study of arrhythmia during SWL in 50 patients [15].

19.5 Analgesics and Sedation

There are no universal guidelines on analgesia for SWL. A wide range from oral analgesics to intravenous sedation or even spinal and general anesthesia has been described. A meta-analysis [16] compared the efficacy and tolerability of simple analgesics, non-steroidal anti-inflammatory drugs (NSAID) and opioids in SWL patients. It showed no significant difference in terms of adequate pain control or side effects among the three classes of drugs.

Sorensen et al. compared intravenous sedation with general anesthesia in 295 patients receiving

SWL for a solitary renal or proximal ureteric stone less than 2 cm [17]. It was found that the SFR was significantly better in the general anesthesia group (87% vs. 55%) after three months.

Therefore, increasing the depth of sedation appears to improve the efficacy of stone clearance by minimizing patients' movement at the expense of higher cost and sedative risk. Clinicians must strike a balance between efficacy and safety when choosing the optimal mode of analgesia.

19.6 Ramping Protocol

Ramping refers to starting SWL with a lower power setting, followed by a stepwise increase in power. Conners et al. showed that ramping might achieve renal vasoconstriction and prevent renal injury in a porcine model [18].

A number of clinical studies have assessed the impact of ramping on stone fragmentation and renal injury. Ng et al. randomized 300 patients who received SWL for renal stones into either a ramping group (first 1000 shocks at lower energy followed by two rounds of 1000 shocks with successively higher energy) or a fixed voltage group (all 3000 shocks at high energy) [19] using a Modulith® SLX-F2. It was found that despite similar treatment success rates, the ramping group outperformed the other group by significantly reducing the incidence of grades 1 and 2 perinephric hematoma (23.8% vs. 43.8%).

There has been no strong evidence to suggest that ramping improves stone-free rates. While a significantly better SFR (96% vs. 72%) was reported in a 50-patient randomized trial [20], more recent randomized controlled trials [19, 21] have reported similar SFR when comparing ramping to fixed voltage SWL.

19.7 Shockwave Rate

A meta-analysis [22] compared the treatment outcomes among low-frequency (60 to 70 waves per minute), intermediate-frequency (80 to 90 waves per minute) and high-frequency SWL (100 to 120 waves per minute). Low-frequency and intermediate-frequency SWL were shown to have higher success rates than high-frequency SWL (odds ratios 2.2 and 2.5, respectively). Moreover, low-frequency SWL was also found to have the lowest complication rates by rank-probability tests.

Therefore, lowering shockwave frequency from 120 to 60–90 waves/min improves stone fragmentation and reduces tissue damage.

19.8 Coupling

Proper acoustic coupling between the generator head and the patient's skin in an air-tight manner is essential to maximize energy delivery to the stone. Defects (air pockets) in the coupling gel would block up almost 99% of shockwaves energy [23]. Pishchalnikov et al. found that poor coupling would result in air pockets that cover up to 19% of the treatment area (contact area), thereby decreasing shockwave energy by 20% [24]. On top of that, patient repositioning during SWL, which would increase bubbles entrapped in coupling gel, would further decrease energy by another 57%. Jain et al. showed that the efficacy of SWL was associated with the amount of air bubbles inside the coupling gel and that elimination of air bubbles from the coupling agent significantly improved success rates [25].

The correct use of coupling media is important to reduce this interference. Ultrasound gel is the most prevalent lithotripsy coupling agent in current practice. Generous amount of gel, elimination of air bubbles during application, avoiding coupling-decoupling and a stationary patient will help to ensure good coupling.

19.9 Procedural Control

Proper stone targeting is indispensable for the success of SWL, either by fluoroscopic or ultrasonic guidance. In general, such techniques are operator-dependent, and more experienced urologists tend to give better outcomes. Improved treatment outcomes have been shown with more frequent use of fluoroscopy [26]. A randomized controlled trial [27] showed that ultrasound is non-inferior to fluoroscopy in terms of treatment success rates. Ultrasound has the added benefits of continue real-time monitoring, locating radiolucent stones and also avoiding radiation hazards.

Throughout SWL, stone targeting is to be checked at regular intervals to maximize its efficiency.

19.10 Auxillary Measures

The use of alpha-blockers after SWL has been shown by meta-analyses to improve stone clearance and reduce pain [28, 29].

Ureteral stenting is not routinely recommended for SWL. Two meta-analyses [30, 31] reported that stenting might decrease steinstrasse rates, although it has no effect on SFR and causes more lower urinary tract symptoms. Its use may be considered for solitary functioning kidneys and large renal stones (>20 mm).

Pace et al. advocated "percussion, diuresis and inversion" (PDI) after SWL, with an aim to improve SFR from 3% to 40% [32]. In a randomized controlled trial of 108 patients, four sessions of PDI plus SWL improved SFR at 3-months from 35.4% to 62.5% ($p = 0.006$) [33].

References

1. Lingeman JE, Siegel YI, Steele B, Nyhuis AW, Woods JR. Management of lower pole nephrolithiasis: a critical analysis. J Urol. 1994;151(3):663–7. https://doi.org/10.1016/s0022-5347(17)35042-5.
2. European Association of Urology Guidelines 2020.
3. Ng CF, Siu DY, Wong A, Goggins W, Chan ES, Wong KT. Development of a scoring system from noncontrast computerized tomography measurements to improve the selection of upper ureteral stone for extracorporeal shock wave lithotripsy. J Urol. 2009;181(3):1151–7. https://doi.org/10.1016/j.juro.2008.10.161.
4. Sahinkanat T, Ekerbicer H, Onal B, et al. Evaluation of the effects of relationships between main spatial lower pole calyceal anatomic factors on the success of shock-wave lithotripsy in patients with lower pole kidney stones. Urology. 2008;71(5):801–5. https://doi.org/10.1016/j.urology.2007.11.052.
5. Elbahnasy AM, Clayman RV, Shalhav AL, et al. Lower-pole caliceal stone clearance after shockwave lithotripsy, percutaneous nephrolithotomy, and flexible ureteroscopy: impact of radiographic spatial anatomy. J Endourol. 1998;12(2):113–9. https://doi.org/10.1089/end.1998.12.113.
6. Ghoneim IA, Ziada AM, Elkatib SE. Predictive factors of lower calyceal stone clearance after Extracorporeal Shockwave Lithotripsy (ESWL): a focus on the infundibulopelvic anatomy. Eur Urol. 2005;48(2):296–302. https://doi.org/10.1016/j.eururo.2005.02.017.
7. Ng CF, Wong A, Tolley DA. A single-center experience of the usefulness of caliceal-pelvic height in three different lithotripters. J Endourol. Jul 2008:1409–16. https://doi.org/10.1089/end.2006.0448.
8. Pareek G, Armenakas NA, Panagopoulos G, Bruno JJ, Fracchia JA. Extracorporeal shock wave lithotripsy success based on body mass index and Hounsfield units. Urology. 2005;65(1):33–6. https://doi.org/10.1016/j.urology.2004.08.004.
9. Tran TY, McGillen K, Cone EB, Pareek G. Triple D Score is a reportable predictor of shockwave lithotripsy stone-free rates. J Endourol. 2015;29(2):226–30. https://doi.org/10.1089/end.2014.0212.
10. Ng CF, Wong A, Tolley D. Is extracorporeal shock wave lithotripsy the preferred treatment option for elderly patients with urinary stone? A multivariate analysis of the effect of patient age on treatment outcome. BJU Int. 2007;100(2):392–5. https://doi.org/10.1111/j.1464-410X.2007.06909.x.
11. Ng CF, Luke S, Chiu PK, Teoh JY, Wong KT, Hou SS. The effect of renal cortical thickness on the treatment outcomes of kidney stones treated with shockwave lithotripsy. Korean J Urol. 2015;56(5):379–85. https://doi.org/10.4111/kju.2015.56.5.379.
12. El-Nahas AR, El-Assmy AM, Mansour O, Sheir KZ. A prospective multivariate analysis of factors predicting stone disintegration by extracorporeal shock wave lithotripsy: the value of high-resolution noncontrast computed tomography. Eur Urol. 2007;51(6):1688–94. https://doi.org/10.1016/j.eururo.2006.11.048.
13. Lu Y, Tianyong F, Ping H, Liangren L, Haichao Y, Qiang W. Antibiotic prophylaxis for shock wave lithotripsy in patients with sterile urine before treatment may be unnecessary: a systematic review and meta-analysis. J Urol. 2012;188(2):441–8. https://doi.org/10.1016/j.juro.2012.04.014.
14. Bierkens AF, Hendrikx AJ, Ezz el Din KE, et al. The value of antibiotic prophylaxis during extracorporeal shock wave lithotripsy in the prevention of urinary tract infections in patients with urine proven sterile prior to treatment. Eur Urol. 1997;31(1):30–5. https://doi.org/10.1159/000474414.
15. Zeng ZR, Lindstedt E, Roijer A, Olsson SB. Arrhythmia during extracorporeal shock wave lithotripsy. Br J Urol. 1993;71(1):10–6. https://doi.org/10.1111/j.1464-410x.1993.tb15871.x.

16. Aboumarzouk OM, Hasan R, Tasleem A, et al. Analgesia for patients undergoing shockwave lithotripsy for urinary stones – a systematic review and meta-analysis. Int Braz J Urol. 2017;43(3):394–406. https://doi.org/10.1590/S1677-5538.IBJU.2016.0078.
17. Sorensen C, Chandhoke P, Moore M, Wolf C, Sarram A. Comparison of intravenous sedation versus general anesthesia on the efficacy of the Doli 50 lithotriptor. J Urol. 2002;168(1):35–7.
18. Connors BA, Evan AP, Blomgren PM, Handa RK, Willis LR, Gao S. Effect of initial shock wave voltage on shock wave lithotripsy-induced lesion size during step-wise voltage ramping. BJU Int. 2009;103(1):104–7. https://doi.org/10.1111/j.1464-410X.2008.07922.x.
19. Ng CF, Yee CH, Teoh JYC, et al. Effect of stepwise voltage escalation on treatment outcomes following extracorporeal shock wave lithotripsy of renal calculi: a prospective randomized study. J Urol. 2019;202(5):986–93. https://doi.org/10.1097/JU.0000000000000344.
20. Demirci D, Sofikerim M, Yalçin E, Ekmekçioğlu O, Gülmez I, Karacagil M. Comparison of conventional and step-wise shockwave lithotripsy in management of urinary calculi. J Endourol. 2007;21(12):1407–10. https://doi.org/10.1089/end.2006.0399.
21. Skuginna V, Nguyen DP, Seiler R, Kiss B, Thalmann GN, Roth B. Does stepwise voltage ramping protect the kidney from injury during extracorporeal shockwave lithotripsy? Results of a prospective randomized trial. Eur Urol. 2016;69(2):267–73. https://doi.org/10.1016/j.eururo.2015.06.017.
22. Kang DH, Cho KS, Ham WS, et al. Comparison of high, intermediate, and low frequency shock wave lithotripsy for urinary tract stone disease: systematic review and network meta-analysis. PLoS One. 2016;11(7):e0158661. Published 2016 Jul 7. https://doi.org/10.1371/journal.pone.0158661
23. Lingeman J, McAteer J, Gnessin E, et al. Shock wave lithotripsy: advances in technology and technique. Nat Rev Urol. 2009;6:660–70. https://doi.org/10.1038/nrurol.2009.216.
24. Pishchalnikov YA, Neucks JS, VonDerHaar RJ, Pishchalnikova IV, Williams JC Jr, McAteer JA. Air pockets trapped during routine coupling in dry head lithotripsy can significantly decrease the delivery of shock wave energy. J Urol. 2006;176(6 Pt 1):2706–10. https://doi.org/10.1016/j.juro.2006.07.149.
25. Jain A, Shah TK. Effect of air bubbles in the coupling medium on efficacy of extracorporeal shock wave lithotripsy. Eur Urol. 2007;51(6):1680–7. https://doi.org/10.1016/j.eururo.2006.10.049.
26. Logarakis NF, Jewett MA, Luymes J, Honey RJ. Variation in clinical outcome following shock wave lithotripsy. J Urol. 2000;163(3):721–5.
27. Van Besien J, Uvin P, Hermie I, Tailly T, Merckx L. Ultrasonography is not inferior to fluoroscopy to guide extracorporeal shock waves during treatment of renal and upper ureteric calculi: a randomized prospective study. Biomed Res Int. 2017;2017:7802672. https://doi.org/10.1155/2017/7802672.
28. Zhu Y, Duijvesz D, Rovers MM, Lock TM. alpha-Blockers to assist stone clearance after extracorporeal shock wave lithotripsy: a meta-analysis. BJU Int. 2010;106(2):256–61. https://doi.org/10.1111/j.1464-410X.2009.09014.x.
29. Bhagat SK, Chacko NK, Kekre NS, Gopalakrishnan G, Antonisamy B, Devasia A. Is there a role for tamsulosin in shock wave lithotripsy for renal and ureteral calculi? J Urol. 2007;177(6):2185–8. https://doi.org/10.1016/j.juro.2007.01.160.
30. Shen P, Jiang M, Yang J, et al. Use of ureteral stent in extracorporeal shock wave lithotripsy for upper urinary calculi: a systematic review and meta-analysis. J Urol. 2011;186(4):1328–35. https://doi.org/10.1016/j.juro.2011.05.073.
31. Wang H, Man L, Li G, Huang G, Liu N, Wang J. Meta-analysis of stenting versus non-stenting for the treatment of ureteral stones. PLoS One. 2017;12(1):e0167670. Published 2017 Jan 9. https://doi.org/10.1371/journal.pone.0167670
32. Pace KT, Tariq N, Dyer SJ, Weir MJ, D'A Honey RJ. Mechanical percussion, inversion and diuresis for residual lower pole fragments after shock wave lithotripsy: a prospective, single blind, randomized controlled trial. J Urol. 2001;166(6):2065–71.
33. Chiong E, Hwee ST, Kay LM, Liang S, Kamaraj R, Esuvaranathan K. Randomized controlled study of mechanical percussion, diuresis, and inversion therapy to assist passage of lower pole renal calculi after shock wave lithotripsy. Urology. 2005;65(6):1070–4. https://doi.org/10.1016/j.urology.2004.12.045.

Laparoscopic Stone Surgery

20

Sridhar Panaiyadiyan, Prabhjot Singh, and Rajeev Kumar

Abstract

Endourology is the standard of care in the contemporary management of urolithiasis. However, in certain special situations, laparoscopic stone surgery offers a minimally invasive option to achieve stone-free status rapidly. With the laparoscopic approach, most series have shown a high stone-free rate in a single setting. This highlights the limited yet important role of laparoscopy in providing a minimally invasive alternative in the management of urinary stones. Laparoscopy for stone surgery is a challenging procedure and requires advanced laparoscopic skills in achieving successful outcomes. In this chapter, we discuss the role of laparoscopy in urolithiasis, various procedures performed with specific indications, technical tips and published outcomes of individual procedures.

Keywords

Urolithiasis · Laparoscopy · Pyelolithotomy · Ureterolithotomy · Laparoscopic-assisted

S. Panaiyadiyan · P. Singh · R. Kumar (✉)
Department of Urology, All India Institute of Medical Sciences, New Delhi, India
e-mail: rajeev.urology@aiims.edu

20.1 Introduction

In the era of endourology, most urinary stones can be dealt with advanced endoscopic techniques. The American Urological Association (AUA) guidelines 2016 on stone management actually advises that laparoscopy should not be preferred for managing stones [1]. However, in certain circumstances that may be related to the stone or unusual anatomy, an endourological approach may not be ideal to achieve stone-free status with minimal complications such as bleeding, sepsis and absorption of a large amount of irrigation fluids.

Although open surgery is the traditional next step, a minimally invasive approach using laparoscopy decreases surgical morbidity and is safe and feasible. While robotic-assisted procedures can be an advantage to the surgeon, it is limited in its availability and provides little added benefit in terms of outcomes. Hence, laparoscopic stone surgery bridges the gap between endourology and traditional open surgery, not only in terms of decreased morbidity but also in achieving a stone-free rate in a single setting. In this chapter, we discuss the scope of laparoscopy in urolithiasis with the primary focus to understand the role of laparoscopic surgery, various surgical techniques and technical tips in the contemporary management of urolithiasis.

A. C.F. Ng et al. (eds.), *Practical Management of Urinary Stone*,
https://doi.org/10.1007/978-981-16-4193-0_20

20.2 Laparoscopic Stone Surgery

Laparoscopic stone surgery can be of two types, reconstructive or ablative, which can be either transperitoneal or retroperitoneal approach. Figure 20.1 shows the various laparoscopic stone surgery options described in the management of urinary stones.

20.3 Reconstructive Laparoscopic Stone Surgery

20.3.1 Renal Stones

Based on the renal stone burden, abnormal anatomical abnormalities and surgeon's expertise, various laparoscopy procedures are performed for renal stones. Table 20.1 describes the current indications for laparoscopy in renal stones.

Table 20.1 Indications for laparoscopy in renal stones

The following are the contemporary indications for laparoscopy surgery in renal stones [2, 3] 1. Renal stones either previously failed or not amenable to endourologic management. 2. Large stone burden with unfavourable pelvicalyceal system, i.e. non-dilated calyces with the dilated extrarenal pelvis.
Special situations which merit laparoscopic surgery in renal stones 1. Renal stone with a concomitant need for the reconstructive procedure (UPJ repair). 2. Anatomical abnormalities in the shape or location of the kidney (horseshoe kidney, pelvic kidney, crossed fused ectopia or malrotated kidney). 3. Symptomatic stones in diverticula not amenable to endourological intervention can be treated with laparoscopy.

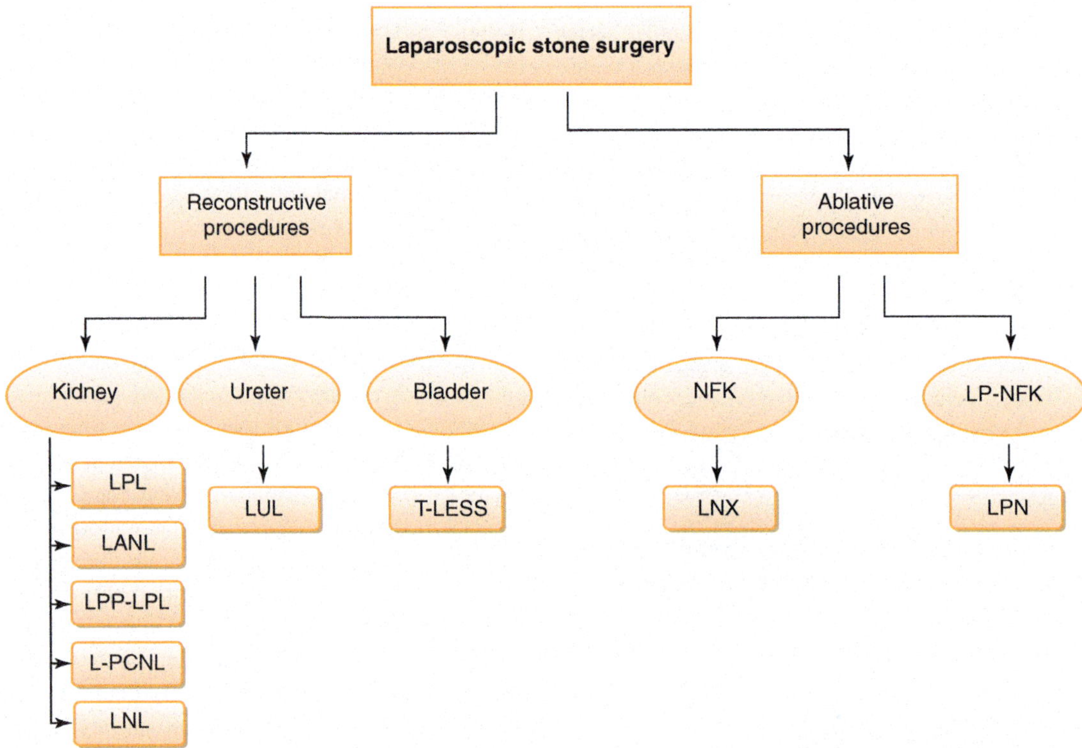

Fig. 20.1 Surgical options for laparoscopic stone surgery. *LPL* laparoscopic pyelolithotomy; *LANL* laparoscopic anatrophic nephrolithotomy; *LPP-LPL* laparoscopic pyeloplasty with concomitant laparoscopic pyelolithotomy; *L-PCNL* laparoscopic assisted percutaneous nephrolithotomy; *LNL* laparoscopic nephrolithotomy; *LUL* laparoscopic ureterolithotomy; *T-LESS* transvesical laparoendoscopic single-site surgery; *NFK* nonfunctioning kidney; *LP-NFK* lower-pole non-functioning kidney; *LNX* laparoscopic nephrectomy; *LPN* laparoscopic partial nephrectomy

20.3.1.1 Laparoscopic Pyelolithotomy (Transperitoneal)

Performing percutaneous nephrolithotomy (PCNL) in patients with large stone burden is not only associated with decreased the stone-free rate (SFR) but also with increased risk of bleeding and blood transfusion rate. Factors associated with severe bleeding are solitary kidney, staghorn calculus, multiple punctures and inexperienced surgeon. Such stones can be approached by laparoscopic transperitoneal pyelolithotomy (LPL), which is reported to have lower bleeding and blood transfusion rates due to avoidance of injury to renal parenchyma [4]. However, one of the prerequisite for successful LPL is the presence of stone in the extrarenal pelvis.

Since its initial description by Gaur et al. [5] in five patients with pelvic stones not amenable to extracorporeal shock wave lithotripsy (ESWL) or PCNL in 1994, multiple series reported LPL either by retroperitoneal or transperitoneal approach with an SFR of 71–100% and conversion rate of 0–27% [2].

20.3.1.2 Technique

A preoperative intravenous urography (IVU) or CT urogram is helpful in delineating the pelvicalyceal system (PCS) anatomy for intraoperative identification of the ureter. The patient is placed in 45° lateral decubitus position, and ports are placed as for any renal surgery following the principle of triangulation (Fig. 20.2a and b).

The white line of Toldt is incised, and the colon is reflected. The ureter-gonadal complex is identified over the psoas and traced to the pelvis with stone. With meticulous dissection, the pelvis is exposed, and stone is 'felt' with the laparoscopic instrument. An incision is made in the pelvis in the shape of 'V' away from the ureteropelvic junction (UPJ). The incision is made preferably using a stone knife or cold scissors. A hook electrode may be used for a relatively bloodless operative field. Care is taken not to break the stone with graspers, as it may dislodge into the calyces. The stone spatula helps in delivering the stone intact, especially when the stone is large. After stone retrieval, antegrade ureteral double-J (DJ) stent is placed either through 5 mm assistant port or through 16 gauge intravenous cannula placed percutaneously in addition to ports. The pyelotomy is closed in a water-tight fashion using 3–0 or 4–0 absorbable sutures, either an interrupted or a continuous fashion. The stone can be placed in an endo-catch bag or indigenously made polyethylene bag.

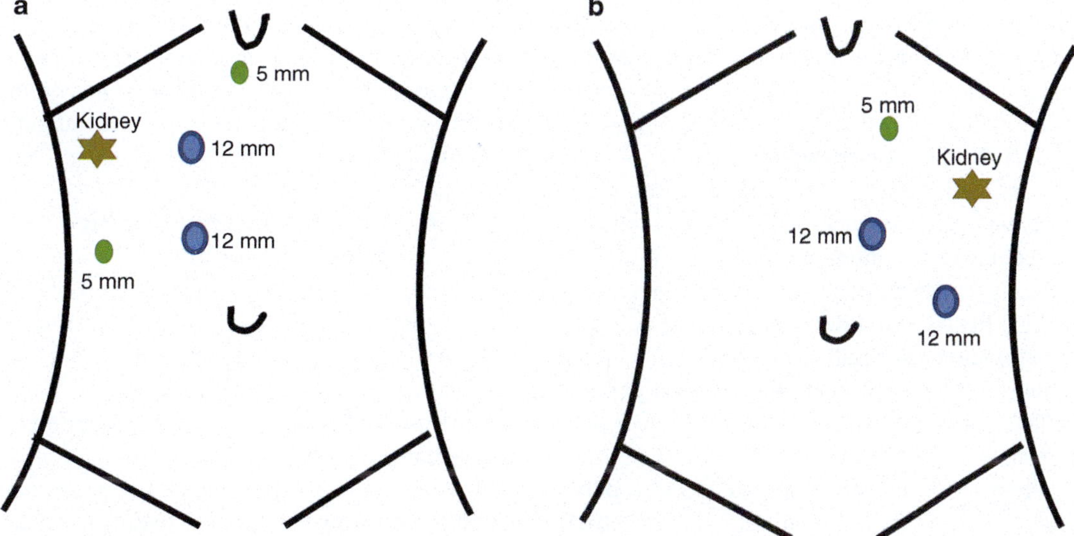

Fig. 20.2 Standard port positions for laparoscopic kidney surgery (**a**) right and (**b**) left

A pelvic stone with an extension to one of the calyces can be technically challenging. Mirroring open Gil Vernet's extended pyelolithotomy technique, the extension of the pyelotomy incision into upper or lower calyces can help in retrieving the partial staghorn stone. Auxiliary use of flexible nephroscopy can also be considered for remaining calyceal stones if extending pyelolithotomy is not feasible. A rigid nephroscope can also be introduced from one of the laparoscopy ports using a second camera system. The pneumoperitoneum may have to be desufflated to decrease the distance from the port to the pelvis. Simultaneous continuous suction in the intraperitoneal cavity avoids the accumulation of irrigation fluid. Such hybrid technique ensures SFR in the same setting, and the surgeon should be well prepared for it [3]. All measures should be taken to retrieve the stone intact or with minimal disintegration. Avoid extensive breakage with lithotripters to avoid urosepsis because of endotoxins released from infected stones, which can lead to septicaemia.

20.3.1.3 Advantages

The main advantage of LPL over PCNL is decreased risk of bleeding as it avoids renal parenchymal damage. This is particularly important for patients with already impaired renal function who require a procedure with the best chance of stone-free status in a single procedure [2].

20.3.1.4 Disadvantages

LPL is difficult or not suitable in cases of the intrarenal pelvis or small pelvis. Specifically, the dissection of the intrarenal pelvis is limited by difficult retraction of the overlying renal parenchyma. In addition, limited exposed pelvis, stone manipulation via small pyelotomy and intracorporeal pyelotomy closure of such renal pelvis is difficult, which can increase the chances or postoperative urine leak [6].

Presence of calyceal stones besides pelvic stones, sometimes results in difficulty in retrieving the calyceal stones. Flexible instrumentation through the 12 mm laparoscopic port is required in such situations for stone clearance [6, 7].

Patients with prior renal surgery can have significant perinephric adhesions, which may affect the successful outcomes or complication rate in LPL [4]. Prior placement of DJ stent or an intraoperative RGP aids ureteral identification in these cases.

20.3.1.5 Literature on LPL

In a metanalysis, Bai et al. [4] compared the outcomes of LPL and PCNL in 901 patients with the large renal stone of size ≥2 cm. Analysing 14 studies with 432 patients undergoing LPL and 469 patients with PCNL, the authors showed a higher SFR with LPL. In addition, LPL was associated with lower incidence of bleeding, blood transfusion and postoperative fever. Moreover, the need for an auxiliary procedure and re-treatment rates were lower with LPL. However, LPL was associated with prolonged urine leakage and longer operative time (OT) and length of hospital stay (LOS) as compared to PCNL. The authors concluded that LPL is safe and feasible in experienced hands, and it should not replace PCNL, which remains the gold standard for kidney stones greater than 2 cm [4].

Thus, LPL is considered an alternative therapy for PCNL in selected cases with renal stones either previously failed or not amenable to endourologic management or in large renal stone with unfavourable (non-dilated) collecting system but with extrarenal pelvis without a history of previous surgery. Table 20.2 describes some of the largest series of laparoscopic stone surgery, including LPL.

20.3.1.6 Laparoscopic Anatrophic Nephrolithotomy

Mirroring the open technique, Kaouk et al. [13] first showed the feasibility of laparoscopic anatrophic nephrolithotomy (LANL) in a survival porcine model. A synthetic staghorn calculus was created by retrograde injection of polyurethane (Fomo Products, Inc., Norton, Ohio) into the renal pelvis through a ureteral catheter and allowed to mature over two weeks. LANL was successfully performed in all ten animals involving hilar vessel control with laparoscopic Satinsky clamp, in situ renal hypo-

Table 20.2 Large series of laparoscopic stone surgeries

Parameters	LPL [8]	LPP-LPL [9]	L-PCNL [10]	LANL [11]	LUL [12]
Sample size (n)	56	20	15	11	126
Mean stone size (mm)	27.5	15	8–45*	52	13.6
Approach (TP/RP)	RP	TP	TP	TP	RP
Mean OT (min)	81	168	55	139	88
SFR	96%	75%	100%	90.9%	97.6%
Conversion rate	3.6%	10%	–	–	2.4%
Urine leak.	–	–	6.6%	27.3%	2.4%
LOS (days)	4.0	4.9	4.8	–	2.8

*Range

Abbreviations: *LPL* laparoscopic pyelolithotomy, *LPP-LPL* laparoscopic pyeloplasty with concomitant laparoscopic pyelolithotomy, *L-PCNL* laparoscopic-assisted percutaneous nephrolithotomy, *LANL* laparoscopic anatrophic nephrolithotomy, *LUL* laparoscopic ureterolithotomy, *RU* renal units, *TP* transperitoneal, *RP* retroperitoneal, *OT* operative time, *SFR* stone-free rate

thermia with ice slush (in one animal), lateral renal parenchymal incision, stone extraction and closure of the collecting system and renal parenchyma. The mean OT, blood loss and warm ischemia time were 125 min, 68 ml and 30 min, respectively [13]. LANL can be considered as a reasonable therapeutic option for large staghorn calculus, which cannot be removed with a reasonable number of access and sessions of PCNL [14].

Technique

The kidney is de-fatted, and the lateral parenchyma is completely exposed. Intraoperative laparoscopic ultrasonography (USG) can help in localisation of the renal stones. The Brödel's line along the lateral aspect is marked with electrocautery. With the help of a laparoscopic Satinsky clamp, renal pedicle control is achieved. The procedure can be done with or without hypothermia, with the help of ice slush placed in a polyethylene bag. After the renal parenchymal incision along the avascular Brödel's line, PCS is opened, followed by extraction of the staghorn stone. The collecting system can be closed with absorbable sutures followed by complete renorrhaphy [3].

Literature on LANL

Deger et al. [15] were the first to report LANL for a staghorn calculus in an adult female. The authors closed the collecting system with a polyglactin 3–0 continuous suture and, in addition, applied gelatin-matrix thrombin tissue sealant (FloSeal®; Baxter BioScience, Deerfield, IL) to seal the system. The cold ischemia time was 45 min.

Later, Simforoosh et al. [14] reported a few modifications in the LANL technique in five patients with large staghorn renal stones unsuitable for PCNL. In contrast to Deger et al. [15], the authors clamped the renal artery alone using a bulldog clamp and Brödel's line nephrotomy incision sutures were buttressed by hemostatic clips instead of knots. There was no incidence of urine leakage after surgery, and they concluded that LANL is a promising alternative for patients who are candidates for open surgery, with an acceptable SFR.

20.3.2 Special Situations with Renal Stones

20.3.2.1 UPJO with Secondary Stones

Renal stones secondary to UPJ obstruction requires relief of the obstruction besides stone clearance. The gold standard treatment has been open pyeloplasty with pyelolithotomy with reported success rate of 90% [6]. Although, endopyelotomy has been described either by antegrade [16] or retrograde [17] access, their success rate is low. With expertise, the goal of stone clearance and correction of congenital abnormality can be dealt with laparoscopy. Thus, laparoscopic pyeloplasty with concomitant pyelolithotomy (LPP-LPL) can be a safe option in the hands of surgeons with advanced laparoscopic skills.

20.3.2.2 Laparoscopic Pyeloplasty with Concomitant Pyelolithotomy

Technique

After positioning and ports placement, the renal pelvis and proximal ureter are dissected. Placing an appropriate pyelotomy incision is specifically important in these cases as this incision is subsequently incorporated in the pyeloplasty. Larger stones can be retrieved with a forceps. Frequently, small pebble-type secondary stones can be found, which can be aspirated/flushed out with the help of laparoscopic irrigator-aspirator system. All stones in the vicinity must be completely retrieved as dropped out stones can cause intense inflammatory reactions around the anastomosis. After stone retrieval, the planned technique of laparoscopy pyeloplasty is completed in a standard manner [3, 6].

Literature on LPP-LPL

Stein et al. [18] in their series of 117 laparoscopic pyeloplasties, noted 15 patients had undergone LPP-LPL for associated renal stones. They performed a transperitoneal approach in 86.7% of patients, and the combined procedure took an average of 174 min. They reported a success rate of 80% with no open conversion or any complication [18].

Later, Ramakumar et al. [19] reported a 90% SFR in 19 patients with transperitoneal LPP-LPL. In one of the largest series, Srivastava et al. [9] did LPP-LPL in 20 patients with a 75% stone clearance rate at the initial surgery. However, the authors reported 100% SFR in the follow-up with additional procedures. Also, 90% improved in their follow-up diuretic renography while the rest 10% had symptomatic improvement.

20.3.2.3 Renal Pelvic Stone in Kidney with Anatomical Abnormalities

Pelvic Ectopic Kidney with Stones

Although LPL can be a suitable option in an anteriorly rotated renal pelvis [20], complex cases like staghorn calculus in pelvic ectopic kidneys require more than one treatment modality to achieve SFR. Laparoscopic-assisted percutaneous nephrolithotomy (L-PCNL) has been described as available option for such stones. Here, the role of laparoscopy is to allow safe bowel retraction and enable direct vision guiding controlled percutaneous access to the collecting system [2, 6].

20.3.2.4 Laparoscopic Assisted Percutaneous Nephrolithotomy

Technique

In approaching a pelvic kidney with stones, the primary surgeon stands on the side of the affected kidney and the assistant on the opposite side, both facing the patient's foot end [21]. L-PCNL was first described by Eshghi et al. [22] in a pelvic kidney with a staghorn calculus. They used a co-axial system comprising a 5F curved-tip angiographic catheter sheathed within a 9F catheter to obtain percutaneous access via retrograde approach. Simultaneous laparoscopy was used to displace the bowel and direct the catheter towards the anterior abdominal wall. Later several modifications of the original description were proposed by various authors [23–25]. Notably, Goel et al. [26] described two different methods of access to the stone in ectopic kidneys. After pneumoperitoneum, the patient is placed in 30 degrees Trendelenburg position. Based on the body habitus and abdominal fat, either colon reflecting or transmesocolic approach to the desired calyx was made under simultaneous fluoroscopic and laparoscopic control with partial desufflation. The tract was serially dilated with Teflon dilators to admit 30F Amplatz sheath, and the abdomen was desufflated. The stone was fragmented and retrieved as in any standard PCNL. After stone clearance, a DJ stent and nephrostomy were placed. At the end of the surgery, pneumoperitoneum was re-established for intraperitoneal drain placement.

Previous Studies

El-Kappany et al. [21] reported L-PCNL in 5 patients after failed ESWL. In their series, the targeted calyx was percutaneously accessed under simultaneous fluoroscopy and laparoscopy control. They reported 80% SFR with their technique with a mean OT of 141 min. In one of the largest series, Holman and Toth [1, 4, 5] reported L-PCNL in 15 patients (Table 20.2). They successfully cleared the stone in all cases with minimal morbidity. D'souza et al. [27] described a modified technique of L-PCNL in 9 patients where a mini PCNL (tract size 15 F) was performed with Holmium laser to dust the stone in ectopic kidneys. They reported a comparable SFR of 88.9%. Recently, Soylemez et al. [28] described L-PCNL with two different laparoscopic (transmesocolic and dissection of mesocolon) and four different PCNL techniques (standard, mini-, micro- and a direct renal pelvic PCNL) for treating stones in pelvic ectopic kidneys and showed an SFR of 75%.

Horseshoe Kidney with Stones

The management of a horseshoe kidney (HSK) with stones poses a difficult problem. The abnormal location, aberrant vessels, proximity to vital structures such as bowel, iliac vessels add difficulty in accessing the stone via percutaneous approach. Also, acute angulation of the ureter makes retrograde access to the stones difficult even in the hands of an expert endourologist [3]. With anteriorly placed renal pelvis in HSK, few reports showed the feasibility of LPL for stone removal.

Various other surgical options such as the open approach to more minimally invasive USG-guided PCNL are available [29]; however, laparoscopic assistance in the form of L-PCNL is a safe alternative provided availability of the expert laparoscopic surgeon [3].

20.3.2.5 Laparoscopic Assisted Percutaneous Nephrolithotomy for HSK

Technique

The technique of L-PCNL for HSK is the same as for pelvic ectopic kidney except for the port placement and orientation to access the more cephalad position of the HSK. In the first description of L-PCNL for HSK with isthmic calyceal stone, the patient was positioned supine with the elevation of the left flank [30]. An 11-mm suprapubic port was placed for the laparoscope. Under the vision, two 5-mm working ports were placed, one in the left iliac fossa and the other in the left anterior axillary line above the umbilicus. The overlying bowel was retracted after locating the bulge of HSK. The targeted calyx is opacified under fluoroscopy, and puncture needle is directed under laparoscopy. The tract serially dilated up to 30F with metallic dilators and Amplatz sheath positioned. Simultaneous fluoroscopy and laparoscopy ensured controlled access to the collecting system with no injury to the intraperitoneal structures [30].

20.3.2.6 Renal Calyceal Diverticular Stone

Another situation where laparoscopy can be applied is in the treatment of calyceal diverticular calculi. The incidence of stones within a calyceal diverticulum ranges from 1 to 10% [31]. Although PCNL is associated with high SFR (>80%), [32, 33] access can be difficult for small and anteriorly located lesions where laparoscopic nephrolithotomy (LNL) and robotic-assisted interventions are feasible alternatives. Van Cangh et al. [34] showed the feasibility of LNL in a patient who had failed ESWL for an anteriorly located stone-bearing calix which also precluded percutaneous approach. Intraoperative USG and colour-Doppler helped them to localise and select the optimum site of nephrotomy. Koopman et al. proposed an algorithm for minimally invasive management of such calyceal stones. In this, they proposed laparoscopy for the management of anteriorly located calyceal diverticula that have failed prior endourologic attempts or primarily for anteriorly located stones of size >3 cm [35].

20.3.3 Ureter Stones

With the introduction of ESWL and ureteroscopy (URS) for the management of ureter stones, the traditional open approach for ureter stone removal has drastically decreased. However, large ureter calculi can still be challenging for modern endourological techniques. Importantly, the SFR decreases from 84% to 42% when the size of the ureteral stone is >1 cm [36]. Thus, in the era of modern endourology, laparoscopic ureterolithotomy (LUL) can be of use in large, impacted ureteral stones not amenable by ESWL or URS [6].

20.3.3.1 Laparoscopic Ureterolithotomy

The earliest report of laparoscopic ureterolithotomy (LUL) was a retroperitoneal approach by Wickham in 1979 [2]. Until the mid-1990s, LUL was limited with only sporadic case reports [37, 38] when the improvement in the technology-enabled wider adoption.

Technique

Patient position and ports placement are as same for upper tract surgery as described before. However, if the stone is in the lower ureter, ports should be shifted caudally. The ureter is exposed after the colon is reflected. At times, the location of the stone is difficult due to periureteral adhesions. In such situations, intraoperative laparoscopic USG or fluoroscopic assistance aid in localising the exact stone position. The surgeon should be cautious about stone migration during manipulation. Ureter proximal to the stone can be controlled with laparoscopic Babcock forceps or by vascular loops to prevent proximal migration of the stone. Once the stone is precisely localised, a vertical ureterotomy is made in over the stone with a laparoscopic knife or hook electrode [6]. Instead of grasping, levering the stone out of the ureter (Fig. 20.3) can prevent the crushing of stone into small pieces and helps in intact removal. The ureter is sutured with 4–0 polyglactin and a drain placed after suturing over a double-J stent. However, if the area of stone impaction is narrow, spatulation of ends and an uretero-ureterostomy is to be considered [3].

Advantages

High SFR after a single procedure with comparable complication rates is the major advantage of LUL over URSfor large upper ureteric stones [39, 40].

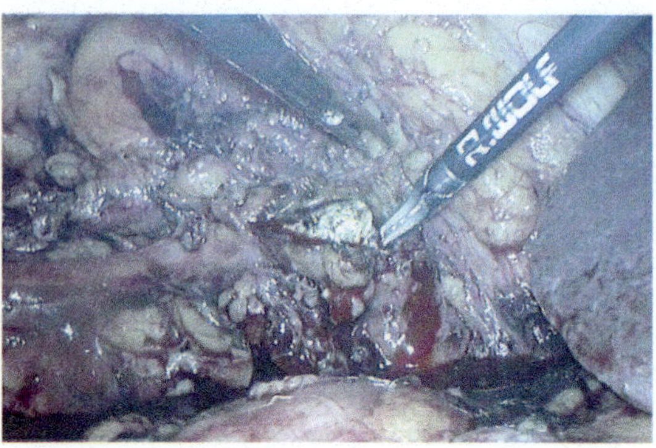

Fig. 20.3 Levering with a ureteral stone with Maryland forceps for extraction during laparoscopic ureterolithotomy

Disadvantages

The disadvantages include a longer LOS, the risk of injury to surrounding structures and open conversion [6]. The most common postoperative complication is urine leak (0–20%), followed by stricture formation (1.4–5.2%) [12, 41–43]. Many authors suggest limiting the ureterotomy length as short as possible to allow stone extraction and using a cold knife instead of electrocautery for ureterotomy to decrease stricture formation [41, 44, 45].

Literature on LUL

In one of the few randomised studies comparing LUL to URS or PCNL, Basiri et al. enrolled 150 patients with large (>1 cm) upper ureteral stones. They showed that the SFR at the time of discharge was highest with LUL (88%), followed by PCNL (64%) and URS (56%). The requirement of the second stone clearance procedure was least with LUL (10%), followed by PCNL (14%) and URS (22%). The authors concluded LUL might offer better single setting SFR with the least need for additional procedures [41].

20.3.3.2 Controversies: To Close or Not to Close the Ureterotomy?

While most surgeons agree with the placement of DJ stent after LUL [46–50], some prefer to close the ureterostomy [37, 48], while others prefer to leave it open [49, 50]. Gaur et al. [51] reported that operative time for retroperitoneal LUL was reduced to 66 min if the ureterotomy was left open compared with 92 min if the ureterotomy was closed. However, they noted a prolonged (>1 week) postoperative urine leak in 19.8% (20/101) of patients in whom the ureter was not stented. Out of these 20 patients, 70% (14/20) also did not have the ureterostomy closed. The remaining 6 had ureterotomy closure, and the probable reason for prolonged urine leak in them was that these ureters were chronically inflamed, edematous and friable after infection and prolonged impaction [51].

Keeley et al. [52] described the outcomes of LUL in five treatment naïve patients with large ureter stones (mean size 27.2 mm) and nine patients after failed ESWL and/or URS. They reported a 100% success rate with no open conversion and a mean OT of 105 min. In their series, ureterotomy was closed in only five patients, out of which two subsequently developed stricture, whereas none of the nine patients with left open ureterotomy develop stricture formation. Importantly, one patient with neither stented nor ureterotomy closure developed a prolonged urine leak [52].

20.3.4 Bladder Stones

Various methods have been described for the management of bladder calculi, from open surgery to transurethral or percutaneous cystolithotripsy. Based on stone-related, patient-related, resources-related factors, a decision on bladder calculi treatment is considered. The role of laparoscopy in bladder calculi is limited. However, it can be considered as an alternative in selected cases.

20.3.4.1 Transvesical Laparoendoscopic Single-Site Surgery (T-LESS)

Roslan et al. [53] used transvesical laparoendoscopic single-site surgery (T-LESS) for the removal of intravesical erosion of polypropylene mesh from the bladder [54]. Using the same technique, multiple bladder stones were removed intact after previous unsuccessful endoscopic lithotripsy.

Technique

For T-LESS, the patients were placed in lithotomy position, and a 1.5–2.5 cm suprapubic skin incision was made 2–5 cm above the pubic symphysis. A single-port device (Tri-Port+, Olympus, Hamburg, Germany) was placed under vision with simultaneous cystoscopy. A pneumovesicum of 14 mm Hg facilitated intravesical manipulation. The stones were removed intact with the grasper through the Tri-Port. Notably, in two patients, auxiliary procedures like diverticulectomy and ureterocele incision and stone extraction were described by the authors. In their series of 12 patients, all patients had complete stone removal without any serious complications. The mean operative time was 46 min, and LOS was 22 h. In two patients, auxiliary procedures of diverticulectomy and ureterocele incision were performed simultaneously. The authors concluded that the T-LESS technique was a safe, efficient and minimally invasive alternative for intact bladder stone removal in selected patients, which avoid the risk of urethral injury [53].

20.4 Ablative Laparoscopic Stone Surgery

The combination of obstruction and infection caused by the urinary stones has detrimental effects on the affected renal units. In untreated cases, this can lead to loss of function of the kidney [55]. In rare cases, an impacted stone in the calyx results in hydro-calyx with recurrent pyelonephritis rendering non-function. In this section, the role of laparoscopy in such conditions is discussed.

20.4.1 Laparoscopic Nephrectomy

Laparoscopic nephrectomy (LN) is an option for hydronephrotic non-functioning kidneys caused by renal stones. However, recurrent pyelonephritis in such kidneys causes significant perinephric adhesions, sometimes making the laparoscopic approach difficult. This is particularly important in the case of xanthogranulomatous pyelonephritis (XGPN). The majority of such patients might have a prior history of interventions like DJ stent placement or a percutaneous nephrostomy to relieve obstruction and/or infection or sometimes an open surgery for prior stone disease.

In the transperitoneal approach, after standard port placement, the ureter is identified and traced up to the hilum. Harmonic shears or electrocautery helps in the dissection. Renal vessels are clipped and divided. Occasionally, dense adhesions at the hilum prevent the delineation of renal vessels. In such a scenario, *en bloc* stapler ligation of the renal vascular pedicle may be used [56]. Dissection is preferred outside of Gerota's fascia, avoiding entering the infected renal unit. However, a subcapsular nephrectomy may be required in patients with severe perinephric adhesions [57]. The specimen is placed in a specimen-retrieval bag and extracted by extending the 12-mm port or via a separate transverse incision below the beltline [3]. Likewise, in cases of the hydronephrotic non-functioning renal unit following ureteral stones, a similar approach for laparoscopic nephroureterectomy is considered along with the stone retrieval.

Ganpule et al. [3] discuss several strategies to reduce risks during LN. These include preoperative drainage of an infected kidney with a nephrostomy, preoperative computed tomography for anatomical delineation, placement of a ureteric catheter to aid identification of the ureter, subcapsular upper-pole dissection and double clipping of the ureter to avoid spillage of infected contents.

20.4.2 Laparoscopic Partial Nephrectomy

In the rare case of non-functioning pole of the kidney because of calculus pyelonephritis, a polar partial nephrectomy would be the preferred treatment option. Winfield and colleagues, in 1992, reported the first laparoscopic partial nephrectomy for a stone-bearing lower calyx diverticulum [58]. They used a self-made, specially designed laparoscopic tourniquet for lower pole clinching. With the combination of electrocautery and laparoscopic argon beam coagulation probe, they excised the lower pole calyceal diverticulum with the stone. The renal parenchyma was extensively fulgurated with an argon beam, and no attempt was made to close the infundibulum. The Gerota's fascia was folded, backed and tacked with laparoscopic hernia clips to close the renal defect. The whole procedure took over 6 h. Later, they updated their experience with success in 4 of 5 similar patients [59].

20.5 Retroperitoneoscopic Laparoscopy for Stone Surgery

Although the first description of retroperitoneoscopy was by Wickham in 1979, its wide application was realised only after standardisation of the balloon technique for creating the working space by Gaur et al. in 1993 [60]. Various stone procedures have been described in the literature for urinary stones by retroperitoneal approach.

20.5.1 Technique

The patient is placed in the lateral flank position, and the bridge of the table is elevated to flatten the flank region. A slight anterior tilt helps the peritoneal contents to fall forward. A 1.5 cm incision is made 2 cm below the tip of the 12th rib along the posterior axillary line. The incision is deepened, and the thoracolumbar fascia is incised. The retroperitoneum is entered and confirmed by the palpation of psoas posteriorly and, at times, the tip of the lower pole cephalad. A retroperitoneal space is then created using either a commercially available balloon or an indigenously made gloved finger. A 12 mm blunt tip trocar or Hassan cannula is inserted for the camera. Under the vision, two working ports (12 mm and 5 mm) are placed. Once inside the retroperitoneal space, the ureter is identified anterior to the psoas and further dissection proceeds according to the planned procedure [6].

20.5.1.1 Advantages

On a technical note, surgeons tend to prefer the retroperitoneal approach as reaching the renal pelvis posteriorly has the advantage of extending the incision into an infundibulum without risk or hindrance of the renal vessels [2]. Other advantages include avoidance of peritoneal cavity contamination, elimination of postoperative shoulder tip pain and decreased incidence of port-site hernia and bowel obstruction. Moreover, in bowel handling, the risk of inadvertent bowel injury or ileus is minimised [6].

20.5.1.2 Disadvantages

However, retroperitoneal dissection is challenging with unfamiliar surgical anatomy and landmarks in the setting of a restricted working space. There is a potential loss of visualisation because of inadvertent peritoneal tear [43, 61].

20.6 Controversies: Retroperitoneal vs. Transperitoneal, Which Is Better?

In a prospective study, Bove et al. [62] compared transperitoneal to retroperitoneal access for LUL in 35 patients. They showed that the transperitoneal approach required less time to access and identify the ureter (14 vs. 24 min), ureterotomy closure (16 vs. 28 min), and mean operating time (75 vs. 102 min). There were no conversions. They concluded that the transperitoneal approach is better for a novice surgeon, but for those with advanced laparoscopic skills, the approach should be left to the discretion of the surgeon.

20.7 Conclusion

In the hands of experts, laparoscopic stone surgery is a safe and effective alternative in the selected cases of urolithiasis, achieving stone clearance in a single setting. However, in difficult situations, combined endourological techniques may be needed to achieve stone-free status.

20.8 Key Learning Points

- Laparoscopic stone surgery is feasible in the hands of expert.
- Laparoscopic assistance is safe and effective alternative in selected cases.
- In most cases, stone-free rates are achieved in a single setting.
- Transperitoneal or retroperitoneal approach is at the discretion of surgeon's preference.

References

1. Kidney Stones: Surgical Management Guideline – American Urological Association. https://www.auanet.org/guidelines/kidney-stones-surgical-management-guideline#x14229. Accessed 25 Aug 2020.
2. Humphreys MR. The emerging role of robotics and laparoscopy in stone disease. Urol Clin N Am. 2013;40:115–28.
3. Ganpule AP, Prashant J, Desai MR. Laparoscopic and robot-assisted surgery in the management of urinary lithiasis. Arab J Urol. 2012;10:32–9.
4. Bai Y, Tang Y, Deng L, Wang X, Yang Y, Wang J, Han P. Management of large renal stones: laparoscopic pyelolithotomy versus percutaneous nephrolithotomy. BMC Urol. 2017;17:75.
5. Gaur DD, Agarwal DK, Purohit KC, Darshane AS. Retroperitoneal laparoscopic pyelolithotomy. J Urol. 1994;151:927–9.
6. Yadav R, Kumar R, Hemal AK. Laparoscopy in the management of stone disease of urinary tract. J Minim Access Surg. 2005;1:173–80.
7. Micali S, Moore RG, Averch TD, Adams JB, Kavoussi LR. The role of laparoscopy in the treatment of renal and ureteral calculi. J Urol. 1997;157:463–6.
8. Chander J, Suryavanshi M, Lal P, Singh L, Ramteke VK. Retroperitoneal pyelolithotomy for management of renal calculi. JSLS. 2005;9:97–101.
9. Srivastava A, Singh P, Gupta M, Ansari MS, Mandhani A, Kapoor R, Kumar A, Dubey D. Laparoscopic pyeloplasty with concomitant pyelolithotomy – is it an effective mode of treatment? Urol Int. 2008;80:306–9.
10. Holman E, Tóth C. Laparoscopically assisted percutaneous transperitoneal nephrolithotomy in pelvic dystopic kidneys: experience in 15 successful cases. J Laparoendosc Adv Surg Tech. 1998;8:431–5.
11. Zhou L, Xuan Q, Wu B, Xiao J, Dong X, Huang T, Chen H, Zhu Y, Wu K. Retroperitoneal laparoscopic anatrophic nephrolithotomy for large staghorn calculi: Laparoscopic anatrophic nephrolithotomy. Int J Urol. 2011;18:126–9.

12. Farooq Qadri SJ, Khan N, Khan M. Retroperitoneal laparoscopic ureterolithotomy – a single centre 10 year experience. Int J Surg. 2011;9:160–4.
13. Kaouk JH, Gill IS, Desai MM, Banks KLW, Raja SS, Skacel M, Sung GT. Laparoscopic anatrophic nephrolithotomy: feasibility study in a chronic porcine model. J Urol. 2003;169:691–6.
14. Simforoosh N, Aminsharifi A, Tabibi A, Noor-Alizadeh A, Zand S, Radfar M-H, Javaherforooshzadeh A. Laparoscopic anatrophic nephrolithotomy for managing large staghorn calculi. BJU Int. 2008;101:1293–6.
15. Deger S, Tuellmann M, Schoenberger B, Winkelmann B, Peters R, Loening SA. Laparoscopic anatrophic nephrolithotomy. Scand J Urol Nephrol. 2004;38:263–5.
16. Motola JA, Badlani GH, Smith AD. Results of 212 consecutive endopyelotomies: an 8-year followup. J Urol. 1993;149:453–6.
17. Chandhoke PS, Clayman RV, Stone AM, McDougall EM, Buelna T, Hilal N, Chang M, Stegwell MJ. Endopyelotomy and endoureterotomy with the acucise ureteral cutting balloon device: preliminary experience. J Endourol. 1993;7:45–51.
18. Stein RJ, Turna B, Nguyen MM, Aron M, Hafron JM, Gill IS, Kaouk J, Desai M. Laparoscopic pyeloplasty with concomitant pyelolithotomy: technique and outcomes. J Endourol. 2008;22:1251–5.
19. Ramakumar S, Lancini V, Chan DY, Parsons JK, Kavoussi LR, Jarrett TW. Laparoscopic pyeloplasty with concomitant pyelolithotomy. J Urol. 2002;167:1378–80.
20. Gupta NP, Yadav R, Singh A. Laparoscopic transmesocolic pyelolithotomy in an ectopic pelvic kidney. JSLS. 2007;11:258–60.
21. El-Kappany HA, El-Nahas AR, Shoma AM, El-Tabey NA, Eraky I, El-Kenawy MR. Combination of laparoscopy and nephroscopy for treatment of stones in pelvic ectopic kidneys. J Endourol. 2007;21:1131–6.
22. Eshghi AM, Roth JS, Smith AD. Percutaneous transperitoneal approach to a pelvic kidney for endourological removal of staghorn calculus. J Urol. 1985;134:525–7.
23. Zafar FS, Lingeman JE. Value of laparoscopy in the management of calculi complicating renal malformations. J Endourol. 1996;10:379–83.
24. Troxel SA, Low RK, Das S. Extraperitoneal laparoscopy-assisted percutaneous nephrolithotomy in a left pelvic kidney. J Endourol. 2002;16:655–7.
25. Watterson JD, Cook A, Sahajpal R, Bennett J, Denstedt JD. Percutaneous nephrolithotomy of a pelvic kidney: a posterior approach through the greater sciatic foramen. J Urol. 2001;166:209–10.
26. Goel R, Yadav R, Gupta NP, Aron M. Laparoscopic assisted percutaneous nephrolithotomy (PCNL) in ectopic kidneys: two different techniques. Int Urol Nephrol. 2006;38:75–8.
27. Dsouza N, Verma A, Rai A. Laparoscopic-assisted mini percutaneous nephrolithotomy in the ectopic pelvic kidney: outcomes with the laser dusting technique. Urol Ann. 2016;8:87.
28. Soylemez H, Penbegül N, Utangac MM, Dede O, Çakmakçı S, Hatipoglu NK. Laparoscopy assisted percutaneous stone surgery can be performed in multiple ways for pelvic ectopic kidneys. Urolithiasis. 2016;44:345–52.
29. Desai M. Ultrasonography-guided punctures—with and without puncture guide. J Endourol. 2009;23:1641–3.
30. Maheshwari PN, Bhandarkar DS, Shah RS, Andankar MG, Saple AL. Laparoscopy-assisted transperitoneal percutaneous nephrolithotomy for recurrent calculus in isthmic calix of horseshoe kidney. J Endourol. 2004;18:858–61.
31. Torricelli FCM, Batista LT, Colombo JR, Coelho RF (2014) Robotic-assisted laparoscopic management of a caliceal diverticular calculus. Case Reports. 2014:bcr2014205437.
32. Bellman GC, Silverstein JI, Blickensderfer S, Smith AD. Technique and follow-up of percutaneous management of caliceal diverticula. Urology. 1993;42:21–5.
33. Shalhav AL, Soble JJ, Nakada SY, Wolf JS, McClennan BL, Clayman RV. Long-term outcome of caliceal diverticula following percutaneous endosurgical management. J Urol. 1998;160:1635–9.
34. Van Cangh PJ, Abi Aad AS, Lorge F, Wese FX, Opsomer R. Laparoscopic nephrolithotomy: the value of intracorporeal sonography and color Doppler. Urology. 1995;45:516–9.
35. Koopman SG, Fuchs G. Management of stones associated with intrarenal stenosis: infundibular stenosis and caliceal diverticulum. J Endourol. 2013;27:1546–50.
36. Park H, Park M, Park T. Two-year experience with ureteral stones: extracorporeal shockwave lithotripsy *v* ureteroscopic manipulation. J Endourol. 1998;12:501–4.
37. Raboy A, Ferzli GS, Ioffreda R, Albert PS. Laparoscopic ureterolithotomy. Urology. 1992;39:223–5.
38. Wuernschimmel E, Lipsky H. Laparoscopic treatment of an upper ureteral stone. J Laparoendosc Surg. 1993;3:301–7.
39. Torricelli FCM, Monga M, Marchini GS, Srougi M, Nahas WC, Mazzucchi E. Semi-rigid ureteroscopic lithotripsy versus laparoscopic ureterolithotomy for large upper ureteral stones: a meta – analysis of randomized controlled trials. Int Braz J Urol. 2016;42:645–54.
40. Kallidonis P, Ntasiotis P, Knoll T, Sarica K, Papatsoris A, Somani BK, Greco F, Aboumarzouk OM, Álvarez-Maestro M, Sanguedolce F. Minimally invasive surgical ureterolithotomy versus ureteroscopic lithotripsy for large ureteric stones: a systematic review and meta-analysis of the literature. Eur Urol Focus. 2017;3:554–66.
41. Basiri A, Simforoosh N, Ziaee A, Shayaninasab H, Moghaddam SMMH, Zare S. Retrograde, antegrade,

and laparoscopic approaches for the management of large, proximal ureteral stones: a randomized clinical trial. J Endourol. 2008;22:2677–80.
42. Lopes Neto AC, Korkes F, Silva JL, Amarante RDM, Mattos MHE, Tobias-Machado M, Pompeo ACL. Prospective randomized study of treatment of large proximal ureteral stones: extracorporeal shock wave lithotripsy versus ureterolithotripsy versus laparoscopy. J Urol. 2012;187:164–8.
43. Fan T, Xian P, Yang L, Liu Y, Wei Q, Li H. Experience and learning curve of retroperitoneal laparoscopic ureterolithotomy for upper ureteral calculi. J Endourol. 2009;23:1867–70.
44. Kijvikai K, Patcharatrakul S. Laparoscopic ureterolithotomy: its role and some controversial technical considerations. Int J Urol. 2006;13:206–10.
45. Nouira Y, Kallel Y, Binous MY, Dahmoul H, Horchani A. Laparoscopic retroperitoneal ureterolithotomy: initial experience and review of literature. J Endourol. 2004;18:557–61.
46. Skrepetis K, Doumas K, Siafakas I, Lykourinas M (2001) Laparoscopic versus open ureterolithotomy. A comparative study. Eur Urol. 40:32–36; discussion 37.
47. Gaur DD. Retroperitoneal endoscopic ureterolithotomy: our experience in 12 patients. J Endourol. 1993;7:501–3.
48. Sinha R, Sharma N. Retroperitoneal laparoscopic management of urolithiasis. J Laparoendosc Adv Surg Tech A. 1997;7:95–8.
49. Bellman GC, Smith AD. Special considerations in the technique of laparoscopic ureterolithotomy. J Urol. 1994;151:146–9.
50. Kiyota H, Ikemoto I, Asano K, Madarame J, Miki K, Yoshino Y, Hasegawa T, Ohishi Y. Retroperitoneoscopic ureterolithotomy for impacted ureteral stone. Int J Urol. 2001;8:391–7.
51. Gaur DD, Trivedi S, Prabhudesai MR, Madhusudhana HR, Gopichand M. Laparoscopic ureterolithotomy: technical considerations and long-term follow-up. BJU Int. 2002;89:339–43.
52. Keeley FX, Gialas I, Pillai M, Chrisofos M, Tolley DA. Laparoscopic ureterolithotomy: the Edinburgh experience. BJU Int. 1999;84:765–9.
53. Roslan M, Przudzik M, Borowik M. Endoscopic intact removal of medium-size- or multiple bladder stones with the use of transvesical laparoendoscopic single-site surgery. World J Urol. 2019;37:373–8.
54. Ingber MS, Stein RJ, Rackley RR, Firoozi F, Irwin BH, Kaouk JH, Desai MM. Single-port transvesical excision of foreign body in the bladder. Urology. 2009;74:1347–50.
55. Keddis MT, Rule AD. Nephrolithiasis and loss of kidney function. Curr Opin Nephrol Hypertens. 2013;22:390–6.
56. Rapp DE, Orvieto MA, Gerber GS, Johnston WK, Wolf JS, Shalhav AL. En bloc stapling of renal hilum during laparoscopic nephrectomy and nephroureterectomy. Urology. 2004;64:655–9.
57. Tobias-Machado M, Lasmar MT, Batista LT, Forseto PH Jr, Juliano RV, Wroclawski ER. Laparoscopic nephrectomy in inflammatory renal disease: proposal for a staged approach. Int Braz J Urol. 2005;31:22–8.
58. Winfield HN, Donovan JF, Godet AS, Clayman RV. Laparoscopic partial nephrectomy: initial case report for benign disease. J Endourol. 1993;7:521–6.
59. Winfield HN, Donovan JF, Lund GO, Kreder KJ, Stanley KE, Brown BP, Loening SA, Clayman RV. Laparoscopic partial nephrectomy: initial experience and comparison to the open surgical approach. J Urol. 1995;153:1409–14.
60. Gaur DD, Agarwal DK, Purohit KC. Retroperitoneal laparoscopic nephrectomy: initial case report. J Urol. 1993;149:103–5.
61. Flasko T, Holman E, Kovacs G, Tallai B, Toth C, Salah MA. Laparoscopic ureterolithotomy: the method of choice in selected cases. J Laparoendosc Adv Surg Tech A. 2005;15:149–52.
62. Bove P, Micali S, Miano R, Mirabile G, De Stafani S, Botteri E, Giampaolo B, Vespasiani G. Laparoscopic ureterolithotomy: a comparison between the transperitoneal and the retroperitoneal approach during the learning curve. J Endourol. 2009;23:953–7.

Part VI

Practical Advices on Special Situation

Overview of Treatment Selection for Individual Patient

21

Christy W. H. Mak and Anthony C.F. Ng

21.1 Introduction

Different methods of surgical stone removal have been discussed in previous chapters. As a Urologist, suitable stone management should be tailor-made for each patient after discussing the potential benefit and risks of different approaches with them. With consideration of their background, premorbid and medical history, stone characteristics and stone management history, an evidence-based management will definitely benefit our patients. In short, we would like to highlight different indications and special considerations for each treatment in this chapter.

21.1.1 Conservative Management

Conservative management and observation should be one of the options for some patients because not all urinary tract stones are needed to be treated timely. Unfortunately, with the currently available literature, there is no consensus reached on the protocol for expectant management. Individual management decisions should be made jointly by physicians and patients.

For asymptomatic renal stones, incidence of symptomatic episode or need for intervention is around 10–25% per year [1]. Symptoms may include haematuria and renal colic. According to the EAU guideline, stone intervention is indicated in a patient with symptoms or complications like obstruction and infection. For recurrent stone formers, patients with stone size more than 15 mm or with stone growth more than 5 mm per year, active stone intervention should also be considered. Occupations like a pilot or heavy vehicle driver and patient preference are also crucial factors [2].

On the other hand, there is no established stone follow-up protocol for patients under conservative management. For radiopaque stone previously shown in CT scan scout film, regular plain radiography (Kidney–ureter–bladder view, KUB) should be used for reassessment. Ultrasound (USG) of the urinary system can be used for radiolucent stones. However, a non-contrast CT scan will occasionally be needed especially for further anatomical evaluation and surgical planning. Certainly, we also need to monitor the clinical symptom of patients, including pain, haematuria or urinary tract infection during follow-up to see if active treatment is indicated.

C. W. H. Mak
SH Ho Urology Centre, The Chinese University of Hong Kong, Hong Kong, People's Republic of China

A. C.F. Ng (✉)
Department of Surgery, Chinese University of Hong Kong, Hong Kong, Hong Kong
e-mail: ngcf@surgery.cuhk.edu.hk

A. C.F. Ng et al. (eds.), *Practical Management of Urinary Stone*,
https://doi.org/10.1007/978-981-16-4193-0_21

21.2 Pharmacological Treatment

21.2.1 Medical Expulsive Therapy (MET)

MET is referred to the use of alpha-blocker, calcium-channel inhibitor or phosphodiesterase type 5 inhibitor (PDE5I) for ureteric stone expulsion by smooth muscle relaxation in the ureter. It should only be considered if the patient has no urgent need for urinary system drainage. Once the patient develops renal deterioration, infection or refractory pain, another approach should be applied.

The use of MET has been a controversial issue over the past decade. In the randomised controlled trial "SUSPEND" in 2015, there showed no difference in stone-free rate (SFR) for Tamsulosin (81%), Nifedipine (80%) and placebo group (80%) but did show a significant trend of benefit towards larger distal ureteric stone [3]. A meta-analysis by Hollingsworth et al. suggested a 57% higher chance of stone passage for larger stone, which is independent of the stone location [4]. EAU 2020 guideline suggested MET seems to be efficacious in treating patients with ureteric stones who are amenable to conservative management and the greatest benefit might be among those with >5 mm distal ureteric stone [2].

For post ESWL cases, Zhu et al. reported MET has a 20% increase in SFR [5] and Lamb et al. reported it can relieve ureteric stent-related symptoms [6]. Common side effects of alpha-blockers include dizziness and hypotension. In patients with prior cardiac condition, use of PDE5I should be cautious and medical assessment before usage is suggested.

21.2.2 Oral Chemolysis

With prior stone analysis showing uric acid stone, oral chemolysis can be considered. Urine pH and CT characteristics like the Hounsfield unit will also provide extra information. Patients will need self-adjustment of the alkaline citrate dosage, for example, potassium citrate or sodium bicarbonate, to achieve the urine pH of 7.0–7.2 measured with urine test stripe. Oral chemolysis is more effective at a higher urine pH. However, this may promote the formation of calcium phosphate stones.

There is no RCT on oral chemolysis alone. However, a combination of oral chemolysis and tamsulosin will increase the frequency of spontaneous passage of distal ureteric uric acid stone >5 mm, as it was shown in an RCT [7]. Monitor the dissolution of radiolucent stone may need USG or sometimes NCCT. Side effect includes upset in the gastrointestinal system and electrolyte disturbance. Percutaneous irrigation chemolysis is rarely performed nowadays.

21.3 Surgical Treatment (Fig. 21.1)

21.3.1 Extracorporeal Shockwave Lithotripsy (ESWL)

ESWL can be used to manage ureteric stones and renal stones. However, the success has a strong correlation with the habitus of the patient, stone composition and stone location [8]. Fluoroscopy is usually applied to locate stones for targeting. However, USG can also be used for radiolucent stones. In some situations, multiple sessions of ESWL may be required. It is contraindicated in patients with uncorrected anticoagulation status, uncontrolled urinary tract infection, arterial aneurysm close to the stone, pregnancy and distal ureteric obstruction like stricture. Preoperative ureteric stenting is suggested for stone >20 mm. It is controversial for fertile women undergoing ESWL, especially for distal ureteric stone as it may have a theoretical impact on fertility. For details of ESWL, please refer to Chap. 20.

21.3.2 Ureteroscopic Lithotripsy (URSL)/Retrograde Intra-renal Surgery (RIRS)

URSL is a relatively safe operation with mostly minor complications. Serious complication like ureteric avulsion is less than 0.5% [9, 10]. With the technical improvement, stone surgeries with larger stones can now be performed by RIRS. A meta-analysis in 2015 suggested the SFR for renal stone

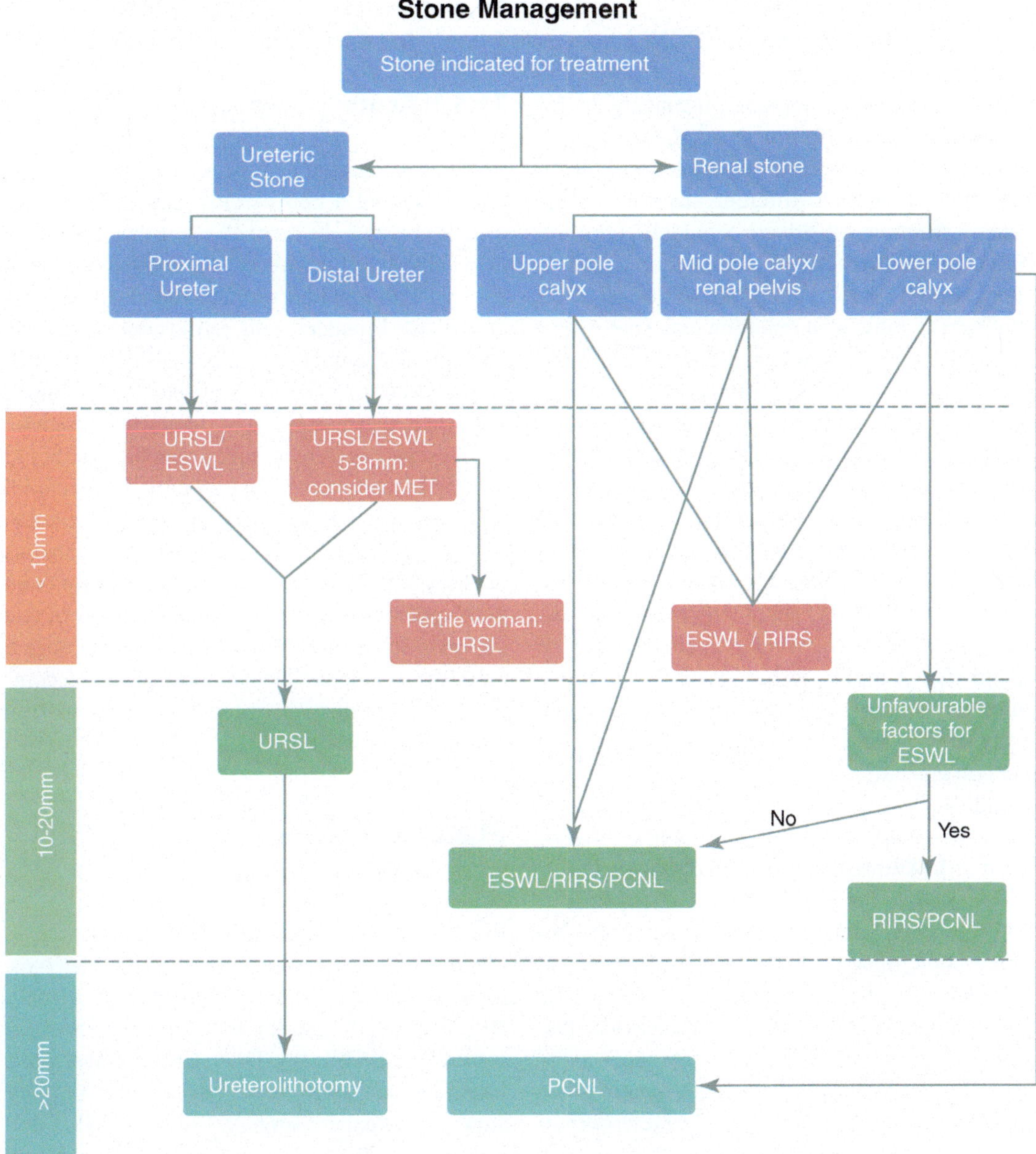

Fig. 21.1 Flowchart for stone management according to size and location

>20 mm by RIRS could be up to 91% with 1.45 procedures [11]. Rate of major complications like subscapular haematoma, ureteric perforation, steinstrasse and severe sepsis were around 4.5% [10].

General anaesthesia is preferred although most of the time it can also be performed under spinal anaesthesia. Ureteric access sheath should be used in RIRS to decrease intra-renal pressure and improve vision. Stone can be managed by dusting or fragmenting technique with a laser fibre. Larger stone fragments can be retrieved by endoscopic basket or forceps. Routine ureteric stenting is not necessary unless in situations with increased risk of complication, like bleeding, residual stones, ureteric injury or sepsis. Further information related to ureteroscopy could be referred to in previous chapters on this topic.

21.4 Percutaneous Nephrolithotomy (PCNL)

PCNL remained the standard management for large renal stones>20 mm or staghorn stone. It may also be considered in lower pole stone >10 mm. Nowadays different sizes of access sheaths from Fr 18–30 are available for mini PCNL to standard PCNL. Fluoroscopic guided punctures are usually done but additional USG may help to reduce the radiation exposure.

In order to understand the perinephric and calyceal anatomy so as to prevent visceral injury, a pre-operative CT scan is suggested. Totally tubeless PCNL is possible but the need for nephrostomy or ureteric stenting should be decided by a surgeon, depends on the presence of residual stone, need for second-look procedure, risk of sepsis or ureteric obstruction and intraoperative bleeding condition. In patient with anti-coagulant, correction of the anticoagulation should be done before the operation. When there is an active untreated urinary tract infection or potential malignant renal tumour, PCNL is contraindicated.

21.5 Laparoscopy/Laparotomy

With the improvement of endourology, open or laparoscopic stone surgery is not common nowadays. Even for large renal stones, PCNL is the first-line treatment. However, in the case of history of unsuccessful endoscopic treatment, laparoscopic surgery may be indicated. In cases with large ureteric stones, laparoscopic ureterolithotomy will be indicated as it can prevent prolonged endoscopic surgery.

Occasionally, for patients with poorly functioned kidneys secondary to staghorn stone or obstructing stones, nephrectomy might be indicated in symptomatic patients or for prevention of future complications.

21.6 Special Considerations for Choice of Treatment

21.6.1 Acute Management

Renal colic management is essential in stone disease. Usage of a non-steroidal anti-inflammatory drug is proven to be more effective than opioids in pain control [12]. However, it is contraindicated in patients with renal impairment and also caution is needed for a patient with cardiovascular risk. In patients with intractable pain, the obstructed urinary system should be drained. Active stone removal is also acceptable in cases without sepsis.

Urosepsis is an emergency. Antibiotics should be started early according to previous bacterial culture results. Emergency urinary decompression should be performed either by percutaneous nephrostomy or ureteric stent. So far, there is no good quality study to prove the superiority of one option over the other. In cases with anuria, severe acidosis or hyperkalaemia, emergency decompression, with or without renal replacement therapy, is also indicated.

21.6.2 Stone Factors: Stone Composition

Brushite, calcium oxalate monohydrate and cystine stones are particular hard stones that have high density in CT scans (Hounsfield unit >1000). It is a predictive factor for significant residual stones after ESWL [8]. These large residual stone fragments may have a negative impact on later stone clearance surgery like PCNL and RIRS. Therefore, endourological management should be considered early as an alternative.

Matrix stone is predominately composed of glucosamines and organic proteins. It is different to other crystalline stones as they are usually ESWL resistant due to the soft composition. PCNL is more effective in cases with large matrix stones.

Uric acid stones are usually homogenously low-density stones in CT scans. This is a favourable factor to predict successful ESWL stone fragmentation. However, most of these stones are radiolucent and therefore imposed difficulties in stone localisation on fluoroscopy during ESWL.

21.7 Stone Factors: Location

21.7.1 Upper/Middle Calyces and Renal Pelvis

ESWL is a good choice for stone <20 mm. It has a good SFR but multiple sessions may be required. RIRS is another good choice as the time from diagnosis to stone clearance is shorter. For larger stones>20 mm, PCNL should be the first-line treatment. ESWL in a patient with large stones may result in steinstrasses. Therefore, preoperative ureteric stenting is suggested. RIRS with a large stone load will be difficult and inefficient. It may cause prolonged operation time, thus increasing the risk of sepsis. However, RIRS may be considered in patients with contraindication for PCNL.

21.7.2 Lower Pole

Stone clearance is more difficult to be achieved with ESWL when there are unfavourable factors for ESWL. Anatomically, steep infundibular-pelvic angle, long calyx and narrow infundibulum will impair the efficacy of ESWL. Also, in obese patients with long skin to stone or shock wave-resistant stone like calcium oxalate monohydrate, brushite or cystine stone, ESWL may be unfavourable.

Moreover, residual stones in calyx may cause recurrent stone formation. If these factors present, RIRS will be a reasonable alternative. Studies showed RIRS had a comparable SFR with ESWL [11, 13, 14], although staged procedures were frequently required in both approaches. PCNL is usually for larger stones (> 20 mm) but with increased invasiveness of operation.

21.7.3 Ureter

Spontaneous ureteric stone (< 4 mm) passage is estimated at 95% within 40 days [14]. However, MET is a possible choice of management especially for distal ureteric stone sized 5-8 mm without significant symptoms or complications [2, 3].

According to the EAU/AUA collaborative guideline project on ureteric stone [15], URSL has a higher SFR for distal ureteric stone than ESWL (94% vs 74%). For proximal ureteric stone <10 mm, ESWL is superior than URSL (SFR: 90% vs 80%). However, for proximal ureteric stone >10 mm, URSL is a better choice (SFR of ESWL: 68% vs URSL 79%).

Overall, URSL is more efficient in larger ureteric stones and obese patients. It has higher SFR in 4 weeks but comparable SFR with ESWL in 3 months [16]. However, it is associated with a higher complication rate, more auxiliary procedures (including stenting and stent removal) and longer hospitalisation. In patients with bleeding disorder or anticoagulation, URSL may be performed with a smaller risk of bleeding than ESWL.

Steinstrasse is referred to as the accumulation of stone fragments in the ureter and resulted as a "street of stones". It happened in 4–7% of cases after ESWL, especially in patients with a large stone load [17]. MET can still be used in asymptomatic cases. Endourology and ESWL are both effective in this situation [18, 19]. However, when there is sepsis, urinary drainage should be performed first before the management of stone, preferably by percutaneous nephrostomy as suggested in the EAU guideline [2].

21.7.4 Patient Factor: Anatomical Consideration

Patients with abnormal urinary tract anatomy are predisposed to stone formation due to urine stasis, abnormal excretory function of urinary tract or abnormal absorption from the gastrointestinal tract. Common examples are patients with urinary diversion by ileal conduit or neobladder, horseshoe kidney, ureteric stricture, duplex urinary system, caliceal diverticulum and renal transplant. The aforementioned principles should be considered together with individual anatomical consideration. Details will be discussed in Chaps. 23 and 25.

21.8 Patient Factor: Pregnancy

Conservative management should be used in pregnant ladies with asymptomatic renal stones as stones treatment may impose potential risks to the foetus, like radiation and drug potential teratogenicity.

USG urinary system remained the first-line investigation due to the safety profile of USG. Moreover, Magnetic resonance imaging (MR Urogram) or low dose NCCT is a potential choice of investigation after discussion with patients. If there are complications like ureteric obstruction, intractable symptoms and sepsis, urinary drainage is suggested either by percutaneous nephrostomy or ureteral stenting. The decision of management should be carefully made with adequate communication among patient, family, obstetrician and urologist.

However, rapid encrustation of the stent or nephrostomy tube is anticipated. Thus, early revision every 4–6 weeks is needed and it should be explained to patients prior to the drainage. In order to reduce the number of revisions, URSL can be safely performed after the second trimester under an experienced hand [20]. However, ESWL remained an absolute contraindication in pregnant ladies. Further discussion on pregnant ladies will be in Chap. 26.

21.9 Patient Factor: Obesity

It is suggested that obesity is associated with a greater risk of renal stone formation [21]. Lifestyle modification should be advocated. Moreover, we will need special consideration for stone management in these patients. During ESWL, targeting stone will be difficult if the skin-to-stone distance (SSD) is large. Also, there was a study suggesting patients with SSD > 10 cm had a higher failure rate for stone clearance [22].

For endourology, URSL remained a safe option for obese patients with BMI > 30 kg/m^2 with a similar SFR and complication rate. However, the complication rate doubles (17%) in morbidly obese patients with BMI > 35 kg/m^2 [23]. For PCNL, preparation of an extra-long instrument is necessary and pre-op CT scan may provide extra information. For patients with poor lung function, supine PCNL may be more favourable than the conventional prone approach.

21.10 Patient Factor: Medical history

It is important that we should consider the premorbid of patients. It is not uncommon that our patient is on multiple medical therapies including anti-coagulant and immunosuppressant. Surgical management should be tailor-made for these patients.

In general, ESWL, PCNL, laparoscopic and open surgery are considered as high-risk bleeding procedures. Prior anticoagulation status should be corrected before performing these procedures. Also, anaesthetic risk is a crucial factor. In patients with high risk for general anaesthesia, PCNL and RIRS may be contraindicated. URSL can be done under spinal anaesthesia or even local anaesthesia for distal ureteric stones in female patients. For patients with ultra-high risk for all anaesthesia, ESWL, long-term ureteric stent or percutaneous nephrostomy and conservative management should be the choice of management. Further discussion will be in Chap. 24.

21.11 Patient Factor: Paediatric Patient

The true incidence of nephrolithiasis in paediatric patients is unclear. All paediatric patients will need metabolic workup as they may have a high risk of recurrence. According to the EAU guideline, expectant management should be adopted for asymptomatic lower pole non-struvite, non-cystine renal stone <7 mm as stone passage may be observed. Otherwise, treatment is indicated for stone located in other calyces and ureter. ESWL is the first-line treatment for most ureteric stones with a high SFR of 70–90% [24]. URSL and RIRS are possible for paediatric patients. Indication for PCNL is also similar to adult. For detailed discussion, please refer to Chap. 26.

21.12 Patient Factor: Recurrent Stone Former

In patients with recurrent stone formation, risk factors should be identified. For example, positive family history, hyperparathyroidism, nephrocalcinosis, abnormal GI tract affecting fat absorption, Genetic diseases like cystinuria, primary oxaluria, type 1 renal tubular acidosis and abnormal urinary tract anatomy mentioned before. Full metabolic workup should be performed including 24-hour urine sampling, stone analysis if possible. Specific pharmacological prevention can be considered in cases with a specific identifiable risk factor. However, in general, we should suggest patients have >2.5 L of daily fluid intake. Moreover, a balanced diet with plenty of vegetables and fibre, reduction in carbonated drink intake, normal calcium intake of 1.2 g/day, limited animal protein intake, weight reduction in obese patients may also prevent stone formation.

References

1. Burgher A, et al. Progression of nephrolithiasis: long-term outcomes with observation of asymptomatic calculi. J Endourol. 2004;18:534.
2. European Association of Urology guideline 2020 on Urolithiasis. https://uroweb.org/guideline/urolithiasis/
3. Pickard R, et al. Medical expulsive therapy in adults with ureteric colic: a multicentre, randomised, placebo-controlled trial. Lancet. 2015;386:341–9.
4. Hollingsworth JM, et al. Alpha blockers for treatment of ureteric stones: systematic review and meta-analysis. BMJ. 2016;355:i6112.
5. Zhu Y, et al. Alpha-blockers to assist stone clearance after extracorporeal shock wave lithotripsy: a meta-analysis. BJU Int. 2010 Jul;106(2):256–61.
6. Lamb AD, et al. Meta-analysis showing the beneficial effect of α-blockers on ureteric stent discomfort. BJU Int. 2011 Dec;108(11):1894–902.
7. El-Gamal O, et al. Role of combined use of potassium citrate and tamsulosin in the management of uric acid distal ureteral calculi. Urol Res. 2012;40:219.
8. El-Nahas AR, et al. A prospective multivariate analysis of factors predicting stone disintegration by extracorporeal shock wave lithotripsy: the value of high-resolution noncontrast computed tomography. Eur Urol. 2007;51:1688.
9. Geavlete P, et al. Complications of 2735 retrograde semirigid ureteroscopy procedures: a single-center experience. J Endourol. 2006;20:179.
10. Castro EP, et al. Differences in ureteroscopic stone treatment and outcomes for distal, mid-, proximal, or multiple ureteral locations: the Clinical Research Office of the Endourological Society ureteroscopy global study. Eur Urol. 2014;66:102.
11. Geraghty R, et al. Evidence for Ureterorenoscopy and Laser Fragmentation (URSL) for large renal stones in the modern era. Curr Urol Rep. 2015;16:54.
12. Pathan SA, et al. A systematic review and meta-analysis comparing the efficacy of nonsteroidal anti-inflammatory drugs, opioids, and paracetamol in the treatment of acute renal colic. Eur Urol. 2018; 73:583.
13. Srisubat A, et al. Extracorporeal shock wave lithotripsy (ESWL) versus percutaneous nephrolithotomy (PCNL) or retrograde intrarenal surgery (RIRS) for kidney stones. Cochrane Database Syst Rev. 2014;11:CD007044.
14. Pearle M, et al. Prospective, randomized trial comparing shock wave lithotripsy and ureteroscopy for lower pole caliceal calculi 1 cm or less. J Urol. 2005;173:2005.
15. Preminger G, et al. 2007 Guideline for the management of ureteral calculi. Eur Urol. 2007;52:1610.
16. Drake T, et al. What are the benefits and harms of ureteroscopy compared with shock-wave lithotripsy in the treatment of upper ureteral stones? A systematic review. Eur Urol. 2017;72:772.
17. Ather MH, et al. Does ureteral stenting prior to shock wave lithotripsy influence the need for intervention in steinstrasse and related complications? Urol Int. 2009;83:222.
18. Sayed MA, et al. Steinstrasse after extracorporeal shockwave lithotripsy: aetiology, prevention and management. BJU Int. 2001;88:675.

19. Rabbani SM, et al. Treatment of steinstrasse by transureteral lithotripsy. Urol J. 2008;5:89.
20. Ishii H, et al. Current status of ureteroscopy for stone disease in pregnancy. Urolithiasis. 2014;42:1.
21. Taylor EN, et al. Obesity, weight gain, and the risk of kidney stones. JAMA. 2005;293:455–62.
22. Gyan P, et al. Shock wave lithotripsy success determined by skin-to-stone distance on computed tomography. J Urol. 2005 Nov;66(5):941–4.
23. Ishii, et al. Outcomes of Systematic Review of Ureteroscopy for Stone Disease in the Obese and Morbidly Obese Population. J Endourol. 2016;30:135.
24. Jee JY, et al. Efficacy of extracorporeal shock wave lithotripsy in pediatric and adolescent urolithiasis. Korean J Urol. 2013;54:865.

22 Challenging Intrarenal Anatomy

Anthony C.F. Ng and Lukman Hakim

22.1 Introduction

While almost everyone has two kidneys, the inner structure of every kidney is not the same. This makes the planning of stone treatment for each patient need to be individualized. Embryologically, while the kidney parenchyma (the metanephric kidney) is developed from the nephrogenic cord (intermediate mesoderm), ureteric bud grows from mesonephric duct. The ureteric bud will grow toward the mesoderm. During the development, the ureteric bud will undergo a series of branching and from the collecting system, including the ureter, the renal pelvis, and calyces. This complicated process resulted in great variation in the collecting system of kidneys, including duplicated system, bifid renal pelvis, as well as variation in caliceal anatomy in individual patients.

22.1.1 Duplicated Urinary System

Duplicated urinary system, or duplex system, is a congenital abnormality of kidney, with an incidence of 1–3%. The underlying pathology is due to abnormal development of ureteric bud during foetal stage. If the bud has early branching, it will result in partial duplex or bifid system, depending on the level of joining of the renal pelvis or ureter. However, if there are two ureteric buds developed in the foetus, then two separate ureters will form, i.e. complete duplex system. Most of the cases, the patients are asymptomatic. However, some of them may also develop complication, including stone formation due to the abnormal anatomy. Also, as in other urinary system, stone could also be formed in the system and some precautions need to be considered during the management of them.

22.1.1.1 Ureterocele

Ureterocele occurs in around 0.1–0.2% patients and is more common in patient with complete duplex system, in which the upper moiety is being affected [1]. Due to the obstruction at the ureteric opening, there is a cystic dilatation of the lower end of the ureter and resulted in the ureterocele. There are subtyping of ureterocele basing on the extend of the ureterocele and also its involvement to the surrounding structure, which will be beyond the discussion here [1]. The obstruction and stasis inside the ureterocele may lead to the formation of stone (Fig. 22.1).

For simple intravesical ureterocele with stone, endoscopic management will be the first line

A. C.F. Ng
Department of Surgery,
Chinese University of Hong Kong,
Hong Kong, Hong Kong

L. Hakim (✉)
Department of Urology, Faculty of Medicine/Rumah Sakit Universitas Airlangga Teaching Hospital,
Universitas Airlangga, Surabaya, Indonesia
e-mail: lukman-h@fk.unair.ac.id

A. C.F. Ng et al. (eds.), *Practical Management of Urinary Stone*,
https://doi.org/10.1007/978-981-16-4193-0_22

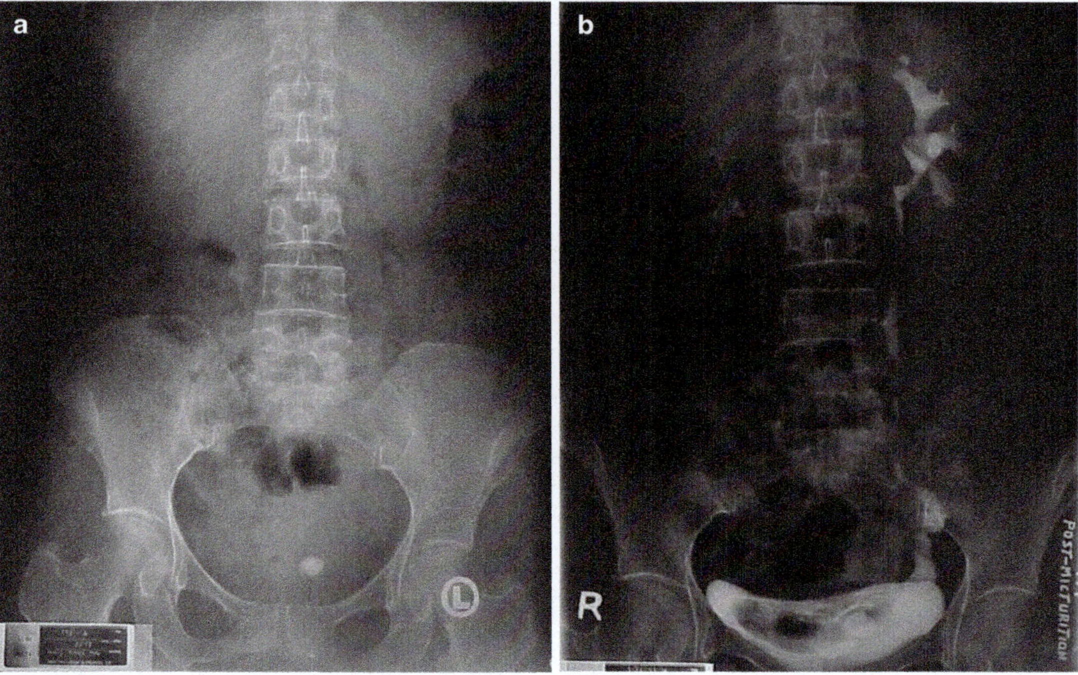

Fig. 22.1 Stone in ureterocele. (**a**) Plain film, (**b**) Post-micturation film

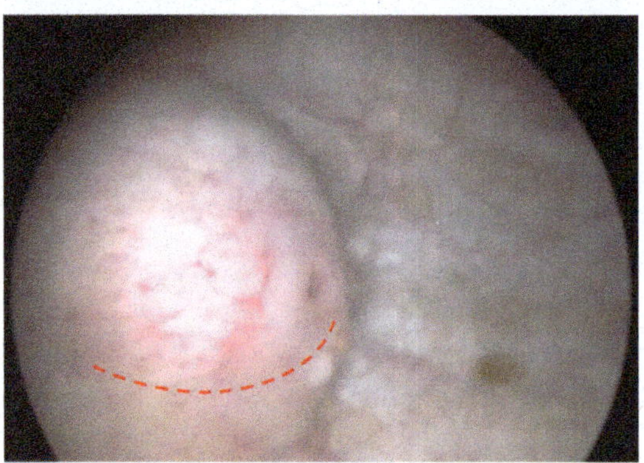

Fig. 22.2 Incision for ureterocele

management. Resection of the enterocele may result in reflux. Therefore, endoscopic transverse incision, either by point electrode or Holmium laser, at the lower level of the ureterocele will help to create a new opening for the relief of obstruction (Fig. 22.2). The upper lip of the new incised opening will also act as a flap to decrease reflux. The stone could then be managed by usual endoscopic approach.

22.1.1.2 Special Precautions in Managing Patients with Duplicated System

Due to the increase risk of vesicoureteric reflux (usually to the lower moiety) and also obstruction (usually to the upper moiety), stone formation is not uncommon in duplicated system. The basic management is similar to other stone disease. However, some special precautions might need to be considered during the planning of treatment.

For small renal stone, SWL could be used as in other situations. However, we need to exclude the possibility of distal obstruction, in particular in patients with dilated ureter on imaging. For patients with an obstructed upper moiety, the lower moiety might be displaced more inferiorly ("drooping lily sign") which might make the drainage of the lower pole stone fragment more difficult and so SWL might not be the preferred choice of treatment.

As in other stone patients, for patients planned for PCNL, a good preoperative imaging is essential for planning of access. Since the upper and lower moieties might not be communicate, even in simple bifid system, and so separate punctures might be needed for patients with stones in different part of the kidney.

When we considering ureteroscopic management or even for ureteric catheter insertion, the Weigert–Meyer rule should be remembered. Due to the congenital abnormality in development, the ureteric orifice of the upper moiety in complete duplicated system is usually located more distal and medial to the one from lower moiety. In female, sometime the ureteric orifice could even go down to urethra, vagina, Gartner's duct, etc., i.e. ectopic ureter. For patient with incomplete duplicated system, care must be taken to cannulate the correct limb at the junction of the ureter of the stone located moiety. Sometimes, the limb might be narrower, and the insertion of ureteric access sheath need to be gentle or may just keep the sheath at the common stem of the ureter. Otherwise, the management of the stone is similar as in other endoscopic treatment.

22.1.2 Lower Pole Caliceal Anatomy and Stone

The observation of the poorer treatment outcome for stones in lower renal calices (LC) had led to studies on the effect of caliceal anatomy on SWL [2]. The impressive cadaveric work of Sampaio had shown there was great variation in the distribution of calices in the lower pole, as well as different infundibular diameter and angle [3]. Since then, many reports on different anatomical factors and their effects had been published [4]. In simple term, the more acute the infundibular angle, the longer and narrower the infundibulum, the poorer the treatment result. The underlying mechanism is probably partly related to the gravitational effect and also the difficulty of the drainage of the caliceal content. Therefore, many adjuvant therapies such as inversion, hydration, and forced diuresis had been proposed to improve the drainage of LC after SWL [5].

Many studies had also been done to compare the outcomes of different treatment modalities for lower caliceal stones. From a network meta-analysis, for stone <20 mm, PCNL has the best treatment efficacy, followed by ureteroscopy, then SWL with adjuvant therapy and then SWL alone [5]. However, adverse effects also followed the same order [5]. Therefore, when deciding treatment for patients, we need to get a balance between efficacy and adverse effects.

Based on all the data, both European Association of Urology (EAU) and American Urological Association (AUA) put LC stone (or Lower pole stone, LP) as one of the parameters in the planning of treatment for patients. In EAU guideline, for intermediate size lower caliceal stone (10–20 mm), if there are unfavourable factors (including poor LC anatomy, long skin to stone distance, shockwave resistant stones) for SWL, RIRS would be the first recommended treatment [6]. For AUA guideline, for LP stone greater than 10 mm, PCNL will be the choice of treatment. For those stone less than 10 mm, if there are any unfavourable factors, such as HU > 1000, skin-to-stone distance >10 cm, or other comorbidities, RIRS should be recommended [7].

The applications of all treatment modalities basically follow the general principles. However, when using RIRS for LC stone, it was recommended to reposition the stone into upper calices or renal pelvis to minimize excessive bending of the ureteroscope during the procedure. Also, it will help to avoid damages in the endoscope during the insertion of laser fibre or other endoscopic accessory instruments.

22.1.3 Caliceal Diverticulum

Caliceal diverticulum (CD) is an out-pocket occurred in calyces. The radiographic incidence ranged from 0.2% to 0.5% and is more common in the upper and middle calyces. It is believed to be a congenital abnormality in the renal parenchyma. CD is usually non-secretory and lined by urothelium with communication ("neck") to the main collecting system. Urine could reflux into the system. Due to the stasis inside, around one to two quarters of CD will harbour stone inside.

While the stones inside CD are usually not big in size, the relative narrowed neck might hinder the passage of stone fragment after SWL. Therefore, the treatment outcomes by SWL were not very satisfactory [8].

PCNL is another option for treatment, as most of the system is dilated and so puncturing the system by imaging guidance (by ultrasound or fluoroscopy using the stone as target) is possible. However, the small space inside the system might lead to some difficulty in stabilizing the guidewire during dilatation. The Amplatz working sheath might also not anchoring well in CD, due to thinner surrounding cortex. Stone clearance is as usual as in other PCNL. After stone treatment, it would be better to also improve the CD drainage, or stone recurrence might occur. If the diverticular neck could be identified, it could be cannulated with guidewire and then subsequently dilatated. However, if the opening is not able to locate, then a neo-infundibulum might need to be created by direct puncturing through the CD toward the renal collecting system. After confirming the puncture, and then guidewire, is in position, the track will then be gently dilated up.

CD stone could also be managed by RIRS approach. The procedure will be done as in usual RIRS. If the opening of the CD could be identified easily, it could then be dilated by balloon or incised by Holmium laser. For cases with small opening that is not readily identified, we could instil the collecting system with methylene blue stained saline. With the whole system filled with the blue stained saline, it will expect some of this will also flow into the CD. Then the collecting system is flushed with clear saline. The retained blue dye in CD will slowly leaking out and allow us to locate the position of the opening of the CD (the "Blue Spritz" test) [9]. After the opening was identified and enlarged, the stone could be easily seen and tackled as usual. At the end of the procedure, a double-J stent could be placed across the dilated CD neck to avoid the closing up of the neck again.

While laparoscopic approach has also been reported, it would be less likely performed in light of the advancement in current endoscopic technique.

References

1. Shokeir AA, Nijman RJ. Ureterocele: an ongoing challenge in infancy and childhood. BJU Int. 2002 Nov;90(8):777–83.
2. Lingeman JE, Siegel YI, Steele B, Nyhuis AW, Woods JR. Management of lower pole nephrolithiasis: a critical analysis. J Urol. 1994 Mar;151(3):663–7.
3. Sampaio FJB, Aragao AHM. Inferior pole collecting system anatomy: its probable role in extracorporeal shock wave lithotripsy. J Urol. 1992;147:322–4.
4. Ng CF, Wong A, Tolley DA. A single-center experience of the usefulness of caliceal-pelvic height in three different lithotripters. J Endourol. 2008 Jul;22(7):1409–15.
5. Lee SW, Chaiyakunapruk N, Chong HY, Liong ML. Comparative effectiveness and safety of various treatment procedures for lower pole renal calculi: a systematic review and network meta-analysis. BJU Int. 2015 Aug;116(2):252–64.
6. EAU guideline.
7. AUA guideline.
8. Turna B, Raza A, Moussa S, Smith G, Tolley DA. Management of calyceal diverticular stones with extracorporeal shock wave lithotripsy and percutaneous nephrolithotomy: long-term outcome. BJU Int. 2007 Jul;100(1):151–6.
9. Chong TW, Bui MH, Fuchs GJ. Calyceal diverticula. Ureteroscopic management. Urol Clin North Am. 2000;27:647–54.

Patients with Special Medical Condition

23

Shuji Isotani

Abstract

The patient who is undergoing surgical treatment for urolithiasis is not always in the same condition; sometimes they are in special condition such as under anticoagulant therapy, chronic urinary infection, or anomaly anatomy. These conditions make challenges for the urologists to perform the surgical treatment. The purpose of this chapter is to summarize the knowledge of the urolithiasis treatment in special condition patients from the clinical point of view. In this chapter, we begin with the situation of the patients who have anticoagulant therapy, then we will discuss the UTI, risk factors of UTI, and antibiotic prophylaxis to prevent postoperative UTI. Then we also summarize the surgical management in the patients who have renal transplantation.

Keywords

Anticoagulant therapy and antiplatelet therapy · Urinary tract infection · Renal transplantation · Antibiotic prophylaxis

S. Isotani (✉)
Department of Urology, Juntendo University, Tokyo, Japan
e-mail: s-isotani@juntendo.ac.jp

23.1 Introduction

Recently, the development of surgical treatment modalities for urolithiasis seems to have changed to be safer and more efficient. For example, in this decade ureteroscopy (URS) have presently become the most beneficial therapeutic option for most of stone with the size and location of kidney stone except the staghorn stone, and the urologist should consider this new treatment. We have many literatures which were published to confirm the effectiveness and safety of URS in the treatment of renal stone. However, the patient is not in the same condition always, sometimes they are in special conditions such as under anticoagulant therapy, chronic urinary infection, or elder patient, these conditions make challenges to the urologist. The purpose of this chapter is to summarize the knowledge of the urolithiasis treatment in special condition patients from the clinical point of view. In this chapter, we begin with the situation of the patients who have anticoagulant therapy, then we will discuss the UTI and how to prevent the UTI by antibiotic prophylaxis.

23.2 Anticoagulant Therapy and Antiplatelet Therapy

There is an increasing population of cardiovascular diseases and an increasing incidence of receiving anticoagulant or antiplatelet therapy. Many of

A. C.F. Ng et al. (eds.), *Practical Management of Urinary Stone*,
https://doi.org/10.1007/978-981-16-4193-0_23

those patients are the high-risk patients who are undergoing anticoagulant therapy by oral warfarin for chronic atrial fibrillation, mechanical heart valve, or prior history of venous thromboembolism on or oral antiplatelet for the patient who suffers the arterial ischemic disorders including cerebrovascular occlusive disease, coronary artery disease, and occlusive peripheral arterial disease [1]. In general, the prior studies indicated the safety and efficacy of discontinuation of warfarin, and replace it as "bridging" therapy by administration of intravenous (IV) heparin or low-molecular-weight heparin for the patient who may have invasive treatment [1].

Today, many urologists have to face more patients who have some vascular-related comorbidities managed by oral anticoagulant or antiplatelet therapy drugs. The perioperative management of patients who receive anticoagulant or antiplatelet therapy is sometimes controversial because the management needs to be careful with maintaining the balance between increased risk of bleeding and thromboembolic events [2–7]. In 2014, AUA (American Urological Association) and ICUD (International Consultation on Urological Disease) construct consensus-based qualitative recommendations based on a systematic literature review [6]. According to AUA recommendation, the anticoagulant or antiplatelet therapy agents should be discontinued and/or reversed before shock wave lithotripsy (SWL). The timing of stopping and resuming the oral anticoagulant or antiplatelet therapy should be decided according to the risks of thrombotic complications and bleeding. Also, about ureteroscopy (URS), the oral anticoagulant or antiplatelet therapy can continue during URS treatment for urolithiasis. For the percutaneous nephrolithotomy (PCNL) for urolithiasis, the oral anticoagulant or antiplatelet therapy medications should be discontinued [6].

23.2.1 Shockwave Lithotripsy (SWL)

Classically, the pregnancy and bleeding diathesis have been two absolute contraindications for SWL. The reason is that the use of anticoagulant therapy or antiplatelet therapy has a high risk of hemorrhagic complications, such as serious postoperative peri-renal hematomas and renal hemorrhage, leading to the protracted postoperative course and possibly requiring drastic measures, such as nephrectomy or renal embolization [8]. Actuary, severe life-threatening complications have been reported in patients who underwent SWL with anticoagulant therapy or antiplatelet therapy [9]. While many studies assessed the SWL complications rates with pathological bleeding diathesis, anticoagulant therapy, or antiplatelet therapy, they were in general small-scaled, retrospective, non-standardized, and of low quality. Despite, in patients with bleeding tendency, URS is usually recommended, SWL is still a possible treatment option instead of being disregarded as an absolute contraindication.

Ideally, SWL should be postponed 6–12 months for the elective cases and only emergent procedures can be considered while maintaining limited patients such as on low-dose antiplatelet agents. Ureteroscopy and laser lithotripsy, while patients are on anticoagulation therapy, remain the safest modalities when treatment need could not be postponed [8]. In general, for the low-risk patients requiring SWL, it is performed to withhold the antiplatelet agents perioperatively (maximum 7 days) after consultation with the prescribing cardiologist and informing patients of risks of hemorrhage and thrombotic events. There is one report that substitution antiplatelet agents by unfractionated heparin; however, it is not recommended because the heparin does not have the completely same preventive effects as antiplatelet agents.

Intermediate- and high-risk patients should be managed individually with a high level of caution. In patients with higher medical risk, it was recommended that unfractionated heparin or low molecular weight heparin was administered and stopped the evening before treatment until stone therapy was completed. Data had shown that there was no significant reduction in hemoglobin, or thromboembolic or hemorrhagic complications in patients managed by this approach [10, 11]. Moreover, the surgeon needs to pay attention to the resumption of anticoagulants, because there were case reports of massive hemorrhage 5 days after shock wave lithotripsy [6].

23.2.2 Endoscopic Surgery (URS)

The antiplatelet agents or anticoagulation therapy was used to be stopped before the endoscopic surgery (URS); however, retrospective reports demonstrated no increase in complications. Therefore, the current AUA/ICUD guidelines state that anticoagulant and antiplatelet therapy during the perioperative period for USR is safe [6]. On the other hand, Daels et al. reported that the URS outcomes among about 12,000 patients worldwide and showed that postoperative bleeding was significantly higher in patients on the antiplatelet agents or anticoagulation therapy compared to those who were not (1.1% vs 0.4%, $P < 0.01$) [5]. Also, Westerman et al. demonstrated that the continuation or temporary alternation (bridging) of anticoagulation sometimes increases the risk of bleeding related to the URS. Therefore, the risks and benefits of proceeding with URS on anticoagulation must be considered carefully. If in the case of severe bleeding from the ureter during operation, placement of a ureteral dilating balloon is useful for making tamponade to stop the bleeding until further intervention. Depending on the damaged levels of the ureter, further treatment options may consist of urgent embolization, endovascular repair, or open surgery.

23.2.3 Percutaneous Nephrolithotomy (PCNL)

According to AUA and ICUD recommendations, oral anticoagulant or antiplatelet therapy medications should be discontinued before PCNL for urolithiasis. In 2012, the CROES (Clinical Research Office of the Endourological Society) Percutaneous Nephrolithotomy Global Study database examined the complications of PCNL in patients on anticoagulant therapy or antiplatelet therapy. It was a large-scale prospective study characterizing risk factors for complications using consecutive patients [12]. They reported that 310 patients in the 5724 patients who underwent anticoagulant medication were associated with a slight increase in the mean modified Clavien–Dindo complication grade. Nevertheless, the use of anticoagulant medications did not increase the risk of complications on multivariate regression analysis. Thus, the largest clinical CROES experience was concluded that the planned discontinuation of anticoagulant therapy and antiplatelet therapy 10 days before the operation and restarting it after 5 days of operation is safe and effective, and the majority of complications in patients on anticoagulant therapy and antiplatelet therapy treated with percutaneous nephrolithotomy are minor. However, this study does not specifically show the results of thromboembolic complications.

In the conclusion, today, Shockwave lithotripsy (SWL) and percutaneous nephrolithotomy (PCNL) are contraindicated in patients who have antiplatelet or anticoagulant treatment, and correction of coagulopathy is recommended before endoscopic procedures (URS) [6]. However, it was suggested that the continuation or bridging of antiplatelet and anticoagulant treatment may increase the risk of perioperative bleeding, and also the replacement of low molecular weight heparin may be able to develop the organ or life-threatening clots [4]. No evidence was shown that anticoagulants are safe to be continued during the stone surgery, and guidelines would recommend consulting an internist and commence bridging therapy [7]. Therefore, we need to consider the balance of the risk of thromboembolic events with that of bleeding complications to know whether to withhold low-dose antiplatelet before the procedure.

23.3 Urinary Tract Infection

23.3.1 Risk Factors

The most common complication of urolithiasis surgery is postoperative urinary tract infection (UTI). Even the reported incidence of postoperative UTI is relatively low from 3 to 5%. However, it could lead to prolonged hospital stay, increased medical costs, unplanned intensive care unit admission, etc. The development of systemic inflammatory response syndrome (SIRS) or systemic sepsis might even be fatal events [13–15]. Therefore, factors associated with the UTI following stone surgery need to be assessed before surgery [2]. The potential mechanism of UTI after urolithiasis surgery involves the migration of bacteria or bacterial products into the bloodstream by elevated intrarenal pressure by the irrigation during endoscopic procedures, and also open up of blood vessels from renal parenchyma during PCNL. In general, the reported risk factors associated with UTI after stone surgical management included female gender, indwelling catheters, urinary diversion, paraplegia, infectious stones, anatomic anomalies, urinary tract obstruction, another infection at other body parts at the time of surgery, significant renal or liver dysfunction, long hospital stay, immunosuppressive status, diabetes mellitus, obesity, chemotherapy or chronic corticosteroid use, voiding dysfunction, and old age [16–21].

For the URS procedure, in 2020, Sun et al. conducted a systematic review and meta-analysis of the existing literature to indicate the risk factors of the infectious complications following URS [2]. From their investigation, preoperative positive urine culture was the most significant risk factor (OR 2.95, $p < 0.01$) for UTI after the URS. Also, the female gender was the second significant risk factor (OR 1.95, $p < 0.01$). Diabetes mellitus (OR 1.55, $p < 0.01$), pre-and postoperative stents (OR 1.53, and OR 1.44, respectively), Extended operative time was associated with infectious complications following URS. However, old age, stone diameter, and renal dysfunction were not correlated with infectious complications.

For PCNL treatment, in 2011, Korets et al. reported the analysis of a total of 204 PCNL with 20 (9.8%) postoperative systemic inflammatory response syndrome (SIRS), including 6 (30%) requiring intensive care (ICU). They demonstrated that multiple stone burden of 10 cm or greater and multiple access tracts were significant predictors of SIRS, and they recommend collecting pelvic urine and stone cultures [22]. Other risk factors associated with post-PCNL UTI including female gender, indwelling catheters, paraplegia, urinary diversion, and voiding dysfunction [16–18]. Struvite stones or staghorn stones were also associated with a significantly high risk of UTI or urosepsis after surgery [23]. In 2017, Dr. Fan reviewed 156 UTI including 21 patients who developed septic shock after minimally invasive percutaneous nephrolithotomy (MPCNL) for upper urinary tract stones. They concluded that postoperative WBC count of less than 2.98 × 109/L, preoperative urine nitrite, and stone size were predictors independently for uroseptic shock after MPCNL [24].

23.3.2 Usage of Antibiotics

In general, for the prevention of postoperative UTI, antibiotic prophylaxis is used before the stone surgery [19, 25, 26]. The administration of the lowest dose of antimicrobials was recommended to decrease the risk of infection for minimizing the risk of drug-resistant organisms.

Current EAU guideline recommends the usage of antibiotic prophylaxis to reduce the rate of symptomatic UTI at the URS treatment as invasive stone therapy even with weak evidence, and also the administration of single-dose antibiotic prophylaxis is recommended to decrease the rate of clinical urinary infection following PCNL with strong evidence [27]. The AUA guideline (2014) recommended the administration of antimicrobial prophylaxis based primarily on prior urine culture results before the invasive stone intervention [25]. However, for SWL, no routine antibiosis is recommended [19]. For URS treatment, the prevalence of fever and UTI after URS treatment was relatively low (≤2.2%) comparing PCNL. In 2015, as CROES URS global study, Dr. Martov reported that the usage of antibiotic prophylaxis was differed widely across all over the countries (13–100%). Also, the factors related to UTI incidence after URS were reported the administration of antibiotic prophylaxis, stone burden, previous history of kidney stones, URS procedure time, post-URS complications, and anticoagulation medication usage [28]. Two meta-analyses demonstrated that there is no evidence of benefit for antibiotic prophylaxis prior to URS in reducing the rate of clinical UTI, but the rate of bacteriuria was reduced significantly with the evidence level Ia [19, 29]. From these results, EAU Guideline recommends the use of antibiotic prophylaxis to reduce the rate of symptomatic urinary tract infection following URS. AUA Guidelines strongly recommend that prophylaxis is indicated in all patients for 24 h. Because RCTs suggesting antibiotic prophylaxis reducing the risk of postoperative bacteriuria, the evidence level is Ib [19, 25, 29].

For PCNL, five meta-analyses of RCTs indicated a moderate level of evidence that antibiotic prophylaxis was associated with a significant decrease in the postoperative UTI following PCNL (Ia); two RCTs concluded that a single dose of a suitable agent was adequate for prophylaxis against clinical infection after PCNL (Ib). Thus, the EAU guideline strongly recommends the use of single-dose antibiotic prophylaxis to decrease the risk of clinical urinary tract infection following PCNL. Also, AUA Guidelines strongly recommended prophylaxis in all patients for 24 h [19, 29, 30].

In addition, the literature suggested that even with maximum caution and the absence of major patient mismanagement, the clinical situation in which the endourologists face the fatal complication after stone surgery still remains possible. For example, urinary tract infections should be treated completely before the surgery, and urinary obstruction with UTI should be drainage several days before the surgery. All the predictable factors should be examined and all efforts should be done to prevent and early recognize and recovery of the postoperative UTI [15, 24, 31]. For general caution, the surgery may be safely performed on good sterile techniques and best surgical practices, such as bathing the skin with soap or an antiseptic agent prior to surgery and preparing non-mucosal skin surfaces with chlorhexidine and alcohol in the operating room. There were no data supporting that hair removal decreases the risk of infection [32].

23.4 Transplanted Kidney

23.4.1 Incidence of Urolithiasis

The reported incidence of transplant urolithiasis varies greatly from 0.3% to 3% among the series of studies [33–35]. In 2016, Cheungpasitporn et al. performed a systematic review and meta-analysis about the incidence of kidney stones in kidney transplant recipients. In their study, they demonstrated that an overall incidence of renal calculi in kidney transplant recipients was 1.0% [36]. The mean age of recipients with kidney stones was 42 years old, and there was no gender difference in the stone formers. Calcium-based (CaOx and CaP) stones were the most common types of renal stones after kidney transplantation, it was followed by struvite stones known as infection stones, and uric acid stones. Sixty-seven percent of kidney stones were calcium-based stones (30% mixed CaOx/CaP, 27%CaOx, and 10%CaP), followed by struvite stones (20%) and uric acid stones (13%) [36, 37]. Urolithiasis in renal transplant may either arise de novo after transplantation or be already present in the donor's kidney. In 2002, Klingler et al. reported nine renal stone cases with renal transplantation [38]. They recommend that the small renal stone (4 mm or less) in the transplanted kidney need to be closely followed up because the stone can pass spontaneously. For both renal stones and ureteral stones greater than 15 mm, they also suggested the antegrade endoscopic procedures (PCNL) as the favorable treatment. New stone formation in transplanted kidneys was reported as the result of many factors, such as gout, secondary hyperoxaluria, secondary hyperparathyroidism supersaturated urine, hypercalciuria, distal renal tubular acidosis, UTI secondary to immunosuppression, ureteric double-pigtail stent, or habitual low oral fluid intake.

Usually, the transplanted patient has metabolic factors such as hypercalciuria, secondary hyperoxaluria, secondary to hyperparathyroidism, or gout [39]. However, the most common urolithiasis of transplanted kidneys is reported in calcium oxalate stones [36]. The reports suggested the risk factors of urolithiasis for transplantedkidneysbypersistenthyperparathyroidism, hypercalcemia, and concomitant hypercalciuria have been identified as major risk factors. The causes of allograft with oxalate stones are is not still fully understood [34]. Patients with allograft calculus will not experience typical renal colic, so the presentation of stone disease in transplanted kidneys is often late [40, 41]. Because the transplanted kidney and ureter are denervated at the operation of transplantation. The diagnosis is suspected if the patient has fever, hematuria, worsening renal function suddenly or transplant pyelonephritis is noticed. The patient only complains the mild discomfort in the iliac fossa where the transplanted kidney lies. The loss of the renal colic but slight pain is derived by the distension of the kidney causing stretching of the overlying renal fascia and abdominal wall musculature. Typically, the patients presented with either oliguria or anuria, and the elevation of serum creatinine concentration by blood analysis. Generally, most of the stones are radiolucent; it is not easy to make a definitive diagnosis by X-ray. The ultrasonography is useful for the diagnosis of urolithiasis as a routine part of follow-up. It is easier and clinically useful to identify the location and size of the allograft stones, and it also can provide the assessment of the hemodynamics of the transplanted kidney. Computed tomography is usually used subsequently for confirming the diagnosis and provide more information for treatment planning. The management of kidney transplant urolithiasis is known to be challenging because of the artificial anatomical relocation of the allografted organs and the complexity of the comorbid disease.

23.4.2 Shockwave Lithotripsy (SWL)

In the transplanted kidney, the spontaneous passage of urolithiasis has been reported; however, close surveillance is recommended to know the evolving obstruction or the possible increase of the stone size [42]. Shockwave lithotripsy is considered as the first-line treatment for non-obstructive stones <1.5 cm in diameter for urolithiasis for the transplanted kidney. The stone-free rate is reported as 78.8% [19] and the surgical technique has been well demonstrated in a large cohort of renal transplant recipients [20], including those with ureteral stones. However, SWL is often challenging for the transplanted kidney, because the location of the kidney in the pelvic can cause difficulty in positioning for SWL treatment. The transplanted kidney is located in close to bony landmarks, and it is usually difficult to use fluoroscopic imaging to know the location of the stone, and also, the overlying bowel may cause difficulty with shock wave delivery. Thus, it is better to be the patient in a prone position to perform the SWL treatment.

23.4.3 Endoscopic Surgery (URS)

Even the flexible URS is reported to be more effective in treating ureteral calculi in the transplanted kidney, URS in the transplanted kidney is technically challenging [43–45]. The difficulties of URS in transplanted kidney are related to the place where the allograft ureter is implanted, it is usually located in high on the posterior or anterior wall. The angle between the new ureteral orifice for the transplanted kidney and the urethra becomes <120°, and it makes it technically difficult to insert the URS to the transplanted ureter, even flexible scope.

In small case series, the reported stone-free rate is of 60–70% [42]. Flexible URS can be used for most patients, and semirigid URS is used to treat ureteric stones. It may be better to approach with a flexible URS, as it provides better maneuverability and efficiency of renal stone fragmentation by the Holmuiun YAG laser fiber [43, 44]. In this situation, attempting only basket extraction without reducing the size of stone by lasering is sometimes dangerous, as significant ureteric damage, and ureteral healing of traumatizing ureter may be reduced by the loss of the vascularity compared to a native ureter. If it is not possible to access the transplant new ureteric orifice, the percutaneous and retrograde combined technique should be considered for accessing the lower ureter. Especially, the long, twisted ureter such as the grafted ureter has been anastomosed to the native ureter is going to be a particular problem.

23.4.4 Percutaneous Nephrolithotomy (PCNL)

The use of PCNL to extract a calculus from a transplanted kidney was first described by Hulbert et al. in 1985. In his report, the renal stone of two cases was reported about the removal of the renal stone using grabber and ultrasonic lithotripsy for each case with making the renal access and sheath dilatation up to 28 F. After his report, this PCNL technique was reported from a variety of institutions. Today, the PCNL is the recommended treatment option for the transplanted renal calculi >1.5 cm in diameter, especially those located in the calyces and renal pelvis.

The transplanted kidney is located in the pelvic position with a relatively superficial location. It makes the limitation of the access to the stone percutaneously. The only anterior access to the allograft kidney using ultrasound-guided or CT-guided puncture with supine position is allowed. Moreover, usually after the transplantation, the kidney was encased by tough fibrous capsule fibrous, which makes it more difficult to dilate the percutaneous access of PCNL, and increases the risk of bleeding by traumatic injury [38, 45]. It may also limit the use of the rigid nephroscope; it is better to prepare flexible instruments to inspect all parts of the kidney and ureter [33, 37]. Using a combined approach with PCNL and flexible URS, the higher stone-free rates (66–100%) were reported [46]. Immunosuppression medication is also suggested that it may potentially impair wound healing, and increase the risk of severe infections or sepsis after percutaneous nephrolithotomy.

23.4.5 Open Surgery

Open surgery has an important role as the surgical treatment for urolithiasis of the transplanted kidney. It may be performed for the cases in which the other treatment modalities have already failed, and it may contain the case with ureteric reimplantation for associated stricture disease [45, 47].

References

1. Larson BJG, Zumberg MS, Kitchens CS. A feasibility study of continuing dose-reduced warfarin for invasive procedures in patients with high thromboembolic risk. Chest. 2005 Mar;127(3):922–7.
2. Sun J, Xu J, OuYang J. Risk factors of infectious complications following ureteroscopy: a systematic review and meta-analysis. Urol Int. 2020 Apr 2;104(1–2):113–24.
3. De Coninck V, Keller EX, Somani B, Giusti G, Proietti S, Rodriguez-Socarras M, et al. Complications of ureteroscopy: a complete overview. World J Urol. 2019 Nov 20;192(5):1–20.
4. Westerman ME, Scales JA, Sharma V, Gearman DJ, Ingimarsson JP, Krambeck AE. The effect of anticoagulation on bleeding-related complications following ureteroscopy. Urology. 2017 Feb;100:45–52.
5. Daels FPJ, Gaizauskas A, Rioja J, Varshney AK, Erkan E, Ozgok Y, et al. Age-related prevalence of diabetes mellitus, cardiovascular disease and anticoagulation therapy use in a urolithiasis population and their effect on outcomes: the Clinical Research Office of the Endourological Society Ureteroscopy Global Study. World J Urol. 2015 Apr 15;33(6):1–6.
6. Culkin DJ, Exaire EJ, Green D, Soloway MS, Gross AJ, Desai MR, et al. Anticoagulation and antiplatelet therapy in urological practice: ICUD/AUA review paper. JURO. 2014 Oct;192(4):1026–34.
7. Türk C, Petřík A, Sarica K, Seitz C, Skolarikos A, Straub M, et al. EAU guidelines on interventional treatment for urolithiasis. Eur Urol. 2016;69:475–82.
8. Alsaikhan B, Andonian S. Shock wave lithotripsy in patients requiring anticoagulation or. CUAJ. 2011 Feb 1:53–7.
9. Sare GM, Lloyd FR, Stower MJ. Life-threatening haemorrhage after extracorporeal shockwave lithotripsy in a patient taking clopidogrel. BJU Int. 2002 Sep;90(4):469–469.
10. Zanetti G, Kartalas-Goumas I, Montanari E, Federici AB, Trinchieri A, Rovera F, et al. Extracorporeal shockwave lithotripsy in patients treated with antithrombotic agents. J Endourol. 2001 Apr;15(3):237–41.
11. Schnabel MJ, Gierth M, Bründl J, Chaussy CG, Burger M, Fritsche H-M. Antiplatelet and antico-

agulative medication during shockwave lithotripsy. J Endourol. 2014 Sep;28(9):1034–9.
12. Labate G, Modi P, Timoney A, Cormio L, Zhang X, Louie M, et al. The percutaneous nephrolithotomy global study: classification of complications. J Endourol. 2011 Aug;25(8):1275–80.
13. La Rosette DJ, Denstedt J, Geavlete P, Keeley F, Matsuda T, Pearle M, et al. The clinical research office of the endourological society ureteroscopy global study: indications, complications, and outcomes in 11,885 patients. J Endourol. 2014 Feb;28(2):131–9.
14. De S, Autorino R, Kim FJ, Zargar H, Laydner H, Balsamo R, et al. Percutaneous nephrolithotomy versus retrograde intrarenal surgery: a systematic review and meta-analysis. Eur Urol Eur Assoc of Urol. 2015 Jan 1;67(1):125–37.
15. Cindolo L, Castellan P, Scoffone CM, Cracco CM, Celia A, Paccaduscio A, et al. Mortality and flexible ureteroscopy: analysis of six cases. World J Urol. 2016 Mar;34(3):305–10.
16. Chen L, Xu QQ, Li JX, Xiong LL, Wang XF, Huang XB. Systemic inflammatory response syndrome after percutaneous nephrolithotomy: an assessment of risk factors. Int J Urol. 2008 Dec 1;15(12):1025–8.
17. Draga ROP, Kok ET, Sorel MR, Bosch RJLH, Lock TMTW. Percutaneous nephrolithotomy: factors associated with fever after the first postoperative day and systemic inflammatory response syndrome. J Endourol. 2009 Jun;23(6):921–7.
18. Troxel SA, Low RK. Renal intrapelvic pressure during percutaneous nephrolithotomy and its correlation with the development of postoperative fever. JURO. 2002 Oct;168(4 Pt 1):1348–51.
19. Wollin DA, Joyce AD, Gupta M, Wong MYC, Laguna P, Gravas S, et al. Antibiotic use and the prevention and management of infectious complications in stone disease. World J Urol. 4th ed. Springer, Berlin; 2017 Sep;35(9):1369–79.
20. Chugh S, Pietropaolo A, Montanari E, Sarica K, Somani BK. Predictors of urinary infections and urosepsis after ureteroscopy for stone disease: a systematic review from EAU Section of Urolithiasis (EULIS). Curr Urol Rep. 2020 Mar 24;21(4):759–8.
21. Uchida Y, Takazawa R, Kitayama S, Tsujii T. Predictive risk factors for systemic inflammatory response syndrome following ureteroscopic laser lithotripsy. Urolithiasis. 2017 Jul 11;46(4):375–81.
22. Korets R, Graversen JA, Kates M, Mues AC, Gupta M. Post-percutaneous nephrolithotomy systemic inflammatory response: a prospective analysis of preoperative urine, renal pelvic urine and stone cultures. J Urol. 2011 Nov;186(5):1899–903.
23. Gao X, Lu C, Xie F, Li L, Liu M, Fang Z, et al. Risk factors for sepsis in patients with struvite stones following percutaneous nephrolithotomy. World J Urol. 2020 Jan;38(1):219–29.
24. Fan J, Wan S, Liu L, Zhao Z, Mai Z, Chen D, et al. Predictors for uroseptic shock in patients who undergo minimally invasive percutaneous nephrolithotomy. Urolithiasis. 2017 Dec;45(6):573–8.
25. Lightner DJ, Wymer K, Sanchez J, Kavoussi L. Best practice statement on urologic procedures and antimicrobial prophylaxis. JURO. 2020 Feb;203(2):351–6.
26. Desai M, Sun Y, Buchholz N, Fuller A, Matsuda T, Matlaga B, et al. Treatment selection for urolithiasis: percutaneous nephrolithomy, ureteroscopy, shock wave lithotripsy, and active monitoring. World J Urol. 2017 Sep;35(9):1395–9.
27. Lo C-W, Yang SS-D, Hsieh C-H, Chang S-J. Effectiveness of prophylactic antibiotics against post-ureteroscopic lithotripsy infections: systematic review and meta-analysis. Surg Infect. 2015 Aug;16(4):415–20.
28. Martov A, Gravas S, Etemadian M, Unsal A, Barusso G, D'Addessi A, et al. Postoperative infection rates in patients with a negative baseline urine culture undergoing ureteroscopic stone removal: a matched case-control analysis on antibiotic prophylaxis from the CROES URS global study. J Endourol. 2015 Feb;29(2):171–80.
29. Schnabel MJ, Wagenlehner FME, Schneidewind L. Perioperative antibiotic prophylaxis for stone therapy. Curr Opin Urol. 2019 Mar;29(2):89–95.
30. Potretzke AM, Park AM, Bauman TM, Larson JA, Vetter JM, Benway BM, et al. Is extended preoperative antibiotic prophylaxis for high-risk patients necessary before percutaneous nephrolithotomy? Investig Clin Urol. 2016;57(6):417–417.
31. Scotland K, Lange D. Prevention and management of urosepsis triggered by ureteroscopy. RRU. 2018;10:43–9.
32. Tanner J, Norrie P, Melen K. Preoperative hair removal to reduce surgical site infection. Cochrane Wounds Group, editor. Cochrane Database Syst Rev. Wiley; 2011 Nov 9;71(11):CD004122.
33. Cassini MF, Cologna AJ, Andrade MF, Lima GJ, Albuquerque UM, Martins ACP, et al. Lithiasis in 1,313 kidney transplants: incidence, diagnosis, and management. TPS. 2012 Oct 1;44(8):2373–5.
34. Harper JM, Samuell CT, Hallson PC, Wood SM, Mansell MA. Risk factors for calculus formation in patients with renal transplants. Br J Urol. 1994 Aug;74(2):147–50.
35. Abbott KC, Schenkman N, Swanson SJ, Agodoa LY. Hospitalized nephrolithiasis after renal transplantation in the United States. Am J Transplant. 2003 Apr;3(4):465–70.
36. Cheungpasitporn W, Thongprayoon C, Mao MA, Kittanamongkolchai W, Sathick IJJ, Dhondup T, et al. Incidence of kidney stones in kidney transplant recipients: a systematic review and meta-analysis. WJT. 2016;6(4):790–9.
37. Cicerello E, Merlo F, Mangano M, Cova G, Maccatrozzo L. Urolithiasis in renal transplantation: diagnosis and management. Arch Ital Urol Androl. 2014 Dec 30;86(4):257–60.
38. Klingler HC, Kramer G, Lodde M, Marberger M. Urolithiasis in allograft kidneys. Urology. 2002 Mar;59(3):344–8.

39. Evenepoel P, Lerut E, Naesens M, Bammens B, Claes K, Kuypers D, et al. Localization, etiology and impact of calcium phosphate deposits in renal allografts. Am J Transplant. 2009 Nov;9(11):2470–8.
40. Sarier M, Duman I, Yuksel Y, Tekin S, Demir M, Arslan F, et al. Results of minimally invasive surgical treatment of allograft lithiasis in live-donor renal transplant recipients: a single-center experience of 3758 renal transplantations. Urolithiasis. 2019 Jun;47(3):273–8.
41. Cho DK, Zackson DA, Cheigh J, Stubenbord WT, Stenzel KH. Urinary calculi in renal transplant recipients. Transplantation. 1988 May;45(5):899–902.
42. Verrier C, Bessede T, Hajj P, Aoubid L, Eschwege P, Benoit G. Decrease in and management of urolithiasis after kidney transplantation. J Urol. 2012 May;187(5):1651–5.
43. Yuan H-J, Yang D-D, Cui Y-S, Men C-P, Gao Z-L, Shi L, et al. Minimally invasive treatment of renal transplant nephrolithiasis. World J Urol. 2015 Dec;33(12):2079–85.
44. Swearingen R, Roberts WW, Wolf JS. Ureteroscopy for nephrolithiasis in transplanted kidneys. Can J Urol Can J Urol. 2015 Apr;22(2):7727–31.
45. Challacombe B, Dasgupta P, Tiptaft R, Glass J, Koffman G, Goldsmith D, et al. Multimodal management of urolithiasis in renal transplantation. BJU Int. 2005 Aug;96(3):385–9.
46. Streeter EH, Little DM, Cranston DW, Morris PJ. The urological complications of renal transplantation: a series of 1535 patients. BJU Int. 2002 Nov;90(7):627–34.
47. Rizvi SA, Sultan S, Ijaz H, Mirza ZN, Ahmed B, Saulat S, et al. Open surgical management of pediatric urolithiasis: a developing country perspective. Indian J Urol. 2010 Oct;26(4):573–6.

24 Patients with Special Anatomy

Selvalingam Sothilingam and Kay-Seong Ngoo

Abstract

Urolithiasis in renal anomalies, such as horseshoe kidney, cross-fused ectopia and malrotated kidneys and in special situations, such as scoliosis and transplanted kidneys, present multiple challenges in terms of surgical approach to the stones, patient positioning during surgery and optimal urinary drainage, in order to achieve excellent stone-free rates. With appropriate imaging, the stones can be accessed using minimally invasive techniques. A combination of PCNL and Flexible URS usually results in good stone clearance. RIRS is also favoured in reasonably-sized stones. The success rate of stone clearance using ESWL is generally low.

Keywords

Pelvic kidney · Renal anomaly · Spinal deformity · Urolithiasis

S. Sothilingam
Pusat Perubatan Sunway Velocity, Kuala Lumpur, Malaysia

K.-S. Ngoo (✉)
Department of Surgery, Hospital Angkatan Tentera Tuanku Mizan, Kuala Lumpur, Malaysia

24.1 Introduction

There will be challenges when a urologist is confronted with urolithiasis in special situations especially with renal anomalies such as horseshoe, crossed fused ectopia, ectopic (pelvic) and malrotated kidneys. Similar difficulties may be encountered in situations where there are skeletal abnormalities and with transplanted kidneys.

These renal anomalies are associated with an increased risk of recurrent urinary tract infection and altered urinary drainage giving rise to an increased risk of stone formation. Furthermore, the renal anomaly will result in altered calyceal orientation, abnormal vasculature and aberrant spatial orientation with respect to other visceral organs [1].

Although in the past open surgery was the mainstay of treatment, urolithiasis in abnormal kidneys can now be successfully and safely managed by endourological procedures. Various procedures such as the standard PCNL, Mini PCNL, URS, RIRS and even ESWL have been described with varying degrees of success. Additional procedures such as laparoscopic pyelolithotomy may have a role as well. There are however no clear guidelines in the preferred choice of treatment in these cases. It is imperative that the procedure chosen is individualised based on the following factors:

1. Stone characteristics (size, location and density)

A. C.F. Ng et al. (eds.), *Practical Management of Urinary Stone*,
https://doi.org/10.1007/978-981-16-4193-0_24

2. Renal anatomy (calyceal orientation, vasculature, drainage of kidney, kidney mobility)
3. Associated skeletal deformities (kyphosis, scoliosis)
4. Orientation of surrounding organs especially bowel
5. Technical expertise/facilities available

24.2 Renal Anatomy

24.2.1 Horseshoe Kidney (HK)

This is one of the most common congenital malformations. It has a prevalence of 1:400–800 in the normal population [2]. The abnormalities associated with HK include malrotation of the kidney. The kidney is located more caudally with high insertion of the ureter which is forced superior and laterally and in 30% of cases may be associated with ureteropelvic obstruction. Therefore, these patients will have a higher risk for urinary tract infection, urolithiasis and urinary stasis. The incidence of stone disease in HK is 20% [3].

24.2.2 Crossed Fused Ectopic Kidney (CFE)

This is where one kidney is shifted from one side to the opposite side, and the two kidneys fusing together during the period of growth more often on the right side. However, the ureter descends to its normal position in the bladder. It is more common in males. The exact incidence is unknown as many patients are asymptomatic, but authors have reported its incidence as 1 in 7500 autopsy cases [4]. CFE may be associated with renal tumours or cystic dysplasia. Symptomatic patients may present with recurrent urinary tract infection, urolithiasis, abdominal mass or hydronephrosis. Ultrasound imaging is a good screening tool and further anatomy can be defined using CT Scan, MRU or radionuclide scintigraphy. Some of these patients may have associated vesicoureteric reflux.

24.2.3 Ectopic/Pelvic Kidney

Pelvic kidney has an incidence of 1 in 2000 cases [5]. The position of the kidney in the pelvis leads to an abnormal ureteric insertion and a tortuous ureter, coupled with kidney malrotation that can lead to urinary stasis and stone formation. It may also be associated with a higher risk of trauma. The majority of patients with pelvic kidneys remain asymptomatic.

24.3 Choice of Treatment

24.3.1 Horseshoe Kidney (HK)

24.3.1.1 PCNL

HK is associated with aberrant vessels entering the isthmus dorsally and a retrorenal colon. The renal pelvis is located anterior and medial. The upper calyx is situated more medially and is usually infracostal. The anteroposterior tilt of the kidney is prominent, and this makes the upper pole calyx more superficial and posteriorly located. In 1973, Fletcher and Kettlewell [6, 7] reported the first PCNL in HK. The puncture is best done in the prone position although the access tract may be longer. Ultrasonography would be the preferred method of visualisation of the calyx and best used with Doppler to avoid puncturing into aberrant vasculature. The upper pole calyx is frequently punctured below the 12th rib on the posterior axillary line with a caudal angle of puncture as has been described by Janetschek and Kuanzel [7, 8]. The puncture is usually more medial, and this should safely avoid the colon which is more posterolaterally related to the kidney. However, a more medial puncture through the paraspinal muscle may be associated with a more difficult dilatation and bleeding.

For a better stone-free rate (SFR), PCNL combined with antegrade flexible ureteroscopy is a safe way to approach stones in multiple calyces and in staghorn calculi. Many studies showed SFRs of the primary PCNL procedure in HK ranging from 81% to 87% [7] PCNL is best suited for stones >15 mm especially with a high stone density (>1000HU). Miller et al. reported an SFR of 84.1% in 35 patients with HK and 97.7% of cases handled with one access including 82.2% of kidneys accessed by the upper pole [7, 9].

The complication associated with this approach is no more than for PCNL in a normal kidney. The complication rates can further be reduced by the use of miniaturised PCNL procedures using the mini-Perc and ultra mini perc for smaller stones and in combination with the standard PCNL for stones that require multiple access.

24.3.1.2 RIRS

RIRS may be an option for stones<15 mm and may be considered for stones >15 mm with density <1000HU. In the larger stones, it may be a staged procedure. The success of RIRS is also dependent on the drainage of the kidney. SFR vary between 75% and 88% [10, 11].

The complication rates for RIRS in HK are no different from those in normal kidneys. However, kidneys with poorer drainage may have a higher incidence of residual stones.

24.3.1.3 ESWL

ESWL may be difficult due to localisation problems in relation to bony anatomy and overlying bowel. Poor results may also be associated with poor drainage of the kidneys. The success rate of 79% for stones <15 mm (HU < 1000) drops to 25–53% for stones >15 mm [11, 12]. If failure occurs due to ESWL, RIRS should be considered as the secondary procedure.

24.3.2 Crossed Fused Ectopia (CFE)

Three-dimensional reconstruction of the kidney by computerised tomography would be an ideal pre-requisite in planning the approach to treating urolithiasis in crossed fused ectopia. Vascular anomalies are usually associated with this condition. There are no standard guidelines in treating stones in CFE.

Based on the literature search of the 35 cases reported [13], treatment methods included open surgery in 4 cases, conservative treatment in 5 patients, ESWL in 7 patients, PCNL in 10 patients, RIRS in 4 patients and laparoscopic pyelolithotomy in 1 case. In another 5 patients, the treatment modality was unknown.

ESWL failed in 3 of the 7 patients treated and they required secondary treatment. Resorlu et al. reported the first use of RIRS in a patient with a 15 mm stone which confirmed that RIRS was safe and feasible in CFE [14].

24.3.3 Pelvic Kidney

PCNL in such kidneys requires a supine oblique position. The kidney is elevated by placing a bolster behind the pelvis. The challenge would be avoiding punctures into the overlying bowel. Some techniques that can assist in the puncture include displacing the bowel by compression using the ultrasound probe (ultrasound-guided puncture) [15] and the use of laparoscopy in displacing the bowel and guiding the puncture needle [7, 16]. However, ultrasound-guided puncture may be challenging in the presence of pneumoperitoneum. Furthermore, due to the potentially deep position of a pelvic kidney, a longer Amplatz sheath and nephroscope may be required. The use of a colour Doppler ultrasound during the puncture may further prevent vascular injury. Dilatation may be a challenge with a higher risk of tract loss.

RIRS and URS will also have their own set of difficulties in the pelvic kidney. The ureter may be tortuous with angulations making it difficult to negotiate the scope. It is important to place a Urethral Access Sheath (UAC) in all cases of RIRS. However, unlike in the normal kidney where the UAC is placed at the pelvi-ureteric junction, in a pelvic kidney, the sheath will be placed at mid or lower ureter to allow for better deflection of the flexible ureteroscope [11, 17].

In a recent paper on managing pelvic kidney stones, the authors concluded that flexible URS and PCNL had equivalent success rates (81.25% vs 86%) and that RIRS was associated with shorter operating time (46 vs 95 min). The stone volume in patients selected for RIRS was notably smaller [11, 17].

ESWL may be an option in pelvic kidneys but although stone fragmentation may occur, the SFR may still be low due to poor kidney drainage.

Another viable option in pelvic kidneys is laparoscopic pyelolithotomy especially in kidneys with a large extrarenal pelvis. The risk of bleeding, bowel, and nephron injury is much lower and the SFR would be much higher.

24.3.4 Algorithm of Stone Management in Anomalous Kidneys [17]

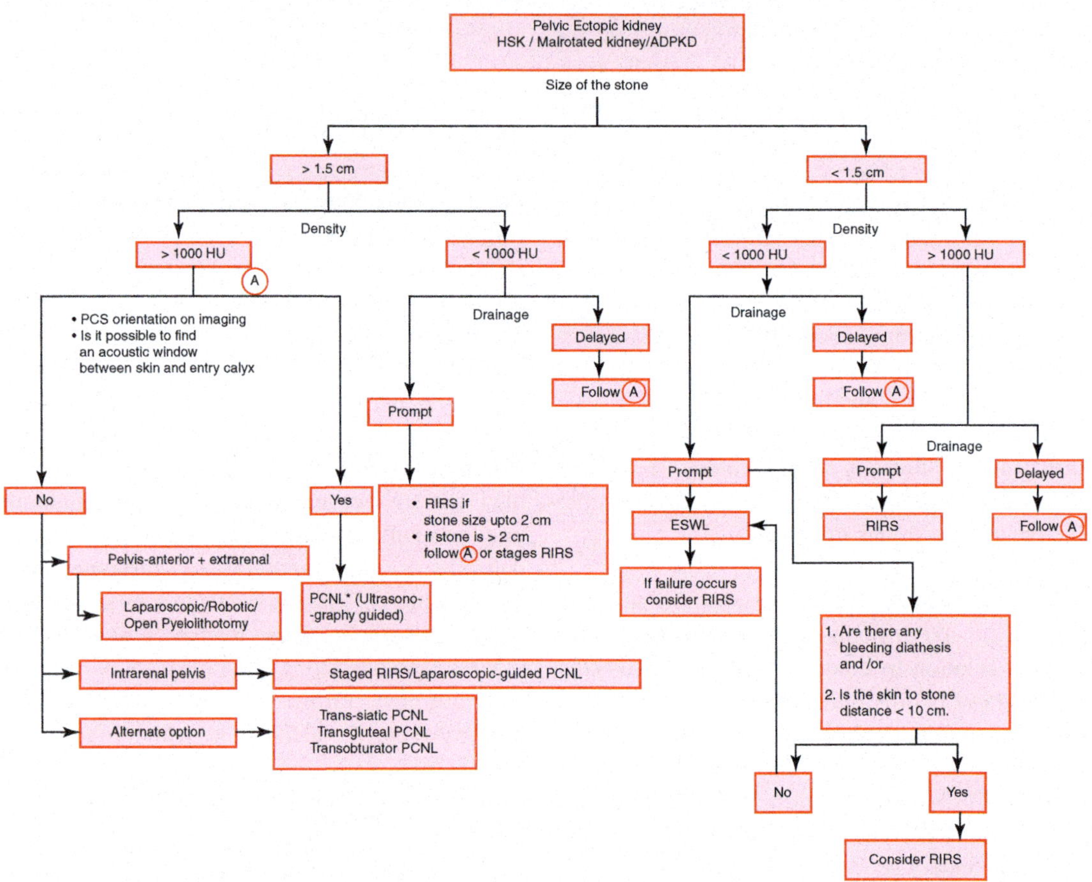

24.4 Stones in Other Special Situations

24.4.1 Skeletal Deformities

Patients with skeletal deformities such as scoliosis and kyphosis also run a risk of urolithiasis due to immobility causing hypercalciuria, urinary tract infection and urinary stasis [18].

ESWL is a feasible option for smaller stones. However, there may be difficulties in locating the stone through imaging, especially with the ultrasound. Furthermore, SFR may be lower due to poorer drainage of the kidneys especially if there is associated malrotation of the kidney. The success of ESWL will also depend on the density of the stone. There would also be added difficulty in the positioning of these patients with spinal deformity.

PCNL would carry similar disadvantages especially since there may be a distortion of the usual bony landmarks. There may also be displacement of surrounding organs especially the bowel and lung. Patient positioning may also be challenging be it supine or prone position. Ultrasound-guided puncture or even CT-guided puncture (with the assistance of an interventional radiologist) may be required. With PCNL in such patients, stone-free rates (SFR) are in the range of 60–88% in most studies [18, 19]. RIRS may also be a challenge with SFR ranging from 35.7% to 75% [11, 20, 21].

24.4.2 Transplanted Kidney

ESWL for smaller stones may be challenging and has to be done prone due to the overlying pelvic bone. It is also imperative to monitor the stone fragments as it is passed out, due to the potential of causing obstruction and tipping the patient to renal failure. Overlying bowel may also make it difficult to localise the stone. Stone clearance up to 66% has been reported [22].

URS/RIRS would also be technically difficult due to the position of the ureteroneocystostomy at the dome of the bladder.

An antegrade approach with PCNL is a reasonable option in these kidneys. Either ultrasound or CT-guided puncture can be done especially since the graft kidney is anteriorly located. Care must be taken when dilating the tract to avoid graft injury and bleeding. High SFR can be obtained especially using flexible scopes, laser and baskets and this has been reported in several series [22].

This is one area where open surgery may also be a choice of treatment if other endoscopic measures are not feasible or fail.

24.5 Conclusions

There are currently no standard guidelines in the management of urolithiasis in anomalous kidneys and in special situations of skeletal deformities. Most recommendations are derived from the literature based on case series. Many authors have proposed various algorithms to aid in decision-making. Each case, however, should be treated individually and the best approach that is safe and yet gives the best SFR should be chosen.

Evaluation in these special situations may require additional imaging techniques such as MRU, CT IVU, 3D-reconstructed CT Scan or Radionuclide Scintigraphy to better define the anatomy and drainage of the kidney. The choice of treatment will also depend on the relationship of the kidney with surrounding organs especially the bowel and will take into consideration any bony anomalies overlying the kidney.

Although historically stones in anomalous kidneys were removed through open surgery, it is now standard of care to approach these stones through a minimally invasive approach. This is especially made possible with smaller and better endoscopes, the availability of laser technology and better imaging techniques.

Procedures that may work well in normal kidneys may not have similar outcomes in anomalous kidneys. One good example is ESWL for small stones in the pelvicalyceal system. Although ESWL may fragment the stone, SFR may remain low in anomalous kidneys due to poor drainage. Stone localisation may also be challenging due to overlapping bowel or due to skeletal abnormalities.

The way in which a procedure is done will also need to be modified and a good example of this is PCNL. Puncture into the calyceal system may require a combined approach of using ultrasound (with or without Doppler), fluoroscopy and sometimes even laparoscopy.

In summary, management of these cases is best done in centers with adequate facilities and experience to ensure not only a good SFR but also safe surgery. These are the appropriate cases where a combined multidiscipline meeting may be useful in coming to a consensus and in choosing the right treatment for the patient.

Nomenclature

PCNL	Percutaneous nephrolithotomy
RIRS	Retrograde intra renal Surgery
URS	Uretero renoscope
ESWL	Extracorporeal Shock Wave Lithotripsy
SFR	Stone Free Rate

References

1. Rana AM, Bhojwani JP. Percutaneous Nephrolithotomy in renal anomalies of fusion, ectopia, rotation, hypoplasia and pelvicalyceal aberration: uniformity inheterogeniety. J Endourol. 2009;23:609–14.
2. Glenn JF. Analysis of 51 patients with horseshoe kidney. N Engl J Med. 1959;261:684–7.
3. Raj GV, Auge BK, Weizer AZ, Denstedt JD, Watterson JD, Beiko DT, et al. Percutaneous management of calculi within horseshoe kidneys. J Urol. 2003;170:48–51.
4. Mudoni A, Cacceta F, Caroppo M, Musio F, Accogli A, Zacheo MD, et al. Crossed fused renal ectopia: case report and review of the literature. J Ultrasound. 2017;20:333–7.
5. Zafar FS, Lingeman JE. Value of laparoscopy in the management of calculi complicating renal malformations. J Endourol. 1996;10:379–83.
6. Fletcher EW, Kettlewell MG. Antegrade pyelography in a horseshoe kidney. Am J Roentgenol Radium Therapy, Nucl Med. 1973;119:720–2.
7. Xiaofeng G, Ziyu F, Chaoyue L, et al. Management of Staghorn stones in special situations. Asian J Urol. 2020;7:130–8.
8. Janetschek G, Kunzel KH. Percutaneous nephrolithotomy in horseshoe kidneys. Applied anatomy and clinical experience. Br J Urol. 1988;62:117–22.
9. Miller NL, Matlaga BR, Handa SE, Munch LC, Lingeman JE. The presence of horseshoe kidney does not affect the outcome of percutaneous nephrolithotomy. J Endourol. 2008;22:1219–25.
10. Weizer JE, Springhart WP, Ekeruo WO, Matlaga BR, Tan YH, Assimos DG, Preminger GM. Ureteroscopic management of renal calculi in anomalous kidneys. Urology. 2005;65:265–9.
11. Mordechal D, Stavros S, Karim B, Benoit P, Amy K, Sanjay K et al. Stones in special situations. World J Urol. 2017.
12. Sheir KZ, Madbouly K, Elsobky E, Abdelkhalek M. ESWL in anomalous kidneys: 11 years of experience in with two second generation lithotripters. Urology. 2003;62:10–5.
13. Yalei C, Yinan Z, Weiting K, Ning S, Zilian C, Yuanman L, Xunbo J. Crossed fused renal ectopia with renal calculi, two case reports and a review of literature. Medicine. 2019;98:48.
14. Resorlu M, Kabar M, Resorlu B, et al. Retrograde intrarenal surgery in cross-fused ectopic kidney. Urology. 2015;85:e5–6.
15. Otano N, Jairath A, Mishra S, Ganpule A, Sabnis R, Desai M. Percutaneous nephrolithotomy in pelvic kidneys: is ultrasound guided puncture safe? Urology. 2015;85:55–8.
16. Cinman NM, Okeke Z, Smith AD. Pelvic kidney; associated diseases and treatment. J Endourol. 2007;21:836–42.
17. Abhishek GS, Ankush J, Sudharshan SB, Gopal T, Arvind P, Ganpule MV, Ravindra S, Desai M. Changing trends in the endourological management of urolithiasis in anomalous kidneys. BJU Int. 2019;123:318–27.
18. Kara C, Resorlu B, Ozyuvali B, Unsal A. Is percutaneous nephrolithotomy suitable for patients with scoliosis: single center experience. Urology. 2011;78:37–42.
19. Goumas-Kartalas I, Montanari E. Percutaneous nephrolithotomy in patients with spinal deformities. J Endourol. 2010;24:1081–9.
20. Colangelo CJ, Kaplan G, Palazzi K, Holmes N, Chiang G. Ureteroscopy in pediatric patients with spinal abnormalities. J Endourol. 2013;27:545–8.
21. Resorlu B, Ozyuvali E, Oguz U, Bozkurt OF, Unsal A. Retrograde Intrarenal surgery in patients with spinal deformities. J Endourol. 2012;26:1131–5.
22. Challacombe B, Dasgupta P, Tiptaft R, Glass J, Koffman G, Goldsmith D, Khan MS. Multimodal management of urolithiasis in renal transplantation. BJU Int. 2005;96:385–9.

25 Management of Stone Diseases in the Special Patient Population

Wonho Jung and Hyung Joon Kim

25.1 Pregnancy

- Ultrasound is recommended as the primary imaging method if urinary tract stones are suspected in pregnant women. MRI without contrast medium can be a second option.
- Low-dose computer tomography should be saved as the last imaging tool in pregnant women. The absorbed dose shall not exceed 50 mGy.
- The primary treatment of non-complicated urinary stones during pregnancy is conservative management.
- Interventional procedures such as ureteral stent indwelling or percutaneous nephrostomy would be necessary. Still, the possibility of encrustation is higher than that of the control, so frequent replacement is recommended every 4–6 weeks at least.
- If the spontaneous passage of urethral stones fails in pregnant women, the URS may be performed.

It is estimated that urinary stones in pregnant women are between 1 in 200 and 1 in 1500, a rate similar to that of nonpregnant women of the same age [1]. Eighty to ninety percent of the cases are detected during the second and third trimesters. One-third of the patients have a previous history of urinary stone disease.

Symptom caused by a urinary stone during pregnancy is not so different as in the general population. Flank pain (85–100%), gross hematuria (15–30%), and lower urinary tract symptoms are common complaints, but due to the special situation, preeclampsia or premature labor may occur in a small number of cases. Acute abdominal or flank pain during pregnancy can be a diagnostic challenge for clinicians. Diagnosis may be delayed due to difficulties in distinguishing hematuria and physiological hydronephrosis caused by pregnancy. Physiological hydronephrosis is observed around 90% during pregnancy. Decrease in the peristalsis of the urinary tract due to progesterone during pregnancy, and the pressure of the urinary tract by the fetus and the enlarged uterus is considered the reason. Physiological hydronephrosis is expected on the right side. It is induced by the uterine dextrorotation and the pressure-reducing effect of the sigmoid colon on the left side. It develops between 6

W. Jung
Department of Urology, Keimyung University Dongsan Hospital, Keimyung University School of Medicine, Daegu, Republic of Korea
e-mail: wjung@dsmc.or.kr

H. J. Kim (✉)
Department of Urology, Konyang University, Daejeon, Republic of Korea
e-mail: hjkim@kyuh.ac.kr

A. C.F. Ng et al. (eds.), *Practical Management of Urinary Stone*,
https://doi.org/10.1007/978-981-16-4193-0_25

and 10 weeks of gestation and can be maintained for up to 4–6 weeks of childbirth. If the patient has a history of urinary stones and pre-pregnancy images, it can help for diagnosis [2].

25.1.1 Diagnosis

The biggest concern in diagnosing urinary stones in pregnant women is exposure to ionizing radiation, which comprises a potential teratogenic effect. In general, all imaging methods used to diagnose urinary stones are well below the absorption safety threshold of 50 mGy. Still, when considering the use of imaging tools, especially if the amount of radiation absorbed by the fetus is expected to exceed 0.5 mGy, there must be sufficient explanation to justify its use. The efforts must be taken to reduce the delivered dose of radiation as low as possible, while the quality of the achieved diagnostic image should be fair enough for use. The fetal effect of radiation depends on the gestational age. Fetal tissues are susceptible to ionizing radiation the most during the first trimester when organs are being developed.

25.1.1.1 Ultrasonography

If urinary stones are suspected in pregnant women, ultrasound is used as primary imaging, with a positive prediction of 77% [3]. However, ultrasound is highly operator-dependent. There are limitations in that it is difficult to distinguish between physiological hydronephrosis and the obstruction caused by the urinary stone. Typical ultrasonic findings suspected of urinary stone obstruction include dilatation of ureter above the lower ureter, high-grade left hydronephrosis, absence of jetting from the ureteral orifice, and an increased renal resistance index (RI). By measuring RI, one can increase the accuracy of ultrasonography in distinguishing physiological dilation and stone-related obstruction. An RI of 0.70 demonstrates 87% accuracy with 45% sensitivity and 91% specificity for diagnosis. If the difference in RI value between the affected kidney and the normal contralateral counterpart exceeds 0.06, the accuracy can be up to 100% with 95% sensitivity and 100% specificity [4, 5]. The bladder should be fully filled to confirm the absence of the distal ureteral stone. Transvaginal ultrasonography can be effective in detecting stones located below the pelvic brim [4, 6, 7].

25.1.1.2 MRI

Although the MRI encompasses the limitation of the inability to visualize the stone, it is considered a second imaging modality for providing useful information. MRI helps to delineate the pathologic obstruction from pregnancy-induced hydronephrosis, determine the degree of urinary obstruction, or indirectly diagnose the stones' location. The positive predictive value of MRI for diagnosing urinary stones is around 80% [3]. The stone's presence can be inferred from signs such as "signal voids," "double kink," and perinephric and periureteral edema. At present, 1.5 T is recommended for use because there is a lack of evidence for the effects of 3.0 T magnetic resonance imaging on pregnant women. The use of Gadolinium for contrast enhancement shall be limited in consideration of its possible impact on the fetus, particularly during the first trimester [8].

25.1.1.3 CT

Computer tomography has a high positive predictive value of 95% or more, but due to fetal effects from radiation exposure, conventional CT is contraindicated during pregnancy [3]. A low-dose CT scan protocol has recently been described, which delivers minimal radiation exposure to the fetus. The judicious use of low-dose CT scans in pregnant women with flank pain, and negative initial ultrasound is advocated. Even so, CT should be prohibited during the first trimester [6].

25.1.2 Management

Although there are limitations in diagnostic tests, the spontaneous passage of urinary stones from pregnant women is 48–80%, similar to that of nonpregnant women. Up to 50% of the remaining stones will pass during the postpartum period. Therefore, conservative management using hydration and pain control is the initial treatment of choice. Nonsteroidal anti-inflammatory drug (NSAID), commonly used to control colic pain caused by stones, is contraindicated in pregnant women. Low-dose morphine can be used for severe pain. For moderate pain, acetaminophen can be effective [9]. Alpha-blockers, commonly used for medical expulsive therapy, are not recommended due to lack of evidence in pregnant women [10]. Conservative management will fail in 15–30%. Ureteral stent indwelling or percutaneous nephrostomy is required if there is a high chance of complications like severe hydronephrosis, sepsis, and premature labor onset [11]. However, during pregnancy, there is a high possibility of encrustation in the urinary stents, which may require frequent replacement every four to six weeks [12]. If the ureteral stent or nephrostomy tube needs to be maintained for a long period, URS may be a reasonable alternative [13–15]. URS under anesthesia is relatively safe during the second trimester. The selection of anesthesia methods requires discussion with an anesthesiologist. Features distinguished from general urinary stone operations include monitoring fetuses during the surgery, positioning patients 15–20° left semi-lateral, and inserting the urinary stent or guidewire image-guided by ultrasound. It is recommended to insert a ureteral stent after the surgery. If childbirth is imminent, delaying treatment to postpartum may be an alternative. In pregnant women, ESWL is contraindicated. PCNL could be performed in highly selected cases. There is a risk of premature birth at 4–10%, related to the insertion of a urinary stent or the URS [16–18]. Where active treatment is necessary, care should be provided at an experienced institution that can respond quickly to fetuses and mothers [16].

25.2 Children

- In children. Ultrasonography is a first-line imaging tool for those suspected of urinary stone.
- KUB or low-dose non-contrast CT could be an alternative option if the US is not enough for diagnosis.
- Asymptomatic renal stones without obstruction may be subjected to active surveillance using periodic ultrasound.
- In children, non-complicated asymptomatic single ureteral stones sized less than 10 mm can be managed conservatively.
- If active treatment is required, ESWL is recommended as the first choice. URS could be performed as the next option.
- For the renal stone sized 10–20 mm, ESWL or RIRS is recommended. If renal stone size exceeds 20 mm, either ESWL or PCNL could be considered.
- When performing ESWL, ureteral stent, or PCN insertion is recommended.

Children (<18 years of age) are indicated for in-depth metabolic investigation since the earlier onset of urolithiasis is relevant to the high risk of stone formation. The risk of renal stone recurrence ranges from 50–70% within 3 years. Besides, functional abnormalities or anatomical anomalies such as vesicoureteral reflux, ureteropelvic junction obstruction, and neurogenic bladder are the second most common causes of urinary stones in children [19]. Correction for such causative factors should also be performed to reduce the chance of recurrence.

Children present with various symptoms depending on the age of diagnosis. For infants younger than 60 days old, irritability is the most common symptom. Children of the mean age of 10 months usually present urinary tract infection and its related symptoms (50%), followed by incidental findings during image workup for other reasons (20%). Children above four years old mostly present diffuse abdominal pain (57%) followed by classical renal colic (44%), urinary tract infection, hematuria, and G-I symptoms as in the adult patient group. In general, puberty begins at the age of nine for girls and ten for boys, and most organs grow to a size similar to adults as they pass puberty. The age of pediatric patients is essential in determining the size of organs and whether they can cooperate with the treatment plan. Therefore, an individualized approach based on these factors would be more appropriate rather than depending on the guideline.

25.2.1 Diagnosis

In children, the cumulative and long-term effects of radiation exposure are the primary concerns as well. Since children have a higher chance of recurrence, the cumulative dose of the radiation can be more significant by repeated imaging. Thus, the carcinogenic risk may be higher for children having more extended life expectancy. Ultrasonography (US) is a first-line imaging tool for those suspected of urinary stones. Its advantage is the avoidance of radiation and not requiring anesthesia. For better diagnosis, it is recommended to include a full-filled bladder view to visualize the adjoining portion of the ureter. Findings such as the absence of ureteral jetting or resistive index of both kidneys' arciform arteries give you a clue on the grade of obstruction. However, ultrasonography fails to identify stones in more than 40% of children. If ultrasonography cannot exclude urinary stone, KUB, or low-dose non-contrast CT could be an alternative option [20]. KUB can help identify radio-opaque stones and for the follow-up. Low-dose CT is sensitive, and sedation or anesthesia is rarely necessary with newer generation high-speed CT scans.

25.2.2 Management

The management option in children is not so much different from those in adults. Pain is managed routinely with NSAID as the first option. Single, asymptomatic lower-pole renal stones can be observed. There is a significantly higher chance of stone passage in patients with non-struvite, non-cystine stones less than 7 mm. Intervention such as SWL, URS, and PNL may be needed for stone stones elsewhere independently of the size.

25.2.2.1 Medical Expulsive Therapy

There is not much evidence on the safety and effectiveness of MET in children as in the adult [21–23]. However, a recent meta-analysis of five trials showed that α-blockers facilitated stone passage with increased SFR compared to control (OR = 2.7, p = 0.001) [24]. Evidence shows alpha-blockers as an effective treatment option in children, especially with distal ureteral stones less than 10 mm [25]. The use of α-blockers was not associated with an increased risk of adverse events than no treatment or placebo. Pills can be taken at about ten years of age or older, but younger children are may not be able to swallow.

25.2.2.2 ESWL

ESWL is an effective treatment method for childhood. It is recommended as a first-line option in children with single ureteral stones less than 10 mm. In children with renal stones, ESWL can be applied to stones with a size up to 20 mm (~300 mm^2). The overall success rate of ESWL in children is 70–90%. Retreatment may be required in 4–50%, and 4–12.5% must undergo additional procedures. However, it may require general anesthesia during the procedure, depending on the patient's age and lithotripter type. It prevents the reduction of treatment effects due to movement during the procedure and reduces radiation exposure due to repositioning. For this reason, general anesthesia is needed during ESWL in most cases under ten years of age [26, 27]. Intravenous sedatives or patient-controlled analgesia may be administered at an age where the child can cooperate [28]. Tuncer et al. compared the effects of ESWL with or without anesthesia in 61 kidney stone children. They reported that in patients over 9 years of age who are well-cooperative, ESWL was successful without anesthesia [29]. Adanur et al. said that the success rate of children under 2 years of age who underwent ESWL reached 99%, while only 2.9% of major complications such as urinary tract infection, steinstrasse were shown [30]. Turna et al. reported a success rate of 84.6% without significant complications in 36 children under 1 year old [31].

25.2.2.3 URS

When choosing invasive procedures such as URS or PCNL in children, it is important to keep in mind that the patient's organ size is small and to the instrument should be chosen accordingly. Recently, the utilization of ureteroscope in children is increasing. The Stone free rate using ureteroscopy is 81–98% for ureteral stone. A flexible ureteroscope can be applied for pediatric renal stones and SFR of 76–100%. Complication rates are relatively low for both semi-rigid and flexible ureteroscopic surgeries (1.9–23% vs. 0–28%). Younger age, cystine composition, large stone size are predisposing factors for treatment failure. Pre-stenting can increase the stone-free rate while decreasing the complication rate. Post-URS stenting is recommended in most cases. Clinicians should keep in mind that additional anesthesia may be needed when inserting or retrieving the stent. Dangle et al. compared the surgical outcome of URS between 64 children under the age of 11 and 40 children over 12. There was no difference in the stone-free rate and the complication rate between the two groups [32]. Atar et al. compared the success rates of URS based on the size of the ureteroscope. Either 4.5Fr or 7.5Fr ureteroscope was used in 69 children under the age of 8. In children under the age of 3, the stone-free rate was significantly higher when using the ureteroscope size of 4.5Fr than 7.5Fr (93.8% vs. 66.7%). There was no difference in the success rates within the two groups between the ages of 4 and 7 [33]. There were also significantly fewer side effects in the 4.5Fr group. In preschoolers who require surgical treatment for ureteral stone, it is advised to use a smaller caliber ureteroscope, the younger they are.

25.2.2.4 PCNL

Large stones with more than 2 cm in size, stones resistant to ESWL or RIRS are indicated for PNL. SFR for pediatric PNL is 71.4–95% after a single session with an overall complication rate of 20%. Dede et al. conducted a PCNL using a 4.85 Fr nephroscope in 24 children aged 1.3 years on average, reporting an average admission of 2.5 days and SFR of 83% [34]. Dow et al. also reported the PCNL outcome using a 14Fr nephroscope in 26 children, 3.6 years of age. In this study, patients had renal stones sized more than 5 cm, but the stone-free rate was 85% [35]. None of the patients in these studies have received blood transfusions. PCNL can be applied to children of various ages. Miniaturization of nephroscope may have benefits in children as for the body configuration being smaller than adults. It reduces the complication rate, length of hospital stay, postoperative pain while increasing the chance of performing tubeless PNL.

References

1. Somani BK, Dellis A, Liatsikos E, Skolarikos A. Review on diagnosis and management of urolithiasis in pregnancy: an ESUT practical guide for urologists. World J Urol. 2017;35:1637–49.
2. Taguchi K, Cho SY, Ng AC, Usawachintachit M, Tan YK, Deng YL, et al. The Urological Association of Asia clinical guideline for urinary stone disease. Int J Urol. 2019;26:688–709.
3. White WM, Johnson EB, Zite NB, Beddies J, Krambeck AE, Hyams E, et al. Predictive value of current imaging modalities for the detection of urolithiasis during pregnancy: a multicenter, longitudinal study. J Urol. 2013;189:931–4.
4. AIUM-ACR-ACOG-SMFM-SRU practice parameter for the performance of standard diagnostic obstetric ultrasound examinations. J Ultrasound Med. 2018;37:E13–E24.
5. Asrat T, Roossin MC, Miller EI. Ultrasonographic detection of ureteral jets in normal pregnancy. Am J Obstet Gynecol. 1998;178:1194–8.

6. Committee on Obstetric P. Committee Opinion No. 723: Guidelines for Diagnostic Imaging During Pregnancy and Lactation. Obstet Gynecol. 2017;130:e210–e2e6.
7. Laing FC, Benson CB, DiSalvo DN, Brown DL, Frates MC, Loughlin KR. Distal ureteral calculi: detection with vaginal US. Radiology. 1994;192:545–8.
8. Safety ACRCoM, Greenberg TD, Hoff MN, Gilk TB, Jackson EF, Kanal E, et al. ACR guidance document on MR safe practices: updates and critical information 2019. J Magn Reson Imaging. 2020;51:331–8.
9. Valovska MI, Pais VM Jr. Contemporary best practice urolithiasis in pregnancy. Ther Adv Urol. 2018;10:127–38.
10. Bailey G, Vaughan L, Rose C, Krambeck A. Perinatal outcomes with tamsulosin therapy for symptomatic urolithiasis. J Urol. 2016;195:99–103.
11. Tsai YL, Seow KM, Yieh CH, Chong KM, Hwang JL, Lin YH, et al. Comparative study of conservative and surgical management for symptomatic moderate and severe hydronephrosis in pregnancy: a prospective randomized study. Acta Obstet Gynecol Scand. 2007;86:1047–50.
12. Ngai HY, Salih HQ, Albeer A, Aghaways I, Buchholz N. Double-J ureteric stenting in pregnancy: a single-centre experience from Iraq. Arab J Urol. 2013;11:148–51.
13. Semins MJ, Trock BJ, Matlaga BR. The safety of ureteroscopy during pregnancy: a systematic review and meta-analysis. J Urol. 2009;181:139–43.
14. Teleb M, Ragab A, Dawod T, Elgalaly H, Elsayed E, Sakr A, et al. Definitive ureteroscopy and intracorporeal lithotripsy in treatment of ureteral calculi during pregnancy. Arab J Urol. 2014;12:299–303.
15. Zhang S, Liu G, Duo Y, Wang J, Li J, Li C. Application of ureteroscope in emergency treatment with persistent renal colic patients during pregnancy. PLoS One. 2016;11:e0146597.
16. Johnson EB, Krambeck AE, White WM, Hyams E, Beddies J, Marien T, et al. Obstetric complications of ureteroscopy during pregnancy. J Urol. 2012;188:151–4.
17. Rosenberg E, Sergienko R, Abu-Ghanem S, Wiznitzer A, Romanowsky I, Neulander EZ, et al. Nephrolithiasis during pregnancy: characteristics, complications, and pregnancy outcome. World J Urol. 2011;29:743–7.
18. Swartz MA, Lydon-Rochelle MT, Simon D, Wright JL, Porter MP. Admission for nephrolithiasis in pregnancy and risk of adverse birth outcomes. Obstet Gynecol. 2007;109:1099–104.
19. Serdaroğlu E, Aydoğan M, Özdemir K, Bak M. Incidence and causes of urolithiasis in children between 0–2 years. Minerva Urol Nefrol. 2016;69(2):181–8.
20. Van Batavia JP, Tasian GE. Clinical effectiveness in the diagnosis and acute management of pediatric nephrolithiasis. Int J Surg. 2016;36:698–704.
21. Aydogdu O, Burgu B, Gucuk A, Suer E, Soygur T. Effectiveness of doxazosin in treatment of distal ureteral stones in children. J Urol. 2009;182:2880–4.
22. Mokhless I, Zahran AR, Youssif M, Fahmy A. Tamsulosin for the management of distal ureteral stones in children: a prospective randomized study. J Pediatr Urol. 2012;8:544–8.
23. Tasian GE, Cost NG, Granberg CF, Pulido JE, Rivera M, Schwen Z, et al. Tamsulosin and spontaneous passage of ureteral stones in children: a multi-institutional cohort study. J Urol. 2014;192:506–11.
24. Tian DLN, Huang W, Zong H, Zhang Y. The efficacy and safety of adrenergic alpha-antagonists in treatment of distal ureteral stones in pediatric patients: a systematic review and meta-analysis. J Pediatr Surg. 2017;52(2):360–5.
25. Barreto L, Jung JH, Abdelrahim A, Ahmed M, Dawkins GP, Kazmierski M. Medical and surgical interventions for the treatment of urinary stones in children. Cochrane Database Syst Rev. 2018;6:CD010784.
26. Landau EH, Shenfeld OZ, Pode D, Shapiro A, Meretky S, Katz G, et al. Extracorporeal shock wave lithotripsy in prepubertal children: 22-year experience at a single institution with a single lithotriptor. J Urol. 2009;182:1835–9.
27. D'Addessi A, Bongiovanni L, Racioppi M, Sacco E, Bassi P. Is extracorporeal shock wave lithotripsy in pediatrics a safe procedure? J Pediatr Surg. 2008;43:591–6.
28. Aldridge RD, Aldridge RC, Aldridge LM. Anesthesia for pediatric lithotripsy. Paediatr Anaesth. 2006;16:236–41.
29. Tuncer M, Çevik B, Eryıldırım B, Faydacı G, Sarıca K. Extracorporeal shock wave lithotripsy management of renal stones in children: does anesthesia affect the treatment outcomes on an age-based manner? Urology. 2017;107:218–22.
30. Adanur S, Ziypak T, Yılmaz AH, Kocakgol H, Aksoy M, Yapanoglu T, et al. Extracorporeal shockwave lithotripsy under sedoanalgesia for treatment of kidney stones in infants: a single-center experience with 102 cases. Int Urol Nephrol. 2014;46:2095–101.
31. Turna B, Tekin A, Yagmur I, Nazh O. Extracorporeal shock wave lithotripsy in infants less than 12-month old. Urolithiasis. 2016;44:435–40.
32. Dangle PP, Bandari J, Lyon TD, Lee A, Ayyash O, Cannon GM Jr, et al. Outcomes of ureteroscopic management of pediatric urolithiasis: a comparative analysis of prepubertal and adolescent patients. Urology. 2016;89:103–6.
33. Atar M, Sancaktutar AA, Penbegul N, Soylemez H, Bodakci MN, Hatipoglu NK, et al. Comparison of a 4.5 F semi-rigid ureteroscope with a 7.5 F rigid ureteroscope in the treatment of ureteral stones in preschool-age children. Urol Res. 2012;40:733–8.
34. Dede O, Sancaktutar AA, Bas O, Daggullu M, Utangac M, Penbegul N, et al. Micro-percutaneous nephrolithotomy in infants: a single-center experience. Urolithiasis. 2016;44:173–7.
35. Daw K, Shouman AM, Elsheemy MS, Shoukry AI, Adoulela W, Morsi H, et al. outcome of mini-percutaneous nephrolithotomy for renal stones in infants and preschool children: a prospective study. Urology. 2015;86:1019–26.

The manufacturer's authorised representative in the EU is Springer
Nature Customer Service Centre GmbH, Europaplatz 3, 69115 Heidelberg,
Germany. If you have any concerns regarding our products, please
contact ProductSafety@springernature.com

Printed and bound by CPI Group (UK) Ltd, Croydon, CR0 4YY
17/07/2026
02170253-0002